Readings in
Pediatric Psychology

Readings in Pediatric Psychology

Edited by

Michael C. Roberts
University of Kansas
Lawrence, Kansas

Gerald P. Koocher
Children's Hospital
Boston, Massachusetts

Donald K. Routh
University of Miami
Coral Cables, Florida

Diane J. Willis
University of Oklahoma
Health Sciences Center
Oklahoma City, Oklahoma

PLENUM PRESS • NEW YORK AND LONDON

Library of Congress Cataloging-in-Publication Data

Readings in pediatric psychology / edited by Michael C. Roberts ... [et
al.].
      p.   cm.
  Consists of articles reprinted from the Journal of pediatric
psychology and its precedessor, Pediatric psychology.
  Includes bibliographical references and index.
  ISBN 0-306-44423-2
  1. Pediatrics--Psychological aspects. 2. Sick children-
-Psychology.   I. Roberts, Michael C.
  [DNLM: 1. Child Psychology--collected works. 2. Pediatrics-
-collected works. 3. Disease--psychology--collected works.   WS 105
R2863 1993]
RJ47.5.R43   1993
618.92'00019--dc20
DNLM/DLC
for Library of Congress   93-7736
                                                                    CIP

ISBN 0-306-44423-2

© 1993 Plenum Press, New York
A Division of Plenum Publishing Corporation
233 Spring Street, New York, N.Y. 10013

Printed in the United States of America

To
Lee Salk and Gail Gardner

This volume is dedicated to the memory of
two pioneers in pediatric psychology.
Lee Salk was a founding committee member and second
president of the Society of Pediatric Psychology.
Gail Gardner was the first editor of *Pediatric Psychology*,
the earliest publication of the Society.

Preface

A number of factors converged to prompt this volume at this particular time. For several years, supervisors in predoctoral and internship programs have noted the need for a compendium of selected articles to illustrate the range of research and practice of pediatric psychology. Although the field is still relatively young, the many new pediatric psychologists in recent years might benefit from a perspective on the history and development of the psychological concepts, the organizational home in the Society of Pediatric Psychology (Section V of the Division of Clinical Psychology of the American Psychological Association), and its publication archive, *Journal of Pediatric Psychology*. Such "classics" help capture the richness and excitement that portrays the field.

Noting the continuing need for resources to serve the specialty, the Executive Committee of the Society of Pediatric Psychology authorized the sponsorship of publication of the *Handbook of Pediatric Psychology* (Routh, 1988) as a synthesis of the field by expert chapter authors. The Society then appointed a committee led by C. Eugene Walker and Annette M. La Greca to develop a series of biennial volumes entitled *Advances in Pediatric Psychology*. A number of discussions among the editorial board of the Journal and with Plenum Publishing Corporation, the *Journal*'s publisher, recognized the value of articles carefully selected to exemplify how pediatric psychology is done.

The four editors of the *Journal* in its history formed a panel to review all articles published and to select those articles for inclusion in this volume representing the various aspects of topic content, problems, populations, and approaches. We quickly recognized that too many excellent articles would not be included by necessity of page constraints. We employed a Delphic procedure to winnow the over 600 articles published in the *Journal* and its predecessor, *Pediatric Psychology*. In addition to reviewing the articles, we considered *Journal* articles most frequently cited in texts and chapters in pediatric psychology. Further, we were provided information on articles referenced in curricula and syllabi on pediatric psychology for predoctoral and internship courses compiled by the Society's Task Force on Curriculum (chaired by Debra Bendell-Estroff and Sheila Eyberg). Starting with 615 articles entering the first round, the panel nominated 216 for consideration in the second round. The third round narrowed the list to 22 articles for inclusion based on consensus of the panel.

(Sixty-two other articles received nomination, but could not be included.) The panel agreed that one additional article, written by Logan Wright and published in 1967 in the *American Psychologist*, should be included because of its seminal value in developing the field of pediatric psychology. We retained the original wording and style for each of the articles. Thus, these articles reflect the times in which they were initially published. All the articles could be nicely categorized into topical sections organizing the book:

  I. Early Development of Pediatric Psychology
 II. Chronic and Life-Threatening Conditions in Childhood
III. Children's Perceptions and Understanding of Pediatrics
 IV. Pain and Distress in Children
  V. Professional Issues and Training

After an introductory chapter on the history of pediatric psychology, overview chapters were prepared for each section by one of the editors to place the topic into perspective from its time of publication, its importance to the field, and to orient the reader to work ongoing in this area.

We thank Eliot Werner and Mariclaire Cloutier of Plenum for their support of the *Journal* and for this volume. We greatly appreciate the contributions of all authors to the *Journal of Pediatric Psychology* through the years. Most importantly, we acknowledge the too-often unheralded contributions of the multitude of editorial board members and ad hoc reviewers who helped shape the field and the *Journal* through their reviews of submitted manuscripts. Their efforts are evident in the pages of the *Journal* and in the reprinted articles here.

As the primary publication of the Society, the *Journal*'s development from a newsletter to a scientific and professional medium parallels the immense growth and increasing contributions of researchers and practitioners in the field. We want this volume to meet the needs and interests of trainers, students and interns, new and experienced professionals. We found the process of selecting these articles, although tedious in some regards, exhilarating in refreshing our perspective on this dynamic, vibrant, and developing field. We hope the readers share our enthusiasm.

Michael C. Roberts
Gerald P. Koocher
Donald K. Routh
Diane J. Willis

REFERENCES

Routh, D. K. (Ed.). (1988). *Handbook of pediatric psychology*. New York: Guilford.

Wright, L. (1967). The pediatric psychologist: A role model. *American Psychologist, 22,* 323–325.

Contents

2028805

5052880S

Introduction to Pediatric Psychology
An Historical Perspective

Michael C. Roberts
The University of Kansas

The history of pediatric psychology is relatively brief, but like developing humans from infancy to adulthood, the early years have been ones of rapid ~~complex growth. In fact, the field's organizational home, the Society~~ of Clinical Psychology

~~of Pediatric Psychology (Section V of the Division~~ rated its twenty-first will provide an over- hology in terms of its d publication archive. the two articles from t. For additional views, istory of pediatric psy- , 1975, 1988a; Walker,

HOLOGY[1]

d early in the separate 975). Anderson (1930), gested that a collabora- ld be a beneficial one. bute particularly to pe- diatrics through intelligence testing and consultation on to parents regarding child-rearing practices. Not much seems to have resulted from this call.

[1]This section relies on several sources: Elkins (1987); Roberts, Quevillon, and Wright (1979); Routh (1975); Salk and Routh (1972); Willis (1977).

1

Later, Kagan (1965), a child psychologist, called for a "new marriage" between psychology and pediatrics. Kagan envisioned that this collaboration would provide pediatricians with an understanding of personality dynamics and research. He suggested that the professionals would work on many childhood problems with an emphasis on prevention, early detection, and treatment. In an important, vitalizing article, Logan Wright (1967) coined the term *pediatric psychology* to describe the psychological practice "dealing primarily with children in a medical setting which is nonpsychiatric in nature" (p. 323). This article, originally published in the *American Psychologist*, is reprinted in Section I in recognition of its significance in outlining the field and proposing what the field needed to accomplish. In his now-classic article, Wright outlined the needs for: (a) establishing a group identity through a formal organization, (b) developing professional training focusing on the specialty, and (c) constructing new bodies of knowledge through applied research. As will be seen in this chapter, these perceived needs led to concrete developments and the current status of the field.

As a foundation of pediatric psychology, Wright operationalized how the psychological professional might function in pediatric settings. This model included roles as a consultant and scientist–practitioner. Schofield (1969) elaborated these roles, suggesting that a more generic psychologist working in medical areas "would be a scientist–clinician . . . with a particular sophistication in physical illness, equipped to research and consult with regard to the psychological concomitants of physical disease" (p. 574). Wright, in a 1969 *Pediatric Psychology* newsletter article, attributed the growth in interest in pediatric psychology at the time to the "increasing importance being assigned to behavioral problems as part of good pediatric care, and to government programs, such as the children and youth projects, and Headstart, which were designed to offer both behavioral and medical care to needy children" (p. 1).

The history of the concept of pediatric psychology parallels the development of its organizational home in the Society of Pediatric Psychology. In 1967, George Albee, the president of the Division of Clinical Psychology of the American Psychological Association (APA), recommended that the Division's Section on Clinical Child Psychology (Section I) attend to the role of psychologists within pediatric settings. A committee was then appointed by Section I consisting of Logan Wright (as chair), Lee Salk, and Dorothea Ross. They sent letters of inquiry to chairs of pediatric departments of all U.S. medical schools. This correspondence revealed 250 names of interested psychologists in medical settings. These became the basis of the interest group the Society of Pediatric Psychology (SPP), which affiliated with the Section on Clinical Child Psychology in 1968 with 75 full members and 22 affiliate members.

The first newsletter, *Pediatric Psychology,* edited by G. Gail Gardner, was distributed in March of 1969. The first symposium was organized by SPP for the 1969 APA convention. At the first business meeting, Wright was elected president, Salk president-elect, and Ross secretary-treasurer. (Table I lists other presidents and editors.) By 1972, membership in SPP had grown to 650 members, but restricted finances limited publication of the newsletter on a regular basis. Indeed, financial concerns for the viability of SPP and its publication flagship plagued the organization for many years until recently (see *Recollections* of past-presidents of SPP collected by Magrab, 1989). Many donations, loans, and fundraisers helped pay for the publications of the *Journal* and its predecessor. Nonetheless, over the years the Society managed to organize programs for the APA convention, publish the newsletter and then a journal, and now both. In 1980, SPP became independent of the Section on Clinical Child Psychology, and it currently functions as Section V of the Division of Clinical Psychology of APA.

Recent activities have expanded the role of the Society into more publications, such as this volume, the *Handbook of Pediatric Psychology* (Routh, 1988b), *Family Issues in Pediatric Psychology* (Roberts & Wallander, 1992), and a continuing book series, Advances in Pediatric Psychology, with the first volume entitled *Stress and Coping in Child Health* (La Greca, Siegel, Wallander, & Walker, 1992). The *Journal* now publishes 800 pages of research and practice information in six issues a year with a commercial publisher (Plenum), and the newsletter (now titled *Pediatric Psychology Progress Notes*) publishes timely organizational information three times a year.

Testimony on behalf of the Society has been presented before the U.S. Senate (regarding the protection of sexual abuse victims while testifying in court hearings). Task forces have focused on critical issues such as curriculum and training, injury control in childhood, professional functioning, and infant mental health, and new ones are appointed as issues arise. The organization has formed liaisons with groups of professionals with related interests (e.g., Society of Behavioral Pediatrics; Division of Child, Youth, and Family Services; Division of Health Psychology). SPP offers awards for research and service to recognize contributions of pediatric psychologists and students in training. It continues to sponsor programming at the APA convention and now cosponsors national and regional conferences in pediatric psychology and child health psychology (e.g., the Florida Conference on Child Health Psychology every other year as a national meeting; regional conferences in alternate years as more local meetings).

The early definition of pediatric psychology remained centered on how and where the psychologists were functioning—in medical (pediatric) settings. The masthead of the *Journal of Pediatric Psychology*, officially established as a journal in 1976, based on a position statement of the Society's

Table I. People and Publications of the Society of Pediatric Psychology

Pediatric Psychology: Newsletter of the Society of Pediatric Psychology

Editors:

G. Gail Gardner (1969–71)   Elizabeth A. Robinson (1985)
Allan Barclay (1972)   Ronald L. Blount (1986–89)
Diane J. Willis (1973–76)   Mary Cerreto (1990)
Michael C. Roberts (1980–83)   Lawrence J. Siegel (1990–1993)
Brian Stabler (1983–84)   Kathleen Lemanek (1994–   )

Journal of Pediatric Psychology

Editors:

Diane J. Willis (1976)   Michael C. Roberts (1988–92)
Donald K. Routh (1977–82)   Annette M. La Greca (1993–1997)
Gerald P. Koocher (1983–87)

Presidents of the Society of Pediatric Psychology

1969–70 Logan Wright   1983 Gary B. Mesibov
1970–72 Lee Salk   1984 Sheila Eyberg
1972–73 Arthur Wiens   1985 Michael C. Roberts
1973–74 Donald K. Routh   1986 Dennis C. Harper
1974–75 David Vore   1987 C. Eugene Walker
1975–76 Thomas J. Kenny   1988 Annette M. La Greca
1976–77 Carolyn S. Schroeder   1989 Sue White
1977–78 Diane J. Willis   1990 Lawrence J. Siegel
1978–79 Elizabeth King   1991 Gerald P. Koocher
1979–80 June M. Tuma   1992 Jan L. Wallander
1980–81 Phyllis R. Magrab   1993 Suzanne Bennett Johnson
1982   Dennis Drotar   1994 Dennis Russo

Recipients of the Lee Salk Distinguished Service Award
(until 1993 the Distinguished Contribution Award)

1977 Lee Salk   1985 Phyllis R. Magrab
1978 Logan Wright   1986 June M. Tuma
1979 Dorothea Ross   1987 Gerald P. Koocher
1980 Arthur Wiens   1989 Dennis Drotar
1981 Donald K. Routh   1990 Gary Mesibov
1982 Diane J. Willis   1991 Annette La Greca
1983 Thomas J. Kenny   1992 Brian Stabler
1984 Carolyn S. Schroeder   1993 Michael C. Roberts

**Recipients of the Special Award for Scholarly Contributions to the Society
of Pediatric Psychology**

1986 Gerald P. Koocher   1992 Michael C. Roberts

**Recipients of the Significant Research Contributions in Pediatric
Psychology Award**

1986 John Spinetta   1991 Barbara Melamed
1988 Lizette Peterson   1993 Karen Matthews

(Continued)

Table I. *(Continued)*

Winners of the Student Research Competition

1982 Sandra Shaheen	"Sequelae of Childhood Lead Poisoning: A Developmental Analysis"
1984 Ann Deaton	"Adaptive Noncompliance in Pediatric Asthma: The Parent as Expert"
1986 David O'Grady	"Resilience in Children at High Risk for Psychological Disorder"
1988 Karen Smith	"Reducing Distress during Invasive Medical Procedures: Relating Behavioral Interventions to Preferred Coping Styles in Pediatric Cancer Patients"
1990 Leilani Greening	"Adolescent Smoking: Perceived Vulnerability to Smoking-Related Causes of Death"
Lenora Knapp	"The Effects of Health Persuasive Appeals on Children's Toothbrushing Behavior"
1992 Jacqueline J. Hutcheson	"Interactional Characteristics of Mothers and Infants with Failure-to-Thrive"

Executive Committee in 1975, stated: "The fields and the content of this Journal, are defined by the interests and concerns of psychologists who work in interdisciplinary settings such as children's hospitals, developmental clinics, and pediatric or medical group practices." This setting-based definition guided much of the early development of the field. Over time, the field continued to evolve and eventually it was recognized that pediatric psychology not only fulfilled its destiny through a firm establishment in the pediatric setting, but had moved out to include improving the health of children outside of medical settings per se through psychological interventions.

One particular development has been the number of other terms and definitions offered for this emerging specialty. For example, Tuma (1982b) discussed the relationship of pediatric psychology with other concepts of medical psychology, behavioral medicine, health psychology and health care psychology, and psychosomatic medicine. These concepts and their definitions are interesting for their relationships with pediatric psychology and for their contribution to the eventual changes in the definition of pediatric psychology. Asken (1975) defined "medical psychology" as "the study of psychological factors related to all aspects of physical health, illness, and its treatment at the individual, group, and systems level" (p. 67). Regarding a related concept, Schwartz and Weiss (1978) stated: "Behavioral medicine is the interdisciplinary field concerned with the development and integration of behavioral and biomedical science knowledge and techniques relevant to health and illness and the application of this knowledge and these techniques to prevention, diagnosis, treatment and rehabilitation" (p. 7). The Division of Health Psychology (undated) presented that

> health psychology is the aggregate of the specific educational, scientific, and professional contributions of the discipline of psychology to the promotion and maintenance of health, the prevention and treatment of illness, and the identification of etiologic and diagnostic correlates of health, illness, and related dysfunctions, and to the analysis and improvement of the health care system and health policy formation. (p. 1)

Levine, Carey, Crocker, and Gross (1983), discussing the developmental mental health relationship with pediatrics, wrote that:

> Developmental pediatrics has concerned itself largely with cognitive competence and the associated physical and mental disabilities that constrain function in childhood. Behavioral pediatrics has emphasized the prevention and treatment of disorders of personality and the effects of family function and social adaptation. *Developmental-behavioral Pediatrics* splices these strands together so as to emphasize their shared themes, their compatible missions, and their complementary contributions to general pediatrics and other disciplines concerned with health and function in childhood. (p. xv)

La Greca and Stone (1985) provided the definition that

> behavioral pediatrics focuses particularly on issues such as psychological factors contributing to the etiology of various childhood diseases (e.g., asthma), the psychological sequelae of various medical problems (e.g., cardiac surgery, leukemia), and psychological factors that contribute to the maintenance of adequate medical care (e.g., compliance in children with juvenile diabetes). (p. 255)

Other terms and definitions have been offered for various aspects of related specialties: behavioral health (Matarazzo, 1980), child health psychology (Karoly, Steffen, & O'Grady, 1982), biosocial pediatrics (Green, 1980), pediatric behavioral medicine (Williams, Foreyt, & Goodrick, 1981), and family health psychology (Akamatsu, Stephens, Hobfoll, & Crowther, 1992).

Recognizing the changing nature of pediatric psychology as a field of research and practice, a panel was formed in 1987 for the *Journal of Pediatric Psychology* to develop a global articulation of pediatric psychology. The final statement proposed by this panel was approved by the Executive Committee of the Society of Pediatric Psychology as the *Journal*'s masthead, beginning in 1988:

Pediatric psychology is an interdisciplinary field addressing the full range of physical and mental development, health, and illness issues affecting children, adolescents, and families. [It encompasses] a wide variety of topics exploring the relationship between psychological and physical well-being of children and adolescents including: understanding, assessment, and intervention with developmental disorders; evaluation and treatment of behavioral and emotional problems and concomitants of disease and illness; the role of psychology in pediatric medicine; the promotion of health and development; and the prevention of illness and injury among children and youth. (Roberts, La Greca, & Harper, 1988, p. 2)

This definition demonstrates the diversity and range of pediatric psychology activities in direct service delivery and research into the behavioral aspects of children's health and illness. These activities are exemplified through the articles in the *Journal of Pediatric Psychology*, especially those reprinted in this volume. Formal definitions aside, what is the field of pediatric psychology? Over time, two elements seem to illustrate the field best: practice and research. Each of these will be discussed for their historical developments. Aspects of training will then be covered.

PEDIATRIC PSYCHOLOGY PRACTICE

Lightner Witmer, the first clinical psychologist in the United States in 1896, likely was the first pediatric psychologist because he worked on pediatric-related problems in a clinical setting and published case studies describing interventions (McReynolds, 1987; Routh, 1975). However, it took many more years to develop the clinical practice of pediatric psychology more fully. Descriptions of clinical practice in pediatric settings were very useful in the early stages for developing psychological consulting and service units and demonstrating what pediatric psychologists do. These early descriptions outlined pediatric psychology practices of intervention and consultation for such units as intensive care nurseries and infant units (Drotar & Malone, 1982; Magrab & Davitt, 1975), oncology (Drotar, 1975; Koocher, Sourkes, & Keane, 1979; O'Malley & Koocher, 1977), neurology (Cerreto, 1980; Hartlage & Hartlage, 1978), renal dialysis and transplantation (Brewer, 1978; Magrab, 1975), plastic surgery (Gluck, 1977), emergency rooms (Axelrod, 1976), private office-based pediatric practice (Fischer & Engeln, 1972; Schroeder, 1979; Smith, Rome, & Freedheim, 1967), and in general pediatrics (Drotar, 1976, 1977; Drotar, Benjamin, Chwast, Litt, & Vajner, 1982; Toback, Russo, & Gururaj, 1975). These descriptive articles, which contain useful information on opportunities, obstacles, and solutions, helped others in establishing similar services and illustrated in concrete ways how the pediatric psychologist practices. They also often portrayed case examples of patients seen on a unit to demonstrate the clinical functioning of the psychologist interacting with patients, problems, families, and other hospital staff. These articles about service units remain some of the richest descriptions of pediatric psychology practice.

Surveys of practicing pediatric psychologists also provide data on the nature of clinical services. For example, Stabler and Mesibov (1984) surveyed members of the Society of Pediatric Psychology and found that pediatric psychologists tend to practice in primary care facilities. A significant part of their time is in direct clinical service with a high proportion of diagnostic testing and consulting. Similarly, Tuma and Cawunder (1983), reporting on a survey of pediatric psychologists, found that more time was spent in assessment than treatment. The contrast of practice patterns for pediatric psychologists versus clinical child psychologists through surveys has found that the latter group attends more to medical disorders and health of children with greater adherence to behavioral assessment and interventions (La Greca, Stone, Drotar, & Maddux, 1988; Tuma & Grabert, 1983).

In a recent survey of the members of the Society of Pediatric Psychology, Drotar, Sturm, Eckerle, and White (in press) examined pediatric psychologists' perceptions of their work settings. They found that clinical activities accounted for almost half of the work time with generally high levels of overall satisfaction with the work environment. Among the sources of satisfaction were included professional autonomy, patient care, and collegial relationships. Sources of dissatisfaction included insufficient time for research, salary, and patient care workload.

Other professionals as researcher–clinicians continued to gather and publish data on the types of cases seen and interventions made in pediatric psychology practices. Mesibov, Schroeder, and Wesson (1977) compiled the various presenting problems for a "Call In/Come In" consultation service of psychologists working in a private pediatric practice. This compilation about this particular service was elaborated on by Schroeder (1979) and later by Kanoy and Schroeder (1985). (Two of these articles are reprinted in Section V of this volume.) In another summary, Walker (1979) compiled cases referred to a pediatric psychology unit within a children's hospital. Ottinger and Roberts (1980) analyzed referrals to a university-based pediatric psychology practicum. Table II depicts a compilation of these case analyses from Roberts (1986; Roberts & Walker, 1989a). As can be seen, these patterns of practice are fairly consistent, with large numbers of referrals for negative behaviors, school-related problems, and personality disorders, followed by physical complaints, adjustment to disease, developmental delays, toileting, and infant management problems. Later

Table II. Referral of Problems to Three Pediatric Psychology Services

	Kanoy & Schroeder (1985)[a]	Ottinger & Roberts (1980)	Walker (1979)
Negative behaviors toward parents Doesn't obey, has tantrums, demanding, cries, whines	15	10	10
Toileting Toilet training, encopresis, enuresis	10	8	5
Developmental delays Perceptual—motor problems, speech problems, slow development, school readiness, overactivity	7	10	16[b]
School problems Dislikes school, poor performance, reading or math problems, child aggression toward teacher	9	15	9
Sleeping problems Resists bedtime, nightmares, naps	8	2	1
Personality problems Lacks self-control, lacks motivation, irresponsibility, overly lies, steals, dependent	10	5	4
Sibling/peer problems Has no friends, aggressive toward peers, siblings, fighting	7	1	<1
Divorce, separation, adoption Custody decisions, appropriate visitation schedule, how to tell child	8	1	2
Infant management Feeding, nursing, cries all the time ("colic"), stimulation	3	6	<1
Family problems Mother feels isolated, conflict over discipline, parents arguing, child abuse	4	3	10
Sex-related problems Opposite-sexed parent's clothing, no same-sexed friends, lack of sex-appropriate interests	2	1	2
Food/eating problems Picky eater, eats too much or too little	1	4	2

(Continued)

Table II. (Continued)

	Kanoy & Schroeder (1985)[a]	Ottinger & Roberts (1980)	Walker (1979)
Specific fears Dogs, trucks, dark	2	—	<1
Specific bad habits Thumb sucking, nail biting, tics	3	2	2
Parent's negative feelings toward child Dislikes child, no enjoyable interactions	2	—	<1
Physical complaints Headaches, stomachaches, fainting	2	16	23
Parent's concerns about school Is child getting what's needed? Does teacher understand child?	2	—	—
Moving Preparation for moving, problems of adjustment afterwards	1	—	<1
Death Understanding and adjusting to death	1	—	1
Guidance of talented child Special programs, proper stimulation	1	1	<1
Adjustment to disease, handicap	—	13	—
Drug/alcohol abuse	—	2	—
Miscellaneous	1	—	11[c]

Blanks indicate category was not used in compilation.
Percentages were rounded to nearest whole number.
[a] A totaled categorization based on Mesibov et al. (1977), Schroeder (1979), and new data in Kanoy and Schroeder (1985).
[b] Combines category with mental retardation and hyperactivity.
[c] Includes depression, hallucinations, suicide, instability.
From Pediatric psychology: Psychological interventions and strategies for pediatric problems by M. C. Roberts, 1986. New York: Pergamon. Copyright 1986 by Pergamon. Reprinted by permission.

descriptions of hospital pediatric psychology units conducted evaluations of the types and outcome of services. Charlop, Parrish, Fenton, and Cataldo (1987) measured outcomes of an outpatient clinic in a children's hospital. Krahn, Eisert, and Fifield (1990) assessed parental perceptions of quality of services for children in a center for children with developmental disability. Olson et al. (1988) evaluated inpatient consultations of a pediatric psychology service. (This article is reprinted in Section V of in this volume.)

Singer and Drotar (1989) analyzed referrals and treatments for a consultation unit in a pediatric rehabilitation hospital.

These evaluations of clinical services continue to demonstrate the efficacy, acceptance, and satisfaction with the professional interventions. As another description of the nature of practice in this field, Roberts and Walker (1989b) published a casebook of 20 chapters of clinical cases describing child and pediatric psychology interventions to depict the range of problems and the process of assessment and intervention.

While these various resources outline practice in the past and present, Kaufman, Holden, and Walker (1989) utilized a Delphic process to determine pediatric psychologists' predictions of the field for the future. Regarding the clinical services aspect of pediatric psychology, these researchers found that the top 10 trends included: applications of pediatric behavioral medicine, developing effective treatment protocols for common problems, professional roles in medical settings, chronic illness, insurance reimbursement for services, compliance with medical regimens, neuropsychology, insurance alternatives such as health maintenance organizations, educating other health professionals, and prevention. These predicted issues for the future relate clearly to the

> professional development of the psychologist in the medical center (e.g., role in the medical center, educating other health professionals), as well as common clinical problems in such a setting (e.g., medical noncompliance; chronic illness) and clinical techniques (e.g., neuropsychology; behavioral medicine). (Kaufman et al., 1989, p. 150)

In summary, the practice of pediatric psychology has evolved a variety of overlapping characteristics including (a) a clinical practice, often in a health care setting, usually at the initial presentation of a problem, not after a series of referrals outside the setting; (b) medically based referral mechanisms and source of patients which include a high proportion of medically related disorders; (c) consultation and collaboration with physicians and allied health services; (d) emphasis on developmental considerations with an orientation to health promotion and problem prevention; and (e) practical orientation to treatment and assessment techniques that can be demonstrated to be effective, economical, and time efficient (Peterson & Harbeck, 1988; Roberts, 1986). Not all of these characteristics can apply at all times because the setting and problems for clinical services are so varied and require new professional relationships and practices (Stabler & Mesibov, 1984; Stabler & Whitt, 1980). The practice aspects of pediatric psychology can be expected to continue evolving, particularly as the research aspects contribute to a stronger knowledge base. These considerations will be reviewed in the next section.

PEDIATRIC PSYCHOLOGY RESEARCH

Wright (1967) asserted that the accumulation of a body of knowledge was essential to the development of the field. He later articulated the following view:

> There are many of us who believe that a scientific approach will be the salvation of the surviving disciplines in behavioral science and mental health, and that disciplines more committed to intuition will face an eventual choice: change or become irrelevant. (Wright, 1969, p. 2)

Early research contributions were made by studying the impact of medical disorders and conditions for measurable psychological effects. For example, Salk, Hilgartner, and Granich (1972) examined the psychosocial effects of hemophilia; Wright and Jimmerson (1971) studied the intellectual sequelae of meningitis; Friedman (1972) considered children with "psychogenic pain." The applications of psychological interventions for medically related problems were also studied and reported. These included applications of conditioning principles for children who refused medication (Wright, Woodcock, & Scott, 1970) and who were addicted to tracheostomies (Wright, Nunnery, Eichel, & Scott, 1968), and puppet therapy for children in the hospital (Cassell & Paul, 1967). These two types of pediatric psychology research, on the impact of disorders and effective intervention, have continued through to the present.

In the formative years, there was no journal specifically oriented to pediatric psychology research. Only a few medical and psychological journals were accepting some articles. The newsletter of the Society of Pediatric Psychology, *Pediatric Psychology*, began to expand in publishing articles about research and practice related to this developing specialty, and eventually became an official journal in 1975. Over time, it increased its emphasis on empirical research articles. In 1975, the *Journal of Clinical Child Psychology* published a special issue, edited by Diane Willis, on the topic of pediatric psychology with articles describing various aspects of this emerging specialty. The recognition from the issue coincided with other events affirming the strength of ideas and interests for pediatric psychology.

Growth in research over time has been rapid and substantial. In addition to the *Journal of Pediatric Psychology*, a number of journals began publishing research articles related to the field. *Health Psychology*, for example, publishes research on the behavioral aspects of children's health and illness as part of its mandate for health psychology over the lifespan. A special issue was published in 1986 giving particular attention to child health psychology. Other journals in psychology and pediatrics, as well as interdisciplinary publications, provide outlets for research (e.g., *Journal of*

Table III. Growth of Pediatric Psychology through Book Publication

Psychological Management of Pediatric Problems (Magrab, 1978)
Encyclopedia of Pediatric Psychology (Wright, Schaefer, & Solomons, 1979)
Behavioral Pediatrics and Child Development (2nd ed.) (Kenny & Clemens, 1980)
Pediatric Psychology: An Introduction for Pediatricians (Lavigne & Burns, 1981)
Handbook for the Practice of Pediatric Psychology (Tuma, 1982a)
Behavioral Pediatrics: Research and Practice (Russo & Varni, 1982)
Child Health Psychology (Karoly, Steffen, & O'Grady, 1982)
Clinical Behavioral Pediatrics (Varni, 1983)
Psychological and Behavioral Assessment: Impact on Pediatric Care (Magrab, 1984)
Pediatric Psychology: Psychological Interventions and Strategies for Pediatric Problems
   (Roberts, 1986)
Child Health Behavior (Krasnegor, Arasteh, & Cataldo, 1986)
Handbook of Pediatric Psychology (Routh, 1988b)
The Pediatric Psychologist (Peterson & Harbeck, 1988)
Handbook of Child Health Assessment (Karoly, 1988)
Casebook of Child and Pediatric Psychology (Roberts & Walker, 1989b)
Handbook of Clinical Behavior Pediatrics (Gross & Drabman, 1990)
Advances in Child Health Psychology (Johnson & Johnson, 1991)
Stress and Coping in Child Health (La Greca, Siegel, Wallander, & Walker, 1992)
Family Health Psychology (Akamatsu, Stephens, Hobfoll, & Crowther, 1992)

Clinical Child Psychology, Children's Health Care, Journal of Behavioral Medicine, Journal of Consulting and Clinical Psychology, Pediatrics, and *Journal of Developmental and Behavioral Pediatrics*). In addition to the rise in journal publications of pediatric psychology articles, the increase in books and chapters summarizing the field, especially its research, has been notable. Some of these are presented in Table III.

Routh (1982) viewed the growth of research as somewhat inevitable because of the foundation of the field in research-based professions. He noted that the early members of the Society of Pediatric Psychology were faculty members in pediatric departments of medical schools and consequently, "scientific research is part of the job definition of many pediatric psychologists" (p. 290).

The history of research in pediatric psychology is isomorphic with the history of the *Journal of Pediatric Psychology*. Journal articles communicate scientific information among professionals and reflect the advancement of science. As noted, the present *Journal* evolved from the *Pediatric Psychology* newsletter published first in March 1969 after the formal establishment of the Society of Pediatric Psychology. The first editor was G. Gail Gardner and issues appeared three to four times a year. Allan Barclay edited the newsletter during 1972. Diane Willis edited *Pediatric Psychology* starting in 1973. Articles in the early issues focused on program descriptions, training, intervention techniques, and the Society organization. To this point, very few articles were research based. The newsletter grew eventually in size and quality to journal standards. In 1976, the new title and emphasis of the publication appeared as the *Journal of Pediatric Psychology* under Willis's editorship. Donald Routh became editor in 1976. At this time, the *Journal* was published by the Society privately but was draining its resources. In 1979, the Society contracted with Plenum Publishing Corporation to publish it. Routh and Mesibov (1979), in an opening editorial, emphasized the need for more original research in addition to reviews and clinically oriented articles. Gerald Koocher assumed the editorship in 1983, followed by Michael Roberts in 1988. Annette La Greca assumed the editorship in 1993.

Several analyses have considered what has been published in the *Journal*, as the field's primary archive, in order to provide information about the nature of research in the field. Routh and Mesibov (1979) considered articles published in the *Journal* up to 1979 and noted that articles were mostly literature reviews and clinically based. They also determined that the journals most cited in the *Journal's* articles were *Pediatrics* and *Child Development*. Routh (1980) compiled a list of individual authors cited most frequently in articles and found their backgrounds to be in psychology, child psychiatry, and pediatrics.

Elkins and Roberts (1988) analyzed the articles published in the *Journal* over the first 10 years as an official journal (1976–1985). The 351 articles published in this time period were categorized according to several variables. Roberts (1992) summarized 212 articles published in the *Journal* from 1988 to 1992 following the same procedure. In terms of the age of the population under study in the articles published, the two analyses demonstrated a relatively equal distribution of ages targeted in the research with more articles relying on combinations of ages. Adolescence specifically had fewer articles over time. With regard to the types of populations under study in the research published in the *Journal*, there was a predominance of articles on medical concerns, followed proportionately by articles on children with developmental/learning disabilities, children with behavioral/emotional disorders, and general or "normal" children. Thus, children with acute and chronic physical conditions were studied related to the management of the medical condition or related to the psychological factors secondary to the physical condition. Along with developmental conditions, these *Journal* articles are clearly consistent with the definitions of pediatric psychology noted earlier.

Considering the types of articles published in the *Journal*, there has been an increasing percentage of applied research with a modest increase in basic research. There was a steady decline over time of *Journal* publication proportionately of articles on professional practice and literature reviews. In the first two years of publication, less than a quarter of the articles reported original research. After 1981 and continuing to the present, more than three-quarters of all articles published were new research. In relatively more articles than others, there has been a variety of viable theoretical orientations guiding research activities including norm-based, multitheoretical, and behavioral, but no one theory predominates. The findings of various theoretical orientations support what might be called the eclectic or multitheoretical nature of the field or what has been called "theoretical ambidexterity" (Roberts, 1986). There have been a few notable changes in the institutional affiliations of the authors of the *Journal*'s articles. Over time, there has been an increase in university-based pediatric psychology researchers and a relative decrease in medical center authors. Overall, however, the largest percentage of authors have been based in medical centers. Pediatric psychology may be becoming more "institutionalized" in university psychology departments leading to increased representation of academic settings (Blount, Roberts, & Santilli, 1987). Finally, in the category of sex of the senior authors, the two analyses found changes from a predominance of male first authors in the early years of articles to an increasing trend of female senior authors over time (from less than 30% to 50% of the articles published). This trend likely reflects the trend in the psychology discipline in general.

Changes in published research can be discerned from the analyses of Elkins and Roberts (1988) and Roberts (1992). The *Journal of Pediatric Psychology,* as the official record, though, provides an historical perspective of the scientific aspects of the field. Elkins and Roberts concluded that their analyses demonstrated an increase in applied research, reflecting a "strong orientation toward solving immediate problems in children's health care" (p. 587). More importantly, original research increased over time in the *Journal,* demonstrating significant growth of the scientific side of the field. In the early years of *Journal* publication, little research was published, with more articles on professional practice descriptions. A predominance of empirical research emerged over time, illustrating a strong research foundation for the field (Roberts, 1992).

As one measure of the effect of the research published in the *Journal of Pediatric Psychology*, the Institute for Scientific Information in the Social Science Citation Index (1986) computed the citation impact factor to be 1.13. This statistic indicates that other journals are publishing articles citing this *Journal*'s articles at a respectable rate, as a measure of the influence this research has had in the scientific community.

Whereas Elkins and Roberts (1988) looked to the past to reflect research publication trends, Kaufman et al. (1989) asked pediatric psychologists to look to the future of research in the field through their Delphic poll. The top 10 important trends in research for the future included: chronic illness, prevention, cost-benefit of interventions, treatment effectiveness, medical compliance, neuropsychology, parenting issues, early intervention with children at risk, research strategies, and child abuse and neglect. These trends are already evident in current *Journal* articles and are projected to require the attention of researchers for the future.

TRAINING IN PEDIATRIC PSYCHOLOGY

Wright (1967) argued for the need to have professional training specifically for pediatric psychology. Specialized training was nonexistent early in the field's development. Most practicing pediatric psychologists brought skills and procedures from a variety of training backgrounds (Mesibov, 1984; Tuma, 1980) and applied them in the pediatric settings to gain experience with the presenting problems (in on-the-job training). In 1980, June Tuma edited a special issue of the *Journal of Pediatric Psychology* focusing on professional training in the specialty. In the opening article she summarized: "There are almost as many differing suggestions of the course to follow for the proper educational background in pediatric psychology as there are authors writing on the subject" (Tuma, 1980, p. 241). Surveys were conducted to provide more definition to the training experiences of pediatric psychologists. These surveys revealed a diversity of backgrounds including developmental, experimental, clinical, school, and counseling psychology. These studies also outlined where professionals did their training and what experiences they endorsed for training (e.g., Stabler & Mesibov, 1984; Tuma & Grabert, 1983).

La Greca, Stone, Drotar, and Maddux (1987), in the official training brochure for the Society of Pediatric Psychology, noted that "there is no single path to becoming a pediatric psychologist" (p. 2). Early in the field's history, any formalized training was primarily obtained through internships or postdoctoral programs. Over time, a majority of pediatric psychologists have had graduate training in clinical psychology (Stabler & Mesibov, 1984). This finding was replicated recently in surveys conducted by the Training Committee of the Society of Pediatric Psychology (La Greca, Stone, Drotar, & Maddux, 1988; La Greca, Stone, & Swales, 1989). These later surveys indicated an endorsement of training in preparation for pediatric psychology research and practice that includes: child development; child psychopathology; child intellectual, personality, emotional, and achievement assessment; child psychotherapy; behavior therapy; developmental disabilities; child and adolescent medical disorders; behavioral assessment; legal and ethical issues; family assessment and therapy. This list is very similar to that outlined by Roberts, Erickson, and Tuma (1985) as minimal training components for psychologists working with children, youth, and families (and endorsed by the National Conference on Training Clinical Child Psychologists; Tuma, 1985). Specific application of this topical curriculum to training the child health psychologist was made by Roberts, Fanurik, and Elkins (1988). Davidson (1988) also discussed training the pediatric psychologist and the developmental-behavioral pediatrician. Other overviews to training are presented in Tuma (1982b) and Routh (1988a). More recently, formal training programs at the predoctoral level have developed experiences in clinical child, health, and applied developmental psychology with considerable related work in pediatric psychology. Tuma (1989) annually publishes a directory of predoctoral internships and postdoctoral programs in pediatric and clinical child psychology. Training for pediatric psychology will remain an important ongoing concern because, as Gary Mesibov (1984) stated in his Presidential Address to the Society of Pediatric Psychology, "the visibility, acceptance, and impact of any group is directly related to its training programs" (p. 9).

SUMMARY

This chapter has reviewed the historical development of the pediatric psychology concept through research, practice, and organizational base. The field is vibrant and vital: Its future is based on a solid progression mastered in its early development.

REFERENCES

Akamatsu, T. J., Stephens, M. A. P., Hobfoll, S. E., & Crowther, J. H. (Eds.). (1992). *Family health psychology.* New York: Hemisphere.

Anderson, J. E. (1930). Pediatrics and child psychology. *Journal of the American Medical Association, 95,* 1015–1018.

Asken, M. J. (1975). Medical psychology: Psychology's neglected child. *Professional Psychology, 6,* 155–160.

Axelrod, B. H. (1976). Mental health considerations in the pediatric emergency room. *Journal of Pediatric Psychology, 1,* 14–17.

Blount, R. L., Roberts, M. C., & Santilli, L. (1987). Pediatric psychologists in academic settings: Signs of the growth and vitality of the field. *Newsletter of the Society of Pediatric Psychology, 11,* 18–22.

Brewer, D. (1978). The role of the psychologist in a dialysis and transplantation unit. *Journal of Clinical Child Psychology, 7,* 71–72.

Cassell, S., & Paul, M. H. (1967). The role of puppet therapy on the emotional responses of children hospitalized for cardiac catheterization. *Journal of Pediatrics, 71,* 233–239.

Cerreto, M. (1980). Training issues: The pediatric psychologist–child neurologist team. *Journal of Pediatric Psychology, 5,* 253–261.

Charlop, M. H., Parrish, J. M., Fenton, L. R., & Cataldo, M. F. (1987). Evaluation of hospital-based outpatient pediatric psychology services. *Journal of Pediatric Psychology, 12,* 485–503.

Davidson, C. V. (1988). Training the pediatric psychologist and the developmental-behavioral pediatrician. In D. K. Routh (Ed.), *Handbook of pediatric psychology* (pp. 507–537). New York: Guilford.

Division of Health Psychology: American Psychological Association. (undated). *Health psychology: New perspectives.* Washington, DC: Author.

Drotar, D. (1975). Death in the pediatric hospital: Psychological consultation with medical and nursing staff. *Journal of Clinical Child Psychology, 4,* 33–35.

Drotar, D. (1976). Mental health consultation in the pediatric intensive care nursery. *International Journal of Psychiatry in Medicine, 7,* 69–81.

Drotar, D. (1977). Clinical psychological practice in a pediatric hospital. *Professional Psychology, 7,* 72–80.

Drotar, D., Benjamin, P., Chwast, R., Litt, C., & Vajner, P. (1982). The role of the psychologist in pediatric outpatient and inpatient settings. In J. M. Tuma (Ed.), *Handbook for the practice of pediatric psychology* (pp. 228–250). New York: Wiley-Interscience.

Drotar, D., & Malone, C. (1982). Psychological consultation on a pediatric infant division. *Journal of Pediatric Psychology, 7,* 23–32.

Drotar, D., Sturm, L., Eckerle, D., & White, S. (1993). Pediatric psychologists' perceptions of their work settings. *Journal of Pediatric Psychology, 18*(2).

Elkins, P. D. (1987). *Journal of Pediatric Psychology: A content analysis reflects the scientific and professional history of pediatric psychology.* Unpublished doctoral dissertation, University of Alabama, Tuscaloosa.

Elkins, P. D., & Roberts, M. C. (1988). *Journal of Pediatric Psychology:* A content analysis of articles over its first 10 years. *Journal of Pediatric Psychology, 13,* 575–594.

Fischer, H. L., & Engeln, R. G. (1972). How goes the marriage? *Professional Psychology, 3,* 73–79.

Friedman, R. (1972). Some characteristics of children with "psychogenic" pain. *Clinical Pediatrics, 11,* 331–333.

Gluck, M. R. (1977). Psychological intervention with pre-school age plastic surgery patients and their families. *Journal of Pediatric Psychology, 2,* 23–25.

Green, M. (1980). The pediatric model of care. *Behavioral Medicine Update, 2*(4), 11–13.

Gross, A. M., & Drabman, R. S. (Eds.). (1990). *Handbook of clinical behavioral pediatrics.* New York: Plenum.

Hartlage, L. C., & Hartlage, P. L. (1978). Clinical consultation to pediatric neurology and developmental pediatrics. *Journal of Clinical Child Psychology, 7,* 19–20.

Institute for Scientific Information (1986). *Social science citation index.* Philadelphia: Author.

Johnson, J. H., & Johnson, S. B. (Eds.). (1991). *Advances in child health psychology.* Gainesville; University of Florida Press.

Kagan, J. (1965). The new marriage: Pediatrics and psychology. *American Journal of Diseases of Childhood, 110,* 272–278.

Kanoy, K. W., & Schroeder, C. S. (1985). Suggestions to parents about common behavior problems in a pediatric primary care office: Five years of follow-up. *Journal of Pediatric Psychology, 10,* 15–30.

Karoly, P. (Ed.). (1988). *Handbook of child health assessment: Biopsychosocial perspectives*. New York: Wiley.

Karoly, P., Steffen, J. J., & O'Grady, D. J. (Eds.). (1982). *Child health psychology*. New York: Pergamon.

Kaufman, K., Holden, E. W., & Walker, C. E. (1989). Future directions in pediatric and clinical child psychology. *Professional Psychology, 20*, 148–152.

Kenny, T. J., & Clemmens, R. L. (1980). *Behavioral pediatrics and child development: A clinical handbook* (2nd ed.). Baltimore: Williams & Wilkins.

Koocher, G. P., Sourkes, B. M., & Keane, W. M. (1979). Pediatric oncology consultations: A generalizable model for medical settings. *Professional Psychology, 10*, 467–474.

Krahn, G. L., Eisert, D., & Fifield, B. (1990). Obtaining parental perceptions of the quality of services for children with special health needs. *Journal of Pediatric Psychology, 15*, 761–774.

Krasnegor, N. A., Arasteh, J. D., & Cataldo, M. F. (Eds.). (1986). *Child health behavior: A behavioral pediatrics approach*. New York: Wiley.

La Greca, A. M., Siegel, L. J., Wallander, J. L., & Walker, C. E. (Eds.). (1992). *Stress and coping in child health*. New York: Guilford.

La Greca, A. M., & Stone, W. L. (1985). Behavioral pediatrics. In N. Schneiderman & J. Tapp (Eds.), *Behavioral pediatrics: The biopsychological approach* (pp. 255–291). Hillsdale, NJ: Lawrence Erlbaum.

La Greca, A. M., Stone, W. L., Drotar, D., & Maddux, J. E. (1987). *Pediatric psychology: Some common questions about training*. Washington, DC: Society of Pediatric Psychology, American Psychological Association.

La Greca, A. M., Stone, W. L., Drotar, D., & Maddux, J. E. (1988). Training in pediatric psychology: Survey results and recommendations. *Journal of Pediatric Psychology, 13*, 121–139.

La Greca. A. M., Stone, W. L., & Swales, T. (1989). Pediatric psychology training: An analysis of graduate, internship, and postdoctoral programs. *Journal of Pediatric Psychology, 4*, 103–116.

Lavigne, J. V., & Burns, W. J. (1981). *Pediatric psychology: An introduction for pediatricians*. New York: Grune & Stratton.

Levine, M. D., Carey, W. B., Crocker, A. C., & Gross, R. T. (Eds.). (1983). *Developmental-behavioral pediatrics*. Philadelphia: Saunders.

Magrab, P. (1975). Psychological management and renal dialysis. *Pediatric Psychology, 3*, 3–6.

Magrab, P. (Ed.). (1978). *Psychological management of pediatric problems* (Vols. 1 & 2). Baltimore: University Park Press.

Magrab, P. (Ed.). (1984). *Psychological and behavioral assessment: Impact on pediatric care*. New York: Plenum.

Magrab, P. (1989). *Recollections*. Washington, DC: Society of Pediatric Psychology.

Magrab, P., & Davitt, M. K. (1975). The pediatric psychologist and the developmental follow-up of intensive care nursery infants. *Journal of Clinical Child Psychology, 4*, 16–18.

Matarazzo, J. D. (1980). Behavioral health and behavioral medicine: Frontiers for a new health psychology. *American Psychologist, 35*, 807–817.

McReynolds, P. (1987). Lightner Witmer: Little-known founder of clinical psychology. *American Psychologist, 42*, 849–858.

Mesibov, G. B. (1984). Evolution of pediatric psychology: Historical roots to future trends. *Journal of Pediatric Psychology, 9*, 3–11.

Mesibov, G. B., Schroeder, C. S., & Wesson, L. (1977). Parental concerns about their children. *Journal of Pediatric Psychology, 2*, 13–17.

Olson, R. A., Holden, E. W., Friedman, A., Faust, J., Kenning, M., & Mason, P. J. (1988). Psychological consultation in a children's hospital: An evaluation of services. *Journal of Pediatric Psychology, 13*, 479–492.

O'Malley, J. E., & Koocher, G. P. (1977). Psychological consultation to a pediatric oncology unit: Obstacles to effective intervention. *Journal of Pediatric Psychology, 2,* 256–260.

Ottinger, D. R., & Roberts, M. C. (1980). A university-based predoctoral practicum in pediatric psychology. *Professional Psychology, 11,* 707–713.

Peterson, L., & Harbeck, C. (1988). *The pediatric psychologist.* Champaign, IL: Research Press.

Roberts, M. C. (1986). *Pediatric psychology: Psychological interventions and strategies for pediatric problems.* New York: Pergamon.

Roberts, M. C. (1992). Vale Dictum: The editor's view of the field of pediatric psychology and its journal. *Journal of Pediatric Psychology, 17,* 785–805.

Roberts, M. C., Erickson, M. T., & Tuma, J. M. (1985). Addressing the needs: Guidelines for training psychologists to work with children, youth, and families. *Journal of Clinical Child Psychology, 14,* 70–79.

Roberts, M. C., Fanurik, D., & Elkins, P. D. (1988). Training the child health psychologist. In P. Karoly (Ed.), *Handbook of child health assessment: Biopsychosocial perspectives* (pp. 611–632). New York: Wiley-Interscience.

Roberts, M. C., La Greca, A. M., & Harper, D. C. (1988). *Journal of Pediatric Psychology:* Another stage of development. *Journal of Pediatric Psychology, 13,* 1–5.

Roberts, M. C., Quevillon, R. P., & Wright, L. (1979). Pediatric psychology: A developmental report and survey of the literature. *Child and Youth Services, 2*(1), 1–9.

Roberts, M. C., & Walker, C. E. (1989a). Clinical cases in child and pediatric psychology: Conceptualization and overview. In M. C. Roberts & C. E. Walker (Eds.), *Casebook of child and pediatric psychology* (pp. 1–15). New York: Guilford.

Roberts, M. C., & Walker, C. E. (Eds.). (1989b) *Casebook of child and pediatric psychology.* New York: Guilford.

Roberts, M. C., & Wallander, J. (Eds.). (1992). *Family issues in pediatric psychology.* Hillsdale, NJ: Lawrence Erlbaum.

Routh, D. K. (1975). The short history of pediatric psychology. *Journal of Clinical Child Psychology, 4,* 6–8.

Routh, D. K. (1980). Research training in pediatric psychology. *Journal of Pediatric Psychology, 5,* 287–293.

Routh, D. K. (1982). Pediatric psychology as an area of scientific research. In J. M. Tuma (Ed.), *Handbook for the practice of pediatric psychology* (pp. 290–320). New York: Wiley.

Routh, D. K. (1988a). A places-rated almanac for pediatric psychology. *Journal of Pediatric Psychology, 13,* 113–119.

Routh, D. K. (1988b). *Handbook of pediatric psychology.* New York: Guilford.

Routh, D. K., & Mesibov, G. B. (1979). The editorial policy of the *Journal of Pediatric Psychology. Journal of Pediatric Psychology, 4,* 13.

Russo, D. C., & Varni, J. W. (Eds.). (1982). *Behavioral pediatrics: Research and practice.* New York: Plenum.

Salk, L., Hilgartner, M., & Granich, B. (1972). The psycho-social impact of hemophilia on the patient and his family. *Social Science and Medicine, 6,* 491–505.

Salk, L., & Routh, D. K. (1972, Spring). An open letter to the Society of Pediatric Psychology. *Newsletter of the Society of Pediatric Psychology,* pp. 1–2.

Schofield, W. (1969). The role of psychology in the delivery of health services. *American Psychologist, 24,* 565–584.

Schroeder, C. S. (1979). Psychologists in a private pediatric practice. *Journal of Pediatric Psychology, 4,* 5–18.

Schwartz, G. E., & Weiss, S. M. (1978). Yale Conference on Behavioral Medicine: A proposed definition and statement goals. *Journal of Behavioral Medicine, 1,* 3–12.

Singer, L., & Drotar, D. (1989). Psychological practice in a pediatric rehabilitation hospital. *Journal of Pediatric Psychology, 14,* 479–489.

Smith, E. E., Rome, L. P., & Freedheim, D. K. (1967). The clinical psychologist in the pediatric office. *Journal of Pediatrics, 71,* 48–51.

Stabler, B., & Mesibov, G. B. (1984). Role functions of pediatric and health psychologists in health care settings. *Professional Psychology, 15,* 142–151.

Stabler, B., & Whitt, J. K. (1980). Pediatric psychology: Perspectives and training implications. *Journal of Pediatric Psychology, 5,* 245–251.

Toback, C., Russo, R. M., & Gururaj, V. J. (1975). Pediatric psychology as practiced in a large municipal hospital setting. *Pediatric Psychology, 3,* 10–11.

Tuma, J. M. (1980). Training in pediatric psychology: A concern for the 1980s. *Journal of Pediatric Psychology, 5,* 229–243.

Tuma, J. M. (Ed.). (1982a). *Handbook for the practice of pediatric psychology.* New York: Wiley.

Tuma, J. M. (1982b). Training in pediatric psychology. In J. M. Tuma (Ed.), *Handbook for the practice of pediatric psychology* (pp. 321–346). New York: Wiley.

Tuma, J. M. (Ed.). (1985). *Proceedings: Conference on training clinical child psychologists.* Baton Rouge, LA: Section on Clinical Child Psychology, American Psychological Association.

Tuma, J. M. (1989). *Directory of internship programs in clinical child and pediatric psychology.* Baton Rouge: Louisiana State University.

Tuma, J. M., & Cawunder, P. (1983). Orientation preference and practice patterns of members of professional child psychology sections and divisions of APA. *The Clinical Psychologist, 36,* 72–75.

Tuma, J. M., & Grabert, J. (1983). Internship and postdoctoral training in pediatric and clinical child psychology: A survey. *Journal of Pediatric Psychology, 8,* 245–260.

Varni, J. W. (1983). *Clinical behavior pediatrics.* New York: Pergamon.

Walker, C. E. (1979). Behavioral intervention in a pediatric setting. In J. R. McNamara (Ed.), *Behavioral approaches to medicine: Application and analysis* (pp. 227–266). New York: Plenum.

Walker, C. E. (1988). The future of pediatric psychology. *Journal of Pediatric Psychology, 13,* 465–478.

White, S. (1991). Pediatric psychology: An abbreviated history of 21 years. *Journal of Pediatric Psychology, 16,* 395–410.

Williams, B. J., Foreyt, J. P., & Goodrick G. K. (1981). *Pediatric behavioral medicine.* New York: Praeger.

Willis, D. J. (Special Editor). (1975). Special topical issue: Pediatric psychology. *Journal of Clinical Child Psychology, 4* (Whole No. 3).

Willis, D. J. (1977). Birth of a journal: Editorial reflections and farewell. *Journal of Pediatric Psychology, 2,* 2–3.

Wright, L. (1967). The pediatric psychologist: A role model. *American Psychologist, 22,* 323–325.

Wright, L. (1969). Pediatric psychology: Prospect and retrospect. *Pediatric Psychology, 1,* 1–3.

Wright, L., & Jimmerson, S. (1971). Intellectual sequelae of hemophilus, influenza meningitis. *Journal of Abnormal Psychology, 77,* 181–183.

Wright, L., Nunnery, A., Eichel, B., & Scott, R. (1968). Application of conditioning principles to problems of tracheostomy addiction in children. *Journal of Consulting and Clinical Psychology, 32,* 603–606.

Wright, L., Schaefer, A. B., & Solomons, G. (1979). *Encyclopedia of pediatric psychology.* Baltimore: University Park Press.

Wright, L., Woodcock, J. M., & Scott, R. (1970). Treatment of sleep disturbance in a young child by conditioning. *Southern Medical Journal, 44,* 969–972.

I

Early Development of Pediatric Psychology

Michael C. Roberts

The University of Kansas

The introductory chapter of this volume discussed the status and definition of pediatric psychology, its history, and future. A number of developmental milestones were noted in the scientific research, clinical practice, professional issues, and organizational home for the field. The progression was not smooth or totally mapped in advance. The field is currently thriving because of the strength of early conceptualization, the vision of its pioneers, the clear need for better understanding of relationships, and the quality of interventions serving children and families.

Two articles have been selected for this section that represent the founding and early conceptualization of psychosocial professionals functioning in pediatric psychologists' activities. Also, as noted, the article by Logan Wright (1967, and reprinted here) was essential in establishing and defining the field. Indeed, it coined the label "pediatric psychology." It remains one of the most cited articles in the field because of its enduring influence and prescience. There were a few psychologists working in pediatric units in 1967, but there was no organization for interaction and no conceptual framework to bind them together. The Wright article and the organizational efforts of Wright, Lee Salk, and Dorothea Ross provided the impetus for getting started and becoming viable. Thinking and practice at the time were also influenced by Salk's (1970) article in *Professional Psychology* describing the functioning of psychology in pediatrics and his (1974) chapter on the pediatrician–psychologist collaboration. Similarly, important conceptual and descriptive articles were published by Fischer and Engeln (1972) and Smith, Rome, and Freedheim (1967).

The article by Marvin Ack (1974) is reprinted here from the *Pediatric Psychology* newsletter as an illustration of how psychosocial conceptualizations and interventions were applied to pediatric settings. At the time of publication, there had been little attention given to the psychosocial needs of children in the hospital. Ack's article and the Children's Hospital in Minneapolis have been cited repeatedly as influential examples for changing hospital practices in general and opening opportunities for psychologists, social workers, and, eventually, child life specialists to provide psychosocial services. Many innovative aspects of this hospital were prompted by a book by Milton Shore, *Red is the Color of Hurting* (1967). Shore and Goldston (1976) later guest edited a special issue of the *Journal of Pediatric Psychology,* "Families, Children, and Hospitalization." In it, Hall (1976), of the Minneapolis Children's Hospital, for example, described the role of the psychologist in an ecologically oriented comprehensive health care program.

Where many psychosocial policies were nonexistent or restrictive not too many years ago, now most pediatric and children's hospitals have formally defined policies and procedures to insure the integrity and support of children and their families (Peterson & Ridley-Johnson, 1980). A comprehensive survey of hospitals serving children in North America (Maieron & Roberts, 1993; Roberts, Maieron, & Collier, 1988) found, for example, that over 70% of the hospitals had written policies delineating a role for families and recognizing the child's developmental and individual needs as priorities in planning care. Ninety-four percent had 24-hour visitation rights for parents and permitted rooming in with the child. Play or recreation rooms were available in 97% of the general and pediatric hospitals, and 82% had professionally staffed play, recreation, or child life programs. These are immense gains from the time in 1974 when Ack noted that "there was one hospital in our country where mental health expertise is a routine part of every decision" (p. 3). Not only does the Minneapolis Children's Hospital continue these then-innovative practices, but now, fortunately, so do most other quality hospitals in the U.S. and Canada.

The results of Roberts et al. (1988) demonstrate how change has occurred in the way children and families are treated in the medical setting. Yet, there is still more room for continued growth in implementing developmentally sound, psychosocially oriented, family-centered care. The Association for the Care of Children's Health, for example, has published a comprehensive set of guidelines for psychosocial care of children and families in hospitals in conjunction with a number of endorsing groups including the Society of Pediatric Psychology (Johnson, Jeppson, & Redburn, 1992). Built on these organizations' histories of effective advocacy and solid research foundation, these guidelines provide the definitive structure for administrators, unit leaders, and on-line professionals to implement such policies as involving parents in the care of their children, designing mental health-conducive medical environments, and training all staff in psychosocial practices. When implemented, the guidelines will help formalize and enhance what Ack envisioned in his descriptive article: Institutions where mental health permeates every structure and function will have beneficial effects for children and families.

Drotar (1991) outlined critical challenges to the future development of pediatric psychology for the future. The five challenges include (a) specialization and professional identity, (b) relationships with other professions, (c) securing resources necessary for effective functioning, (d) the conflict between clinical service delivery and prevention, and (e) development of training models. He described the developments of the past as setting the ground for future growth. In many ways, the pediatric psychology field has eclipsed even Wright's optimism for its growth. The remaining articles and overviews in this volume are, we hope, testimony to the fruits of the efforts of the founders of the field. These later articles reinforce the validity of the early writings (e.g., Ack, 1974; Salk, 1970; Wright, 1967). Many of the later articles published in the *Journal of Pediatric Psychology*, as the publication archive of the field and Society of Pediatric Psychology, might not have been envisioned by these founders, but these changes indicate the exciting evolution and potential for change inherent in research and practice of a dynamic field.

REFERENCES

Ack, M. (1974). The psychological environment of a children's hospital. *Pediatric Psychology, 2,* 3–5.

Association for the Care of Children's Health. (1989). *Caring for children and families: Guidelines for hospitals* (Draft for Field Testing). Washington, DC: Author.

Drotar, D. (1991). Coming of age: Critical challenges to the future development of pediatric psychology. *Journal of Pediatric Psychology, 16,* 1–11.

Fischer, H. L., & Engeln, R. G. (1972). How goes the marriage? *Professional Psychology, 3,* 73–79.

Hall, M. C. (1976). The child psychologist in an ecologically-oriented comprehensive health care program. *Journal of Pediatric Psychology, 1,* 12–13.

Johnson, B. H., Jeppson, E. S., & Redburn, L. (1992). *Caring for children and families: Guidelines for hospitals.* Bethesda, MD: Association for the Care of Children's Health.

Maieron, M., & Roberts, M. C. (1993). Psychosocial policies in hospitals serving children: Comparative characteristics. *Children's Health Care, 22,* 143–167.

Peterson, L., & Ridley-Johnson, R. (1980). Pediatric hospital response to survey on prehospital preparation for children. *Journal of Pediatric Psychology, 5,* 1–7.

Roberts, M. C., Maieron, M. J., & Collier, J. (1988). *Directory of hospital psychosocial policies and programs* (1988 edition). Washington, DC: Association for the Care of Children's Health.

Salk, L. (1970). Psychologist in a pediatric setting. *Professional Psychology, 1,* 395–396.

Salk, L. (1974). Psychologist and pediatrician: A mental health team in the prevention and early diagnosis of mental disorders. In G. J. Williams & S. Gordon (Eds.), *Clinical child psychology: Current practices and future perspectives* (pp. 110–115). New York: Behavioral Publications.

Shore, M. F. (Ed.). (1967). *Red is the color of hurting.* Washington, DC: U.S. Government Printing Office.

Shore, M. F., & Goldston, S. E. (Special editors). (1976). Special topical issue: Families, children, and hospitalization. *Journal of Pediatric Psychology, 1* (Whole No. 4).

Smith, E. E., Rome, L. P., & Freedheim, D. K. (1967). The clinical psychologist in the pediatric office. *Journal of Pediatrics, 71,* 48–51.

Wright, L. (1967). The pediatric psychologist: A role model. *American Psychologist, 22,* 323–325.

1

The Pediatric Psychologist
A Role Model

Logan Wright
University of Oklahoma Medical Center

In a recent article, Kagan (1965) announced a marriage had taken place between pediatrics and psychology. If this union proceeds like most which are happy and productive, then we might soon look forward to a "blessed event." The offspring could be of two sexes: the psychological pediatrician and the pediatric psychologist. The psychological pediatrician will be a scholar-professional who is trained both as a physician and as a behavioral scientist. He will emerge from the growing number of medical school programs which now combine the residency in a medical specialty with the PhD in a related academic area. At least one major program (University of Iowa) now offers the opportunity to combine a pediatric residency with a PhD in child psychology. The purpose of this article, however, is not to make presumptions regarding medical offspring but rather to focus on those of psychological gender.

Presumably a pediatric psychologist is any psychologist who finds himself dealing primarily with children in a medical setting which is nonpsychiatric in nature. Since the prevalence of such workers is apparently increasing, the question must be raised as to whether there is a significant difference in the psychologist's role under psychiatric versus pediatric circumstances.

The basic researcher, utilizing child subjects but with interests in the traditional areas of learning, perception, development, etc., may not be significantly affected by a change in his working environment. However, psychologists who render professional services might best seek to understand the implications of having a clientele which consists of nonpsychiatric referrals and colleagues who are neither exclusively nor primarily interested

Reprinted from *American Psychologist,* 22, 323-325. Copyright 1967 by the American Psychological Association. By permission.

in behavioral problems. The psychologist who is insensitive to the altered requirements of pediatric circumstances, or who is too inflexible to change his role, may wind up like a kind of refrigerator salesman among Eskimos: most pediatricians will resist his offerings and the "buyers" remain bewildered as to just why their purchase was necessary. In this connection, let me venture to sculpture a psychologist's model, which, it is hoped, has goodness of fit with the pediatric setting.

Ideally the pediatric psychologist is a person who is competently trained in both child development and in the child clinical area. Knowledge of child development is an essential part of the understanding necessary in the performance of psychological work as well as a vital ingredient in making the psychologist a valuable teacher and consultant who aids medical colleagues and students in their respective endeavors. Training in the clinical area is, of course, necessary if the psychologist is to be a contributing member of a medical treatment or teaching team.

In the area of psychological testing, the kinds of diagnostic services which the pediatric psychologist is asked to render will not be typical. Requests for developmental and/or cognitive appraisals are disproportionately high by comparison to the requirements of a psychiatric setting. For this reason, the pediatric psychologist should be predisposed toward, and uniquely skilled in, making such evaluations. The damaged prestige, as well as the grossness and lack of precision, which has characterized much intellectual assessment in recent years is highly inappropriate in the pediatric setting. Ideally the pediatric psychologist should feel that cognitive development represents an area in which referral questions can best be answered, and he should welcome the opportunity to respond at a higher level of confidence than is usually achieved in many of the other areas of assessment.

Another area of extensive pediatric concern is that of child rearing. A tremendous claim on the pediatrician's time is made by parents with child-rearing problems. The pediatrician is, of course, uniquely qualified to answer those problems which are biological in nature, however, the pediatric psychologist is in a strategic position to assist in handling behavioral difficulties. He should, therefore, be aware of what constitutes a desirable climate for optimal cognitive, affective, and interpersonal growth. And, he should possess the ability to help parents develop appropriate skills in providing such a climate. Ideally, he should maintain a conviction that the behavioral sciences have uncovered certain principles of human behavior which can benefit parents and seek to generate new knowledge regarding such principles as well as ways of communicating these principles to parents.

The majority of patients seen in pediatric settings are reasonably free of significant psychopathology in the form of neurotic or psychotic disorders. This should not, of course, be interpreted as a justification for inadequate understanding of psychopathology, but must be viewed as a need for increased knowledge and interest in the area of normal personality. Traditionally psychiatry and clinical psychology have been absorbed in the matters of aberrant behavior. What better place than the pediatric setting could one find to fill the gaps of knowledge regarding normal personality and positive mental health. Possibly this is the place where problems of prevention of emotional disorders and even the study of conspicuously effective personality could best be undertaken. It is hoped that pediatric psychology will emerge as a frontier for research in these areas.

In addition to possessing an unusual knowledge concerning child development, cognitive appraisals, and normal personality the pediatric psychologist might best contribute to the effectiveness of our newly wed discipline if he possesses two additional predispositions: toward economy and toward the applied. The pediatrician, and for the most part the entire pediatric setting, is not geared to treatment which involves extensive amounts of professional time being expended with single patients. Time is more limited, and volume is higher. Cases cannot be handled by such techniques as long-term individual psychotherapy. Since the psychodiagnostic and particularly the psychotherapeutic areas of the mental field are in dire need of methods which are more economical, it seems reasonable that pediatric psychology might focus upon research designed to uncover methods which are temporally and financially efficient.

As for the question of applied versus basic research, this also appears to have some significance for pediatric psychology. At this stage of the new relationship, there is likely to be more interest in the application of existing psychological knowledge to pediatric problems than in extending the boundaries of knowledge in the behavioral sciences. Even in the beginning, it would be hoped that basic knowledge might result if only as a byproduct. But, basic knowledge must eventually emerge if the research of pediatric psychologists is to escape the plague of results which cannot be generalized beyond their own area of specialization. Possibly behavioral research in the pediatric setting will not suffer a great deal from an initial exposure to the world of applied problems. The value of such exposure in enabling subsequent research of a basic type to raise the most pertinent and answerable questions would appear to be substantial.

What does the future of pediatric psychology hold? At least three trends need to be firmly set in motion. These involve: (a) a clear delineation of the role of the pediatric psychologist, (b) more specific training for personnel who plan to enter this area, and (c) construction of a new body of knowledge. As a first step in clarifying the role of the pediatric psychologist, a survey of national scope would appear to be in order. Its purposes would be to tally the numbers and kinds of psychological personnel involved in pediatric settings at the present time, to identify the proportion of time these persons spend in various activities such as teaching and consultation with other professionals, various types of diagnostic and therapeutic endeavors, etc., and to solicit the opinions of these people regarding what pediatric psychology should involve.

Role confusion could be more rapidly eliminated if psychologists in pediatric settings could obtain a sense of group identity and increase intragroup communication. In this connection, some formal organization such as a special interest group within existing divisions of the American Psychological Association (for example, Division 7 or Division 12) would seem to be in order. A newsletter or other forms of intragroup communication would also be invaluable in helping to solidify and enhance the pediatric psychologist's role.

If and when a clearer picture of pediatric psychology emerges, it should then be possible to upgrade the quality of training for personnel in this area. It is possible that adjustments could occur in university affiliated clinical training programs as well as at the internship and postdoctoral levels. Initially the internship would appear to be the most practical place to initiate change. Universities of necessity, and appropriately so, emphasize the basics of theory and methodology which are common to all psychologists regardless of specialization. As far as postdoctoral programs are concerned, pediatric psychology will not soon attain either a sufficient identity or an extensive enough body of knowledge to warrant anything like a 1- or 2-year postdoctoral program. Internships in pediatric psychology or regular clinical internships with special emphasis in this area appear most logical as first steps. But, unless something is done at some level of training, the mistake will be made of having personnel who are pediatric psychologists not by training and experience but by experience only. It is hoped that other forms of training in addition to that offered at the internship level can emerge as additional maturation occurs in both pediatric psychology and in psychologists' conceptions of professional training.

Finally no behavioral discipline or subspecialty can justify its existence in the present world unless it has something unique to contribute to knowledge. Initially, pediatric psychology may attempt primarily to apply existing knowledge in child clinical psychology and child development to pediatric problems. The knowledge which will be generated, if the results of such applications are carefully controlled and recorded, will form the embryo of a new body of knowledge. It is hoped that this embryo will grow and be supplemented by certain areas of basic research which will emerge as being unique and of special interest to pediatric psychologists. There is no doubt that journal space will be made available as worthwhile research of this type begins to emerge.

As a prospective movement which hopes to contribute to the quality of psychological activities in the service of children, as well as to the level of understanding in the behavioral sciences, it is hoped that pediatric psychology might develop rapidly. An emerging role and a sense of group identity would facilitate such growth. What appears to be needed at this point are card-carrying members of a militant group set out to destroy inappropriateness and inefficiency in psychological services, as well as the dearth of behavioral information, in pediatric settings.

REFERENCE

Kagan, J. The new marriage: Pediatrics and psychology. *American Journal of Diseases of Children,* 1965, 110, 272-278.

2

The Psychological Environment of a Children's Hospital

Marvin Ack, Ph.D.

Children's Health Center and Hospital, Minneapolis, Minnesota

In most hospitals around the country, psychologists, psychiatrists and social workers devote most of their energy and expertise to the disturbed and disturbing child. While we are so engaged, the reality is that most hospitals are run by administrators who, although bright and dedicated people, are primarily governed by considerations of personnel efficiency and financial stability. The rules, regulations, and procedures of most pediatric hospitals, are in short, established for the convenience of physicians, surgeons, administrators, board members, etc.: for the *adults,* not the children. The very purpose of the hospital—to get children well, may be undermined by these organizational factors which so often affect therapeutic practices.

Despite our increased sophistication in a variety of areas, I do not believe there was one hospital in our country where mental health expertise is a routine part of every decision. The Children's Health Center and Hospital in Minneapolis is committed to change in this limited concept of a health care delivery system. The Center admitted its first in-patient on January 29 of this year. But, the ideas of total and comprehensive health care had been germinating for twenty years. At that time a Board of Trustees was established and has been in continuous existence since. When I was contacted last in 1971 and asked to assume the position of Director of Mental Health, I was told that the Board and the physicians associated with the venture wanted a hospital where the child's emotional state would be given as much weight as his physical condition. Further, mental health was to permeate the entire hospital and I was asked how this could be accomplished.

What follows is the result of the thinking and efforts of myself, a volunteer Mental Health Committee and the mental health staff of the Center.

Reprinted from *Pediatric Psychology,* 2(3)(1974):3–5.

The Committee is composed of community professionals who unstintingly donated their time to develop our plan of action. Our conviction is that if one wishes to produce institutional change, two areas must be attacked simultaneously: the psychological sophistication of the individuals within the organization must be increased so that they meet and treat persons in constructive ways that foster adaptation; and secondly, systems factors must be altered, wherever necessary, to allow that increased sophistication to manifest itself. Too often one hears sensitive employees state "that is what I would like to do, but time doesn't permit it," or "our organizational chart doesn't permit those types of interventions or behaviors."

As a consultant, one can only suggest system changes, whereas an Officer of the organization has the power and responsibility to make such alterations when the welfare of the patient demands it. In our organization, decision-making resides in the Office of the President which consists of the President (a pediatrician), a Vice President for Administration, and a Vice President for Mental Health Ecology. This *troika* operates under the assumption that decisions in one area of the hospital will necessarily have repercussions in all other areas. For example, one cannot make a decision on the nurse-patient ratio solely on the basis of economics. That ratio is determined by and conversely effects the therapeutic programs. Therefore, rules, regulations, procedures, programs and personnel practices are thoroughly discussed, viewed from every point of view and decisions are jointly arrived at. The responsibilities of the Vice President for Mental Health Ecology go from scrutinizing practices and effecting changes in the admitting process through discharge and follow-up. For example, and as a result of the direct input of mental health, for elective hospital admissions, the admitting work is done in advance so that on the day of hospitalization, all the parent needs to do is to sign a form. Almost no one ever spends more than five to ten minutes in the Business Office before being shown to their room. If it is not an elective situation, we will often take the child to his room, make him comfortable, and then fill out the admitting forms at the bedside, or have the parent come down later to the Business Office. In our Emergency Room, the forms first ask for the presenting problems and lastly ask for insurance information. We wanted our Emergency Room personnel to concern themselves with the physical status of the youngster, and all our forms and procedures reflect and reinforce this major concern. In our Outpatient Department all patients are seen by appointment and if anyone has to wait ten minutes beyond his appointment time, nurses have been taught to tell the patient the exact reason for the delay. As a result, we have many patients who prefer our Clinic to private pediatric offices because of the consideration and courtesy they receive.

We have unlimited visiting privileges for both parents and siblings. We feel strongly that the experience should be as normal a one as possible. We have made provisions for and encourage parents of pre-schoolers to spend the night with their child. When they do, they are urged to assume responsibility for the non-medical care of the child. Siblings are prompted to visit their brothers or sisters to allay their feelings and fears that something drastic might have occurred to them. Again, this decision was reached by the mental health staff in consort with all the nursing supervisors and ultimately with all nursing personnel. Parents of pre-school children, fearful of separation can accompany their child through the induction of anesthesia so as to lessen the anxiety of separation. The anesthesiologist who will attend at the operation will visit the child and family the night before. At that time, among other duties, he describes his entire procedure. Because small children are often more fearful of leaving Mother than they are of surgery, the mother will hold the child in her lap while anesthesia is administered. She is often the one to place the mask on her youngster's face. This was a joint decision of the mental health staff and the anesthesiologists. We hope soon to experiment with parents in the post operative recovery area. In discussions with many of our surgical staff, a variety of new procedures were established which we feel lessen the psychic trauma of surgery as well as the potential development of pathogenic fantasies. For example, a child about to have his tonsils removed will wear his pajama bottoms through surgery. A small point, perhaps, but very important to the four to six year old concerned about the integrity of his genitals.

Our efforts have not been limited just to regulations and programs as novel as they may be. We were also consulted in regard to the architecture and decor of the hospital. For example, we have two sets of elevators: one for inpatients going to and from surgery, etc., and another for outpatients and the general public. The purpose of this costly plan is obvious: we did not want to have children coming for routine physical examinations to see severely ill youngsters. And for the severely ill child, we did not want him subjected to the stares and whispers of others. All our departments (which service both in and outpatients) have dual access to maintain this principle. The hospital is carpeted throughout; the walls are painted orange and yellow with some blue and purple mixed in. Other walls are decorated with Peter Max type wallpaper. None of our staff wear traditional hospital uniforms, but rather—wear smocks of different colors to identify them. Nurses wear blue smocks, lab technicians—green, X-ray technicians—orange, office personnel—brown, and so forth. Since traditional hospitals are so stigmatized in the minds of children, we deliberately try to avoid the traditional look. Prior to the opening of the hospital, an art contest was held to which only children attending Minneapolis public schools could participate. From the 1500 pictures submitted, 300 of them were selected, framed and now hang in rooms and on walls throughout the hospital.

Each Saturday morning, children scheduled to enter the hospital the following week, are invited to a preoperative tour. First, they are taken to each area of the hospital they will experience. They visit the rooms, the X-ray department, the anesthesia "holding area," the intensive care unit (if necessary), the playrooms, and so forth. They are shown where their parents will wait while they are being operated upon. Following the tour and some Coke and cookies, a nurse and a mental health staff member will talk with the parents while a group of specially trained volunteers will play a modified version of "the doctor game" with the children. The children get an opportunity to use stethoscopes, measure blood pressure, try on surgical garb, give injections and so forth. While this is going on, parents will have a discussion about the meanings of hospitalization, possible psychological consequences and how they can aid their youngsters to successfully cope with this potentially difficult situation.

Our psychological rationale is twofold: 1. An event is traumatic primarily because it is unexpected. Therefore, to the greatest extent possible, we prepare children and their parents for everything that will occur. The more disturbing and frightening the event, the greater the need for preparation. 2. The natural way children have of "working through" difficult life experiences is to do actively what they have experienced passively; therefore, the doctor game. In addition, once on the ward, nurses have been educated to help the child discuss his operation and his associated feelings. Some children write autobiographies of their stay, others paint pictures of their experiences—whatever technique, the children and parents are assisted in working through the event. In addition, each floor has a well-equipped playroom with a recreational therapist. Recreation is used not primarily as a diversionary activity, but as a therapeutic device.

If a child or parent is excessively apprehensive, they or their physician can request individual preparation by a member of the mental health staff. Although the techniques and interpretations may vary according to the age and illness of the child, the goals of the preparation are the same for all children. First, we attempt to elicit the fantasies the patient has about what is wrong with him and what will be done to him while in the hospital. Then he is helped to understand that no one is at fault, especially him. Following that, he is given a complete and honest description of his anesthesia, surgery, and post-operative care. Depending on his age, this may be done with dolls, clay, drawings or any other device which seems fruitful. Lastly, he will be convinced that only the parts of the body discussed will be operated upon. During this time we are careful to avoid such emotionally laden words as 'cut' or 'put to sleep.' By now, a large proportion of our attending medical staff who are going to hospitalize children for major procedures such as open heart surgery or cancer, will almost routinely refer the child and his family to the mental health unit.

Obviously, one cannot always predict in advance which child will be adversely affected by a hospital stay. Therefore, each ward has assigned to it, a mental health staff person. (I keep using the phrase "mental health staff" because we try hard not to make distinctions between social worker, psychologist, and psychiatrist. Competency, not discipline, determines what an individual can do.) The staff person will make frequent ward rounds, working directly with patients or with their parents or with any of the hospital staff responsible for the child.

The Director of Mental Health was involved in interviewing and hiring all supervisory personnel. This was done to get his assessment of the person's capacity to work with children and in such an atmosphere, and to impress upon the potential employee the central position of the child's "feeling state." For three months prior to our opening and continuing presently, a weekly seminar for supervisors has been held on the "psychology of leadership." We feel strongly that it is difficult to meet the emotional demands children make in a setting as highly charged as a hospital unless each individual felt himself to be a significant and valued member of the organization. This can be accomplished only when persons feel they have a voice in the decisions which govern their functioning. As much as possible, each department determines its own modus operandi, and each person in the department has a voice in that decision. It is ludicrous and naive to expect an institution to function effectively unless employee morale is high. We have worked diligently to apply mental health sensitivity to personnel problems and thereby maintain the atmosphere we created.

I hope the foregoing has given you a feeling for ubiquitousness of the mental health program. By placing the Director of Mental Health in the top echelons of management, an ambassador with portfolio was created. The position itself says to the employees and the public alike, "the mental health of the patient is a crucial concern to this hospital." In addition, it gives mental health an opportunity to contribute input to those hundreds of daily decisions which in most hospitals are made on the basis of financial criteria only. Decisions which nonetheless significantly affect the total ambience of the institution and therefore the ability to deliver health care in a psychologically sound fashion.

Earlier, it was stated that if positive psychological principles were to govern an institution's practices, the sophistication of the staff must be increased. Despite how talented the mental health staff may be, in a pediatric hospital it is really the nurses, doctors, lab technicians, aids and volunteers who dispense the majority of "mental health." It is they who are in constant and prolonged contact with the child and it is they who can make or break such a program. Therefore, from its inception the mental health program accepted as its top priority, the education of other professional health care deliverers. A large proportion of our staff's time is spent in just such educational endeavors. Regularly scheduled seminars on such topics as principles of child rearing, psychology of stress, psychological effects of hospitalization and surgery, management of the dying patient and principles of child development are held or planned for all personnel. Although didactic methods are occasionally used, most of our teaching centers around cases with whom ward personnel are currently contending. The content of these seminars includes not only the psychology of the child, but what feelings or fantasies are going on in the staff. It is the author's belief that a majority of the medical "errors" made, are the result of feelings or attitudes in the physician or nurse which block or distort perception, rather than from a lack of knowledge. A great deal of the content of these seminars is the feelings of the staff when faced with a particular type of child. Such a format assures relevancy rather than dealing only with what is of interest to the teacher, but often considered esoteric by others. By relying on discussion rather than lecture, we keep the participants active rather than passive, and attempt to change unproductive attitudes as opposed to simply conveying knowledge and praying it will be used appropriately. In short, we try to adhere to our own principles of learning.

Another regularly scheduled meeting is our psychiatric grand rounds conference. At this time a patient who has been comprehensively assessed in our mental health clinic is presented. The purpose of this meeting is to demonstrate to others what an intensive examination of a child can reveal and equally important, what it cannot determine. Since so many of our non-psychology colleagues think our tests magic, it is sometimes extremely valuable to reinforce reality and thereby further the respect for the complexity of the human mind.

Another regularly scheduled meeting on some wards is mental health care conferences. These conferences are much shorter, are centered on a single child, involve only those personnel responsible for that youngster, and have as their goal a plan of action for all staff in their dealings with that patient.

Lastly, we have frequent ad hoc meetings with specific persons around particular topics. For example, when we first began to treat seriously burned children, we had major difficulties with their care. This was surmounted by having all of the staff meet together to discuss their feelings about the amount of pain they had to inflict as part of the therapy. This apparently simple expedient proved very successful and ultimately led to the establishment of a "burn team" which included representatives from surgery, physical medicine, occupational therapy, nursing and mental health.

Likewise, when our intensive care unit suddenly had three children expire after months of death-free operation, the mental health staff was called and conducted on-the-spot sessions to help the nursing staff deal with its feelings of frustration and dependence.

Although this is a pediatric medical/surgical hospital, our Outpatient department contains a mental health clinic. The clinic functions as do most child guidance clinics, both diagnostically and therapeutically. Fifty per cent of the mental health professional's time is assigned to clinic activities and 50 per cent to the mental health ecology program. We feel strongly that only persons well versed in clinical skills can do a really sensitive job in the area of prevention. Conversely, the clinician who gets the opportunity to see and deal with children in real situations, as opposed to the artificiality of the psychotherapy room, can only be a better, more realistic and sensitive therapist as a result. It also gives our staff a variety of activities, preventive, educative and therapeutic, which keep them constantly challenged and makes the long days bearable.

What we are attempting at The Children's Health Center and Hospital in Minneapolis, we feel is totally new. In addition, to have a psychologist in such a position in a medical setting, is to say the least—unique. Yet, in the seven short months we have been open, the number of referrals to the mental health unit has increased dramatically. The attendance and involvement of physicians and nurses at our voluntary meetings has risen surprisingly. Most important, we feel we have shortened the hospital stay for many patients, we have reduced the usual trauma of hospitalization for patients and families, and we have rendered more meaningful and satisfying the job of the individual health care attendant. Any novel and difficult event in the life of an individual is bound to have an effect upon the adjustment of that person. We hope we are demonstrating that in an institution where mental health permeates every structure, that effect can be a beneficial one. Equally, we hope our setting will serve to stimulate others to examine their institutions and the role psychology plays in its existence.

II

Chronic and Life-Threatening Conditions in Childhood

Gerald P. Koocher
Harvard Medical School

A natural evolutionary process has led to an increased focus within pediatric psychology on how chronic and life-threatening illnesses affect children and their families. The progress of modern pediatric medicine has driven this progression. Over the past three decades the toll taken by acute infectious illnesses of childhood, such as smallpox, diphtheria, and polio, has been drastically reduced or entirely eliminated. High-dose chemotherapy techniques have led to dramatic progress in the treatment of childhood cancer. Cardiac surgery techniques have improved by leaps and bounds. A wave of new drugs that control immune system functioning have made organ transplantation strikingly more successful than in the past. Genetic mapping holds great promise for predictive testing, preventive medical care, and spectacular new approaches to potentially cure illnesses which were previously untreatable. In some cases treatment is now available in utero for certain congenital conditions. Children who most certainly would have died without hope in the 1960s are destined to be the survivors of the twenty-first century. The net result is that illnesses which were uniformly and swiftly fatal have yielded to a more optimistic but uncertain future as chronic life-threatening conditions.

Consider the most obvious changes in the care of three chronic life-threatening illnesses affecting large numbers of children. Childhood cancer is no longer an automatic death sentence, but the treatments needed to pursue survival are medically intensive, symptomatically stressful, include degrees of anxiety-provoking uncertainty, and pose long-term iatrogenic risks. People with cystic fibrosis are living longer thanks to new antibiotics, and the prospect of new progress through molecular biology and genetics is on the horizon. While lung transplantation is an option for many with cystic fibrosis, this option is not a cure and carries risks of its own including the stresses of waiting for scarce organs and the hazards of chronic immuno-suppressant therapy. Juvenile diabetes is easier to treat than in the past thanks to genetically engineered insulin products, micro-electronic sensing devices, and the promise of islet-cell transplantation, but little is known about the real impact of these new products and techniques on long-range outcome for newly diagnosed children.

As medical techniques evolve, so does the practice of pediatric psychology. Psychotherapeutic intervention aimed at fostering better communication and coping among ill children and their families remains an important service. However, other issues demanding psychological intervention skills include those related to managing symptom control (e.g., pain and nausea), facilitating compliance with problematic medical regimens, fostering adaptation to intensive treatment contexts, and stress buffering for both affected families and professional staff delivering medical care. The papers selected for this section provide excellent examples of how psychological techniques have been successfully applied to keep pace with the evolution of medical care.

AN OVERVIEW OF FAMILY HEALTH PSYCHOLOGY

Reprinted in this section, Drotar's paper (1981) titled "Psychosocial Perspectives in Chronic Childhood Illness" was based on his Presidential Address to the Society of Pediatric Psychology. It presents a masterful overview of the special perspectives required in clinical, consultative, and research work with chronically ill children. Drotar describes the need to focus on the family as the unit of treatment or study in the psychology of chronic childhood illness. He also cautions the reader to view coping processes as a function of treatment, stage, and severity of the physical illness. At the same time, Drotar observes that research on personality factors comparing chronically ill children to healthy controls is not especially useful. Rather, he calls for a research focus on factors which contribute to successful coping in the three major arenas of any child's real-life context: family, school, and peer relations. He recognized perhaps the most significant conceptual change over the years in attending to the coping and adjustment strengths of children with chronic illness rather than focusing on the deficits they might or might not show in comparison to "healthy" control groups. This trend, supported by other writers, guides much of the research and practice in the field of pediatric psychology (e.g., Hanson et al., 1990).

In this article, Drotar also places important emphasis on issues related to the care providers. He notes that the comprehensive care of chronically ill children generally takes place under highly charged interpersonal conditions. These circumstances can lead to significant communication disruptions among and between both staff and family members. In addition, interactional problems between care providers and family members can raise ethical questions and uncertainties that compromise patient care. Drotar emphasizes that dialogue among the key players, both family members and professionals, appears to be the best solution.

Since publishing this paper, Drotar has continued to be highly productive as an investigator, with strong attention to familial factors in coping with chronic childhood illness. He has also developed some interest in cross-cultural aspects of chronic illness and medical care in developing nations. He continues to focus his work on family aspects of health psychology. There is no better corroboration of Drotar's foresight than the special series of 15 papers published in the June and September 1989 issues (Volume 14, Numbers 2 and 3) of the *Journal of Pediatric Psychology* on "Family Issues in Pediatric Psychology" (now published in a separate text; Roberts & Wallander, 1992). An edited volume by Akamatsu, Stephens, Hobfoll, and Crowther (1992) describes similar issues in family health psychology. In the decade following his presidential address, the most meaningful and valuable studies in this arena have followed the template described in Drotar's 1981 paper.

LISTENING TO PARENTS

Deaton's (1985) article "Adaptive Noncompliance in Pediatric Asthma: The Parent as Expert" was based on her doctoral dissertation and won a student research competition award from the Society of Pediatric Psychology. Deaton demonstrated that informed adaptive responding by parents caring for their children with asthma is far more likely to yield better management of childhood asthma than is rote compliance. She also illustrated the importance of recognizing parents as the experts on their children's unique patterns of responses to chronic conditions and related interventions. For example, a parent might properly decide that it is wiser to tolerate a degree of mild wheezing at bedtime, rather than treat immediately with medication that might induce insomnia. Compliance with a complex medical regimen will not succeed without active involvement by the parents and use of their knowledge base. As one parent told Deaton, "Doctors are sometimes right, but they better listen to a mother sometimes too, because she's with these kids 24 hours a day" (p. 11).

Perhaps Deaton's most significant finding was that adaptiveness was a better predictor of more favorable outcome than was compliance. The message for both clinicians and researchers is a need to refocus thinking about medical compliance in pediatric populations to recognize two points. First, parental expertise and awareness have critical value and, second, non-compliance may be adaptive in some cases. The importance of such factors in assuring medical adherence has been well supported by other authors (see e.g., Koocher, McGrath, & Gudas, 1990). Pediatric psychologists have given considerable attention to issues of adherence because of its importance to medical treatment and because of the useful contributions of psychology as a science of behavior. The August 1990 issue of the *Journal of Pediatric Psychology* was a special issue edited by Annette La Greca on "Adherence with Pediatric Regimens" presenting 10 articles dealing with such conditions as asthma (Lemanek, 1990), bone marrow transplantation (Phipps & DeCuir-Whalley, 1990), diabetes (Jacobson et al., 1990), and seizure disorders (Hazzard, Hutchinson, & Kraswiecki, 1990).

A few years later Deaton went on to further detail her work on parents as both experts and decision makers in the care of their children's asthma (Deaton & Olbrisch, 1987). She continues a strong professional focus on enhancing the role of parents in the care of their chronically ill children. More recently she has been at work on a guide for the families of children with traumatic brain injuries. In the interim, a growing body of research has tended to underscore the central point of Deaton's paper: the necessity to capitalize on parental skills, cooperation, and expertise in order to maximize effective care of the chronically ill child. The range of chronic conditions has been investigated particularly regarding family stress and parental roles, adaptation, and varied responses, including conditions of cancer (Sanger, Copeland, & Davidson, 1991), spina bifida (Kronenberger & Thompson, 1992), asthma and diabetes (Auslander, Haire-Joshu, Rogge, & Santiago, 1991; Hamlett, Pellegrini, & Katz, 1992; Hanson et al., 1990; Kovacs et al., 1990), cystic fibrosis (Mullins et al., 1991), juvenile rheumatoid arthritis (Chaney & Peterson, 1989; Ennett et al., 1991), sickle cell disease (Gil, Williams, Thompson, & Kinney, 1991), congenital heart disease (DeMaso et al., 1991), visual impairment (Henggeler, Watson, & Whelan, 1990), physical handicaps (Wallander et al., 1989), as well as general illness behavior (Walker & Zeman, 1992). Siblings and family functioning have also been studied for children with handicaps and chronic disease (Dyson, 1989; Lobato, Faust, & Spirito, 1988).

CHILDHOOD GENDER DISCORDANCE

Many practitioners are not inclined to regard childhood gender dysphoria as a chronic illness condition. Unfortunately, many would view such matters chiefly as a "behavior problem." Money and Russo (1979) helped to address this problem in their paper titled "Homosexual Outcome of Discordant Gender Identity/Role in Childhood: Longitudinal Follow-Up." John Money is probably the most prolific contemporary scholarly writer on gender-identity problems in the world. In this paper, written with his colleague from Johns Hopkins University, Anthony J. Russo, Money reports on a small but impressively followed longitudinal sample of boys with prepubertal discordance of gender. Money has been well known for studies of hermaphroditism and psychological issues related to abnormalities in other sexual anatomy or sexual genetics. As a result, referrals of children with other types of gender identity problems often came to his attention.

Twelve boys had been referred to Money's clinic at Johns Hopkins because of cross-dressing, preferring play activities more typical of girls, or stating an overt wish to be a girl. Nine who were between the ages of 23 and 29 at the time of follow-up were locatable for the 1979 report, and several of these young men had been followed annually. They had also received counseling through the clinic at Johns Hopkins. At the time of the follow-up, all were homosexual in sexual preference, or predominantly so. One more important finding was the lack of secondary psychopathology (i.e., psychopathology unrelated to gender issues) in this group as young adults. Another was the universal report by the now young adult males that they had benefitted from having a nonjudgmental counselor available to them during the difficult juvenile years when discussion of their intimate and sensitive sexual feelings brought scorn, disapproval, and stigmatization from other authority figures in their lives.

Money's long history of integrating the biological and the psychological in understanding gender dysphoria is all the more impressive given recent early reports of neuroanatomy differences between homosexual and heterosexual males. His special contributions were also recognized with a distinguished career contribution award by the American Psychological Association. On an anecdotal level, this study also provides important support for the long-term benefits of counseling this population. It appears that the relationships the young men had with their mental health counselors were islands of support and self-esteem-building experiences, at a time in their lives when they felt different, unaccepted, challenged, and intimidated by other elements in their lives in a homophobic society. His subsequent writings (Money, 1986, 1987) have reinforced these points by looking adaptively at the development of males with a homosexual adjustment pattern from both a psychological and biological perspective. A recent article in the *Journal of Pediatric Psychology* dealt with gender issues. Quattrin, Aronica, and Mazur (1991) reported on the psychosocial management of male hermaphroditism spanning 21 years.

PEDIATRIC PSYCHO-ONCOLOGY

Interestingly, two of the articles selected for this section were independently drawn by the panel of editors from the special *Journal* issue on "Death and the Child," edited by Koocher. Each article addresses a separate psychosocial aspect of pediatric oncology, with one focusing on consultation/liaison issues (O'Malley & Koocher, 1977) and the other discussing the involvement of children in the decision-making process of whether or not to use experimental chemotherapy at the end-stage of the illness (Nitschke, Wunder, Sexauer, & Humphrey, 1977). Both papers marked the early stages of a surge in attention to the psychological needs of children with cancer.

O'Malley and Koocher's (1977) paper, "Psychosocial Consultation to a Pediatric Oncology Unit: Obstacles to Effective Intervention," used actual clinical case material to illustrate typical obstacles encountered in consultation liaison work on a pediatric oncology ward. Differing perspectives of staff members, family members, and children with cancer were described in the context of how consultation requests are generated, how expectations diverge, and how the consultation model should constructively differ from the traditional medical "consult." Subsequent writings described the further evolution of this model (Koocher, Sourkes, & Keane, 1979), burnout prevention in doing such work (Koocher, 1979, 1980), and the problems of long-term cancer survivors (Koocher & O'Malley, 1981). O'Malley has left consultation liaison work and is now a vice president of the Devereaux Foundation. Koocher's recent work has reached into the realms of medical nonadherence and adaptation to bereavement.

Subsequent work published in the *Journal of Pediatric Psychology* (Kazak & Meadows, 1989; Speechley & Noh, 1992) has underscored the factors which facilitate coping with childhood cancer with a special emphasis on social support and coping strategies (Bull & Drotar, 1991; Sanger, Copeland, & Davidson, 1991). Such material is part of a growing literature of value to those doing consultation/liaison work with oncology patients. By identifying the contextual factors bearing on adjustment, staff intervening from the time of initial hospitalization onward will be better able to focus on the known points of vulnerability in long-term adjustment.

The other article reprinted here from the special issue of the *Journal of Pediatric Psychology* on "Death and the Child" is by Nitschke, Wunder, Sexauer, and Humphrey (1977): "The Final-Stage Conference: The Patient's Decision on Research Drugs in Pediatric Oncology." This important paper effectively documents an important turning point in the care of children with terminal cancer. Less than a decade earlier, Evans and Edin

(1968), both pediatric oncologists, had advocated a kind of benign lying to children with cancer. They noted with apparent regret, "A present trend seems to emphasize complete frankness and discussion of death with the fatally ill child" (p. 142). In place of such an approach, Evans and Edin argued in favor of shielding the child from fears of death. In their ground-breaking 1977 paper, Nitschke and his colleagues demonstrated the value of actively involving both the child and family in discussions about experimental chemotherapy, palliative steps, and other aspects of terminal care. It was clear that children as young as 6 years of age could actively participate in this constructive, alliance-building, patient care conference method.

Nitschke and his colleagues followed their *Journal of Pediatric Psychology* paper with a number of elaborations on the same theme. Perhaps the most widely cited one appeared in *The Journal of Pediatrics* five years later (Nitschke et al., 1982). These papers were highly influential in persuading practitioners that the benefits of open communication and active involvement of both the child and family result in better medical care and less emotional strain on all concerned than do secret keeping and concealed decision making. A few of the many subsequent papers providing confirmatory data on the value of such open communications include Claflin and Barbarin (1991), Slavin, O'Malley, Koocher, and Foster (1981), and Spinetta (1980). As a result of this body of work, there are few advocates of keeping children out of the decision-making loop today.

As more and more children survive cancer and its treatment, pediatric psychology researchers have investigated such issues of emotional strain of parenting these children in terms of social support (Kazak & Meadows, 1989; Speechley & Noh, 1992), stressors and coping strategies (Bull & Drotar, 1991), and child-rearing practices (Davies, Noll, DeStefano, Bukowski, & Kulkarni, 1991). Aspects of the children who have survived cancer have also been examined for peer relationships and adjustment (Noll, LeRoy, Bukowski, Rogosch, & Kulkarni, 1991; Spirito et al., 1990).

COPING WITH DEATH AND LOSS

Two papers reprinted in this section focused attention on family coping following the death of a child from cancer, although the findings apply as well to the loss of a child from any cause. Once again, as with most of the papers in this section, Drotar's (1981) advice on the sort of research and intervention planning that is necessary for successful work in pediatric psychology is well illustrated.

Spinetta, Swarner, and Sheposh (1981) addressed, "Effective Parental Coping Following the Death of a Child from Cancer." In this particular paper, Spinetta and his colleagues present data on a semistructured interview schedule as a means of assessing a family's adaptation to loss following the death of a child from cancer. This paper was an important first step in the development of an instrument to test long-standing but inadequately documented hypotheses from the anecdotal clinical literature on parental bereavement.

Important factors related to level of adjustment included a consistent philosophy of life, sources of interpersonal support, and the ability to have open communication with their terminally ill child. Typical of Spinetta's prodigious research on childhood cancer, this paper used creative methods of inquiry to focus on qualitative interpersonal aspects of care for the ill child. In addition to addressing feelings of depression, the instrument also addresses the resumption of normal social contacts, the ability to directly confront reminders of the deceased child, and concealed unresolved feelings.

Spinetta subsequently became the first psychologist to receive a career development award from the American Cancer Society and was honored by the Society of Pediatric Psychology for his significant research contributions. The semistructured interview instrument described in this paper has now been translated into eight languages and is being used in cross-cultural bereavement research under Spinetta's direction and the auspices of the World Health Organization at 15 centers around the world with the families of childhood cancer and thalassemia patients. Data collection sites currently include Italy, Greece, Germany, Austria, Belgium, Holland, France, Hong Kong, Singapore, and Bangkok.

The second paper in this category focused on similar issues, but from a more global and longitudinal perspective. Therese Rando's paper (1983) titled "An Investigation of Grief and Adaptation in Parents Whose Children Have Died from Cancer," like that of Ann Deaton, was a work growing out of a doctoral dissertation that marked the beginning of a substantial and impressive body of writing. In this case the focus has been fairly consistently on bereavement issues, with special attention to coping with the death of a child. In this particular study she reported on the experiences and adaptation of 54 parents interviewed between two months and three years following their child's death from cancer. She discovered a phenomenon of intensification of grief in the third year after the loss, suggesting that for some parents bereavement may actually worsen over time. She also found that there are "optimum" amounts of anticipatory grief, and that previous loss experiences were associated with poorer bereavement outcomes in many cases. Many of her findings seemed paradoxical or surprising at the time, but were subsequently supported by other reports (e.g., Koocher & MacDonald, 1992; Osterweis, Solomon, & Green, 1984).

Rando's continued work on the particular aspect of mourning a child culminated in the highly praised volume titled *Parental Loss of a Child* (Rando, 1986a). Her other books include *Grief, Dying, and Death: Clinical Interventions for Caregivers* (1984), *Loss and Anticipatory Grief* (1986b), and *How to Go on Living When Someone You Love Dies* (1988). She is now internationally known as an expert in adaptation to loss and has proven her talent for integrating scientific findings in a manner that can be used effectively for the general reader.

COMMONALITIES

Each of the papers in this section attempts in some way to link theory to application from a bio-psycho-social perspective in the care of children with chronic or life-threatening conditions. As a group, the papers emphasize the need for a comprehensive contextual approach to understanding and intervening systemically for the benefit of such children. The importance of social support by family members, peers, and care providers is evident in each paper. In addition, the value of thoughtful psychological intervention in improving long-term outcomes is also well illustrated. One aspect of chronic and life-threatening illness not covered in these reprinted articles is the impact of the disease and its medical treatment on other aspects of pediatric patients' functioning. Nonetheless, this consideration has received attention from pediatric psychologists. For example, the effects of medical treatment for cancer (including cranial radiation and chemotherapy) have been studied in terms of cognitive abilities and processing (Copeland et al., 1988; Cousens, Ungerer, Crawford, & Stevens, 1991; Heukrodt et al., 1988; Waber et al., 1990; Williams Ochs, Williams, & Mulhern, 1990). Other diseases and their treatments have also been studied (e.g., neuropsychological functioning after liver transplantation; Stewart et al., 1991).

The articles reprinted in this section exemplify an important characteristic of pediatric psychology—indeed, many would view this work in chronic and life-threatening conditions as the *sine qua non* distinguishing this field from others (Peterson & Harbeck, 1988; Roberts, 1986). Indubitably, the future developments in the field will relate to these types of phenomena as advancements in medicine bring on issues of adjustment, side effects, adherence, and survival. Similarly, the advances in the psychological understanding of these types of pediatric problems will enhance the care and functioning of children and families. The papers reprinted here represent seminally important pieces in the development of effective, comprehensive, and humane treatment of children and families with chronic and life-threatening conditions. They clearly fulfill the mandate for the field noted in the masthead of the *Journal of Pediatric Psychology:* "the relationship between psychological and physical well-being of children and adolescents including . . . evaluation and treatment of behavioral and emotional problems and concomitants of disease and illness . . . "

REFERENCES

Akamatsu, T. J., Stephens, M. A. P., Hobfoll, S. E., Crowther, J. H. (Eds.). (1992). *Family health psychology.* New York: Hemisphere.

Auslander, W. F., Haire-Joshu, D., Rogge, M., & Santiago, J. V. (1991). Predictors of diabetes knowledge in newly diagnosed children and parents. *Journal of Pediatric Psychology, 16,* 213–288.

Bull, B. A., & Drotar, D. (1991). Coping with cancer in remission: Stressors and strategies reported by children and adolescents. *Journal of Pediatric Psychology, 16,* 767–782.

Chaney, J. M., & Peterson, L. (1989). Family variables and disease management in juvenile rheumatoid arthritis. *Journal of Pediatric Psychology, 14,* 389–403.

Claflin, C. J., & Barbarin, O. A. (1991). Does "telling" less protect more? Relationships among age, information disclosure, and what children with cancer see and feel. *Journal of Pediatric Psychology, 16,* 169–192.

Copeland, D. R., Dowell, R. E., Fletcher, J. M., Sullivan, M. P., Jaffe, N., Cangir, A., Frankel, L. S., & Judd, B. W. (1988). Neuropsychological test performance of pediatric cancer patients at diagnosis and one year later. *Journal of Pediatric Psychology, 13,* 183–196.

Cousens, P., Ungerer, J. A., Crawford, J. A., & Stevens, M. M. (1991). Cognitive effects of childhood leukemia therapy: A case for four specific deficits. *Journal of Pediatric Psychology, 16,* 475–488.

Davies, W. H., Noll, R. B., DeStefano, L., Bukowski, W. M., & Kulkarni, R. (1991). Differences in the child-rearing practices of parents of children with cancer and controls: The perspectives of parents and professionals. *Journal of Pediatric Psychology, 16,* 295–306.

Deaton, A. V. (1985). Adaptive noncompliance in pediatric asthma: The parent as expert. *Journal of Pediatric Psychology, 10,* 1–14.

Deaton, A. V., & Olbrisch, M. E. (1987). Adaptive noncompliance: Parents as experts and decision makers in the treatment of pediatric asthma patients. *Advances in Developmental and Behavioral Pediatrics, 8,* 205–234.

DeMaso, D. R., Campis, L. K., Wypij, D., Bertram, S., Lipshitz, M., & Freed, M. (1991). The impact of maternal perceptions and medical severity on the adjustment of children with congenital heart disease. *Journal of Pediatric Psychology, 16,* 137–149.

Drotar, D. (1981). Psychosocial perspectives in chronic childhood illness. *Journal of Pediatric Psychology, 6,* 211–228.

Dyson, L. L. (1989). Adjustment of siblings of handicapped children: A comparison. *Journal of Pediatric Psychology, 14,* 215–229.

Ennett, S. T., DeVellis, B. M., Earp, J. A., Kredich, D., Warren, R. W., & Wilhelm, C. L. (1991). Disease experience and psychosocial adjustment in children with juvenile rheumatoid arthritis: Children's versus mothers' reports. *Journal of Pediatric Psychology, 16,* 557–568.

Evans, A. E., & Edin, S. (1968). If a child must die. . . . *New England Journal of Medicine, 278,* 138–142.

Gil, K. M., Williams, D. A., Thompson, R. J., & Kinney, T. R. (1991). Sickle cell disease in children and adolescents: The relation of child and parent pain coping strategies to adjustment. *Journal of Pediatric Psychology, 16,* 643–663.

Hamlett, K. W., Pellegrini, D. S., & Katz, K. S. (1992). Childhood chronic illness as a family stressor. *Journal of Pediatric Psychology, 17,* 33–47.

Hanson, C. L., Rodriguez, J. R., Henggeler, S. W., Harris, M. A., Klesges, R. C., & Carle, D. L. (1990). The perceived self-competence of adolescents with insulin-dependent diabetes mellitus: Deficit or strength? *Journal of Pediatric Psychology, 15,* 605–618.

Hazzard, A., Hutchinson, S. J., & Kraswiecki, N. (1990). Factors related to adherence to medication regimens in pediatric seizure patients. *Journal of Pediatric Psychology, 15,* 543–555.

Henggeler, S. W., Watson, S. M., & Whelan, J. P. (1990). Peer relations of hearing-impaired adolescents. *Journal of Pediatric Psychology, 15,* 721–731.

Heukrodt, C., Powazek, M., Brown, W. S., Kennelly, D., Imbus, C., Robinson, H., & Schantz, S. (1988). Electrophysiological signs of neurocognitive deficits in long-term leukemia survivors. *Journal of Pediatric Psychology, 13,* 223–236.

Jacobson, A. M., Hauser, S. T., Lavori, P., Wolfsdorf, J. I., Herskowitz, R. D., Milley, J. E., Bliss, R., & Gelfand, E. (1990). Adherence among children and adolescents with insulin-dependent diabetes mellitus over a four-year longitudinal follow-up: I. The influence of a patient coping and adjustment. *Journal of Pediatric Psychology, 15,* 511–526.

Kazak, A., & Meadows, A. (1989). Families of young adolescents who have survived cancer: Social-emotional adjustment, adaptability, and social support. *Journal of Pediatric Psychology, 14,* 175–191.

Koocher G. P. (1979). Adjustment and coping strategies among the caretakers of cancer patients. *Social Work in Health Care, 5,* 141–150.

Koocher, G. P. (1980). Pediatric cancer: Psychosocial problems and the high cost of helping. *Journal of Clinical Child Psychology, 9,* 2–5.

Koocher, G. P., & MacDonald, B. L. (1992). Preventive intervention and family coping with a child's life-threatening or terminal illness. In T. J. Akamatsu, M. A. P. Stephens, S. E. Hobfoll, J. H. Crowther (Eds.), *Family health psychology.* New York: Hemisphere (pp. 67-88).

Koocher, G. P., McGrath, M. L., & Gudas, L. J. (1990). Typologies of non-adherence in cystic fibrosis. *Developmental and Behavioral Pediatrics, 11,* 353–358.

Koocher, G. P., & O'Malley, J. E. (1981). *The Damocles syndrome: Psychosocial consequences of surviving childhood cancer.* New York: McGraw-Hill.

Koocher, G. P., Sourkes, B. M., & Keane, M. W. (1979). Pediatric oncology consultations: A generalizable model for medical settings. *Professional Psychology, 10,* 467–474.

Kovacs, M., Iyengar, S., Goldston, D., Stewart, J., Obrosky, D. S., & Marsh, J. (1990). Psychological functioning of children with insulin-dependent diabetes mellitus: A longitudinal study. *Journal of Pediatric Psychology, 15,* 619–632.

Kronenberger, W. G., & Thompson, R. J. (1992). Psychological adaptation of mothers of children with spina bifida: Association with dimensions of social relationships. *Journal of Pediatric Psychology, 17,* 1–14.

Lemanek, K. (1990). Adherence issues in the medical management of asthma. *Journal of Pediatric Psychology, 15,* 437–458.

Lobato, D., Faust, D., & Spirito, A. (1988). Examining the effects of chronic disease and disability on children's sibling relationships. *Journal of Pediatric Psychology, 13,* 389–407.

Money, J. (1986). Homosexual genesis, outcome studies, and a nature/nurture paradigm shift. *American Journal of Social Psychiatry, 6,* 95–98.

Money, J. (1987). Sin, sickness, or status: Homosexual gender identity and psychoneuroendocrinology. *American Psychologist, 42,* 384–399.

Money, J., & Russo, A. J. (1979). Homosexual outcome of discordant gender identity/role in childhood: Longitudinal follow-up. *Journal of Pediatric Psychology, 4,* 29–41.

Mullins, L. L., Olson, R. A., Reyes, S., Bernardy, N., Huszti, H. C., & Volk, R. J. (1991). Risk and resistance factors in the adaptation of mothers of children with cystic fibrosis. *Journal of Pediatric Psychology, 16,* 701–715.

Nitschke, R. J., Humphrey, G. B., Sexauer, C. L., Catron, B., Wunder, S., & Jay, S. (1982). Therapeutic choices made by patients with end-stage cancer. *The Journal of Pediatrics, 101,* 471–476.

Nitschke, R. J., Wunder, S., Sexauer, C. L., & Humphrey, G. B. (1977). The final-stage conference: The patient's decision on research drugs in pediatric oncology. *Journal of Pediatric Psychology, 2,* 58–64.

Noll, R. B., LeRoy, S., Bukowski, W. M., Rogosch, F. A., & Kulkarni, R. (1991). Peer relationships and adjustment in children with cancer. *Journal of Pediatric Psychology, 16,* 307–326.

O'Malley, J. E., & Koocher, G. P. (1977). Psychosocial consultation to a pediatric oncology unit: Obstacles to effective intervention. *Journal of Pediatric Psychology, 2,* 54–57.

Osterweis, M., Solomon, F., & Green, M. (Eds.). (1984). *Bereavement: Reactions, consequences, and care.* Washington, DC: National Academy Press.

Peterson, L., & Harbeck, C. (1988). *The pediatric psychologist.* Champaign, IL: Research Press.

Phipps, S., & DeCuir-Whalley, S. (1990). Adherence issues in pediatric bone marrow transplantation. *Journal of Pediatric Psychology, 15,* 459–475.

Quattrin, T., Aronica, S., & Mazur, T. (1990). Management of male pseudohermaphroditism: A case report spanning twenty-one years. *Journal of Pediatric Psychology, 15,* 699–709.

Rando, T. A. (1983). An investigation of grief and adaptation in parents whose children have died from cancer. *Journal of Pediatric Psychology, 8,* 3–22.

Rando, T. A. (1984). *Grief dying, and death: Clinical interventions for caregivers.* Champaign, IL: Research Press.

Rando, T. A. (Ed.). (1986a). *Parental loss of a child.* Champaign, IL: Research Press.

Rando, T. A. (Ed.). (1986b). *Loss and anticipatory grief.* Lexington, MA: Lexington Books.

Rando, T. A. (1988). *How to go on living when someone you love dies.* Lexington, MA: Lexington Books.

Roberts, M. C. (1986). *Pediatric psychology.* New York: Pergamon.

Roberts, M. C., & Wallander, J. L. (Eds.). (1992). *Family issues in pediatric psychology.* Hillsdale, NJ: Lawrence Erlbaum.

Sanger, M. S., Copeland, D. R., & Davidson, E. R. (1991). Psychosocial adjustment among pediatric cancer patients: A multidimensional assessment. *Journal of Pediatric Psychology, 16,* 463–474.

Slavin L., O'Malley J. E., Koocher, G. P., & Foster, D. J. (1981). Communication of the cancer diagnosis to pediatric patients: Impact on long-term adjustment. *American Journal of Orthopsychiatry, 139,* 179–183.

Speechley, K. N., & Noh, S. (1992). Surviving childhood cancer, social support, and parents' psychological adjustment. *Journal of Pediatric Psychology, 17,* 15–31.

Spinetta, J. J. (1980). Disease-related communication: How to tell. In J. Kellerman (Ed.), *Psychological aspects of childhood cancer* (pp. 175-182). Springfield, IL: Thomas.

Spinetta, J. J., Swarner, J. A., & Sheposh, J. P. (1981). Effective parental coping following the death of a child from cancer. *Journal of Pediatric Psychology, 6,* 251–264.

Spirito, A., Stark, L. J., Cobiella, C., Drigan, R., Androkites, A., & Hewett, K. (1990). Social adjustment of children successfully treated for cancer. *Journal of Pediatric Psychology, 15,* 359–371.

Stewart, S. M., Silver, C. H., Nici, J., Waller, D., Campbell, R., Uauy, K., & Andrews, W. S. (1991). Neuropsychological function in young children who have undergone liver transplantation. *Journal of Pediatric Psychology, 16,* 569–583.

Waber, D. P., Gioia, G., Paccia, J., Sherman, B., Dinklage, D., Sollee, N., Urion, D. K., Tarbell, N. J., & Sallan, S. E. (1990). Sex differences in cognitive processing in children treated with CNS prophylaxis for acute lymphoblastic leukemia. *Journal of Pediatric Psychology, 15,* 105–122.

Walker, L. S., & Zeman, J. L. (1992). Parental response to child illness behavior. *Journal of Pediatric Psychology, 17,* 49–71.

Wallander, J. L., Varni, J. W., Babani, L., DeHaan, D. K., Banis, H. T., Wilcox, K. T. (1989). Family resources as resistance factors for psychological maladjustment in chronically ill and handicapped children. *Journal of Pediatric Psychology, 14,* 157–173.

Williams, K. S., Ochs, J., Williams, J. M., & Mulhern, R. K. (1991). Parental report of everyday cognitive abilities among children treated for acute lymphoblastic leukemia. *Journal of Pediatric Psychology, 16,* 13–26.

3

Psychological Consultation to a Pediatric Oncology Unit
Obstacles to Effective Intervention

John E. O'Malley
Harvard Medical School and Children's Hospital Medical Center, Boston

Gerald P. Koocher
Harvard Medical School and Sidney Farber Cancer Center

One of the basic services provided by mental health professionals in a pediatric teaching hospital is consultation to the inpatient units. Although there is ample literature concerning the emotional impact of hospitalization in children (Langford, 1961; Oremland & Oremland, 1973; Prugh et al., 1953) and models for intervention (Miller, 1973; Rotmann, 1973), there has been little focus on the obstacles to effective intervention. Schowalter (1971) discusses several problem areas in an adolescent liaison service, particularly as a result of the relationship between mental health professional and pediatrician. The child psychiatrist or psychologist may feel pressured or expected to find rapid success. The consultant often avoids communication and would rather work alone. Pediatricians, on the other hand, may be bored, confused, or threatened by such intervention. Schowalter further suggests that collaboration always involves consultation, but consultation does not always involve collaboration. He sees this as a pitfall to effective intervention. Rothenberg (1968) writes of the need of both the consultant and the person seeking consultation to give up jargon if liaison is to be maintained. Most authors suggest the need for mutual support and knowledge.

During the preparation of this paper the authors were supported in part by National Cancer Institute Grant CA 18429 CCG under the leadership of Norman Jaffe, M.D.
Originally published in *Journal of Pediatric Psychology, 2*(2)(1977):54-57.

THE SETTING

Children's Hospital Medical Center is a 340 bed pediatric teaching hospital of the Harvard Medical School. There are 14 inpatient units, primarily divided by patient age group and type of service (ages 0-2, general medicine, etc.). In 1974, 12,533 inpatients were served, with an average stay of 7.6 days. A total of 8,898 surgical procedures were performed.

One inpatient division which will form the backdrop for this discussion is a children's cancer ward. It is a unit of 18 beds for children of all ages with a variety of cancers. In addition to the usual complement of personnel of Children's Hospital, it is staffed by Oncology senior physicians, fellows, and social workers from the Sidney Farber Cancer Center. Most of the senior staff have been involved in this division 20 or more years. This division, although it is not typical of all the inpatient units, will serve as the example because the authors are intimately aware of its operation, and the obstacles to effective intervention tend to be more exaggerated and glaring than in other units. Children with cancer and those facing death or an uncertain future arouse many intense feelings in all who are involved in the division.

The generation of a consultation within the traditional medical or "disease" model is a reasonably straightforward affair. The house officer or primary care physician calls in a specialist to offer advice on specific diagnostic or treatment issues. The consultant examines the patient, performs indicated tests, and renders an opinion (usually to the primary physician). Mental health problems, on the other hand, do not lend themselves to such clear-cut management.

In the traditional treatment of an "illness," a common etiology, course, and treatment can usually be specified. In the case of a "mental or emotional illness," the origins, symptom picture, and therapeutic approach which is most effective all depend on highly individualized factors. In addition, psychology is founded on the cornerstone of interpersonal relations, which unlike a blood sample, tissue culture, or other material for a physical diagnostic test, cannot be accurately assessed without building a meaningful cooperative relationship between doctor and patient.

In addition, the "psych. consult." per se hardly ever solves the referral problem. In the ideal case some emotional relief and management suggestions may result, but these tend to be chiefly short-term or stop-gap measures, except in rare cases which are purely reactive disturbances.

Keeping these factors in mind, one does not find it surprising that the ways in which pediatric consultations are generated in a teaching pediatric hospital are also quite different from the usual medical model. This will have relevance when obstacles to effective consultation are discussed below.

IMPEDIMENTS TO EFFECTIVE CONSULTATION: STAFF ISSUES

The tumor therapy unit presents many examples of atypical organizational patterns, because of the unique chronic emotional pressure on the staff, the patients, and their families. The medical staff, especially the more junior, may be rather easily overwhelmed by the emotional reactions of patients, no matter how intellectually prepared they are to assist the patient over a difficult course. The staff member with young children at home who must bear the bad news of a poor or uncertain prognosis to other young parents, and the resident who sees mounting depression in an adolescent (not much younger than the resident) as alopecia results from antimetabolite therapy, are both prime candidates for depression themselves. This over-identification, which is common in inexperienced staff, is often recognized by sensitive ward personnel, who realize that such junior staff cannot reasonably be expected to undertake full management of complex and physically devastating drug protocols or differential diagnoses and offer emotional support as well. Thus, the sensitive nurse or the physician involved may request a mental health consultation with the dual charge of getting some support for the patient while taking the pressure off the junior staff. It is a relatively guilt free way to withdraw emotionally and provide protection from the staff member's own feelings and fears. In cases when the house officer is unable to sense his or her own needs to make an emotional separation, it is not uncommon for other members of the floor staff to sense these and initiate the request for consultation.

Bobby is a 10-year-old boy whose treatment for Hodgkins Disease left him virtually no immune defenses, highly susceptible to infection. He was admitted to the hospital with a rash, high fever, mouth sores, and generalized weakness, despite protestations that he wanted "to go home and die." This was his third hospitalization in as many months for acute febrile episodes, and the condition was defying the best diagnostic efforts of the treatment team. After talking with Bobby and listening to his dejection and tearful desperation, the consultant overheard part of the treatment team exuberant with excitement. They had suddenly thought of an alternative diagnosis for Bobby's mysterious fevers. It did not immediately matter that this new alternative (graft versus host reaction) had implications as grave as the others in terms of prognosis. What mattered was a new potential strategy in the struggle for Bobby's life, which hung in the balance. On the one hand it was paradoxical to see rejoicing in contrast to Bobby's utter depression in the next room, but on the other hand the staff could work more effectively without the added burden of having to support Bobby's heavy emotional load.

In such cases the intervention of the psychological consultant quite literally lifted a burden from the primary care staff. While this is fine as far as it goes, an unusual burden on the consultant is often the net result. Failure of the consultant to recognize the origin of the consultation request and the not-so-hidden agenda of such a request will leave the consultant doing only part of the necessary task. Focus on the patient only, without helping the staff with their emotional load, can result in a variety of maladaptive behaviors on the part of the staff (e.g., total emotional withdrawal, isolation from the patient, lack of coordinated effort, etc.).

Another major area of impediment to effective intervention is the often discrepant expectations of the staff originating the request for consultation and the ability of the consultant to identify and meet these expectations. These discrepancies, if not recognized, will lead to distrust, lack of confidence, and under-utilization of the consultant.

One expectation may be for the consultant to "make" the patient conform to treatment protocols or to hospital rules. The sense of lack of control on the part of the staff may lead to intolerable anxiety and precipitate a request for psychological consultation cloaked in misleading jargon.

Jim was referred for psychiatric consultation with the question of "psychotic behavior." There was nothing in the history of his 13 years to suggest psychosis. Talking with the nurse who asked for the consult revealed that Jim refused loudly to have an IV placed which was necessary for delivery of the antimetabolite. It was not conceivable at the time to the nurse that anyone would refuse potential life-giving treatment. This created such disbelief and anxiety that the mental health consultant was called. After a brief interview with Jim, who clearly needed to feel that he had some control over his own destiny, control that was taken away by his cancer, management suggestions were discussed with the nurse to allow for such control. By allowing Jim to choose the time (medicine had to be given only once per day), the site of the IV, and to keep track of the flow (reporting it to the nurse if any deviation occurred), the nurse found that no further difficulties arose.

The same principle can be applied to a number of consultations requested because of "disruptive behavior." Disruption in an inpatient unit may be considerably different than at home. Patients wandering off the floor or not abiding by rules of isolation may create anxiety in the staff, who are used to uncompromising and total control. Again the consultant must recognize these divergent expectations (i.e., who needs to control whom and for what reason).

A patient may be "punished" with a "psych. consult." referral. The consultant must recognize this pitfall or intervention will be useless at best and may at worst aggravate the tense relationship between patient and staff. The staff's anger at any given patient may be due to a number of reasons: (1) a staff person's guilt for not being able to stop the progress of the tumor leads to frustration and anger, and this is projected to the patient, the source of the guilt. The patient is guilty for the staff feelings and therefore must be punished. (2) The staff may react to troublesome behavior not with anxiety as in the previous example, but with anger originating from their impotence to effect change. (3) Anger may result from a patient's rebuff of staff's attention and support or (4) from the patient's selective choice of one staff person to be emotionally close to the exclusion of other staff.

Denise, an 8-year-old girl with acute myelocytic leukemia, was a particularly appealing child who easily engaged adults. The course of her illness was difficult and agonizing, and as she approached the terminal phase of her illness, she maintained close relationships with her parents and her primary physician only. The nursing staff saw this as a retreat and withdrawal and clear evidence of "depression." One staff person who in fact originated the request for consultation felt that she was particularly close to Denise and was now being excluded. The nurse told Denise that since she was no longer responsive that there must be a problem, and the "head shrinker" would have to be called if the situation did not improve. The staff member was hurt and angered by Denise's rejection and thus threatened her by suggesting that something was "wrong with her head." After an interview with Denise and her family, it was clear that Denise had adequate emotional support, was open and direct about her feelings with her parents and the physician, and had no need to share with another person. The task of the consultant then was to help the staff recognize and deal with their feelings about such a "withdrawal" and to see it not as a personal attack or rejection, but as a natural consequence of her emotional maturity in the face of overwhelming stress.

The staff may expect a rapid cure, instant and immediately effective intervention, with the least interruption of the medical management. This notion probably has several origins, including the inexperienced staff's need for activity, action, and magic in the face of anxiety; education in which the medical model is paramount; watching other medical disciplines operate; and the mental health consultant's occasional willingness to be seen in that role. However, the inevitable failure of meeting this expectation will result in dissatisfaction with the consultant and beliefs that he or she is incompetent and therefore someone not to be utilized.

Mary is a 16-year-old adolescent who was very depressed not only about her loss of a limb from osteogenic sarcoma but because of an extremely chaotic family situation. The staff accurately perceived Mary's depression as interfering with her will to live in general and especially her cooperation with treatment. The primary physician called for a psychiatrist, indicating that Mary was due to go home the next day. The consultant saw the patient, arranged to see the family the next day, and asked the primary physician to hold discharge until the evaluation was completed. The physician was angered and asked why the delay was necessary. The notion that one visit should certainly be ample to "cure" Mary prevailed. Education of the physician, and Mary, continues to be followed through her frequent hospitalizations.

IMPEDIMENTS TO EFFECTIVE CONSULTATION: PARENTAL ISSUES

Although many parents welcome psychological consultation and support, this is hardly the universal condition. Even when such a consultation is requested directly by the family, the context is quite different from that of the usual medical model, since the needs being espoused go far beyond the patient alone. The reasons behind the request may range from personal needs of the parent to a search for a parent surrogate as they prepare to abandon emotionally this gravely ill child. A key problem here, and in most consultations with terminally ill children, is keeping the parents involved with the child as much as possible. Given the situation of an eager consultant and uneasy parents, the danger of trying to fill the parents' role is a significant one. The consultant must walk a fine line between the child and the parents, facilitating the emotional supports each may offer to the other.

Reed, a 16-year-old boy with osteogenic sarcoma, was reaching the terminal stage of his cancer. He had multiple metastases including some to the brain. The family had always been close and supportive to Reed, but as death neared they felt Reed was withdrawing, depressed, and unable to cope. The parents requested that the mental health consultant see Reed. Indeed, Reed was depressed and felt unable to talk with his parents about his impending death. In tears, he shared how frightened he was and how distant his parents seemed to be. He read his parents' behavior as their not wanting to talk about death, and so Reed did not want to burden them. After several talks, Reed's spirits improved considerably, and the parents were eager to have the consultant continue—"to make Reed happy," as they put it. To see him smile meant to them that death was not imminent and that their emotional burden was relieved. The parents began to make less frequent and shorter visits. Telephone calls to the consultant were made to have messages relayed to Reed. Reed's desire to talk about how he felt, the psychiatrist's willingness to listen and the parents' difficulty coping with the terminal events all contributed to the effective exclusion of the parents and interference with the relationship that was most important: parent and child.

Once this situation was recognized, the consultant met with Reed and his parents together and helped to facilitate communication between them. Both Reed and his parents had much to say to each other, and as they were more able to do so, the mental health consultant's involvement decreased. Death came for Reed peacefully.

The parents' expectations of a psychological consultant may also parallel those of the staff. The parents need often to be relieved of the emotional burden of a child's uncertain future, or pain, or impending death may likewise be cloaked in the consultation request. The parents are asking for help for themselves in a manner that relieves them of guilt for thinking of themselves. They may need to withdraw and regroup their emotional forces but are unable to do so unless someone relieves them. This "change of shift" is a common expectation parents have and must be acknowledged and sanctioned if it is in the service of their coping mechanisms.

The parents may expect the consultant to make their child happy and not talk of morbid things. If this is unrecognized, effective consultation is impossible. Without clarifying the parents' expectations, the consultant saw *Jane,* a lovely 15-year-old girl with advanced Hodgkins disease, because she was depressed. In the interview, Jane was furious that her parents would not allow her to talk about death, her sadness, nor her grief. "Don't talk like that! Everything will be fine." Jane was able to share these feelings with the consultant and experienced some relief. However, when Jane shared the content of the interviews with her parents, they became very angry and summarily dismissed the consultant. The parents were unable to deal with the finality of the illness and wanted their daughter to help maintain their denial. This was the reason the consultant was called. When this did not happen, and because the consultant failed to clarify their expectations, emotional intervention was abruptly stopped.

Some families are threatened by the notion of a "psych. consult." for many reasons. Some families pride themselves on being emotionally strong, able to overcome all obstacles, and see the need for mental health intervention as a sign of weakness. These are often fears in some families that the psychiatrist will "read their thoughts" and find out that they are angry at their child for being sick or have thoughts of a hope for rapid demise—thoughts that are unacceptable to them. The consultant must clarify his or her role to such parents and provide reassurance to them if a family reluctantly requests such a consultation.

IMPEDIMENTS TO EFFECTIVE INTERVENTION: CHILD ISSUES

Although it initially sounds unlikely, careful observation suggests that many psychological consultations are initiated by children themselves. Recently an angry and unhappy 14-year-old osteogenic sarcoma patient came to the outpatient clinic for examination just prior to admission for chemotherapy. When told that her regular doctor was on vacation, the girl voiced the wish that "his plane should crash to bits in the ocean." This and other such overt hostile comments quickly elicited a call to psychiatry from the staff, who were not used to such open verbal assaults. Talking with the young woman brought out a number of realistic emotional concerns regarding her illness and its impact on the family. Yet it was clear that the lines of communication were not open at home or on the inpatient unit, and that the provocative anger was really intended as a means for getting someone to talk with her about all of this.

It is striking how even young children will quite directly act in "help seeking" ways when they are in need. Failure by the staff to identify such behavior will miss the opportunity for psychological intervention.

When the staff or family request a psychological consultation, adequate preparation for the child will facilitate the intervention. Lack of such preparation and adequate explanation to the child results in ineffective intervention. Adolescents are particularly sensitive to the meaning of having a "head shrinker" visit them. The child, if not told why a consultation is being requested and given an opportunity to clarify the process of such a consultation, may be an unwilling participant. He or she may in fact decide that it is dangerous to share anything with anyone, since they will label you "crazy" and send for the "witch doctor."

Donald is a 17-year-old young man with testicular carcinoma who quietly shared some concern about his manhood to his primary physician. The physician thought it would be appropriate to have Donald talk with the mental health consultant and indicated such to him. When the consultant arrived, Donald rolled over in bed and pretended to be asleep. Several more visits gained no more insight than that he was tired and did not want to talk. Donald shared with his parents the fact that he hated this hospital because everyone was so noisy and because they thought he was "mental." He still has refused psychological intervention.

Children may expect the consultant to be an arbitrator between themselves and the staff. The consultant needs to hear beneath these requests issues of control, anger, and grief about the illness—and issues of uncertainty, death, and despair. Children (as well as adults) may be afraid to be angry at their primary caregiver for fear they may be abandoned. The consultant can be seen as a safe person with whom to share feelings.

CONCLUSION

The nature of psychological consultation on a children's inpatient unit differs significantly from the usual medical mode. The process of such consultation may in itself lead to obstacles preventing effective intervention. Nonetheless, willingness on the part of the consultant to alter some of the stereotypic procedures—working alone, keeping a low profile, sharing with few—must be present if services to hospitalized children are to be provided. The consultant must also be willing to be on public display, and to be tested as to helpfulness, availability, and common sense. Showing respect for the staff's knowledge and insights, being sensitive to their emotional needs, and being available at their request will foster a working alliance in the service of meeting the patient's needs.

The process of effective consultation can be sabotaged in many ways, by staff or consultant. Recognizing how a consultation is generated, by whom, and for what reason and with what expectation is but the first step in the process. Failure to do so leads to dissatisfied consumers of psychological services, tension between staff and consultant, and atrophy or disuse of such services. The consultant must recognize the social and environmental milieu in which he or she must operate, including the personalities of key staff people, the nuances of interpersonal staff relations, and the basis for the highly charged emotional atmosphere. The consultant must recognize the hidden agendas (to punish, to relieve, to arbitrate, etc.) of each consultative request and deal appropriately with them before effective consultation can take place.

This paper outlines only some of the obstacles to psychological consultation, but to recognize these is a start on the road toward meaningful solutions.

REFERENCES

Langford, W. S. The child in the pediatric hospital: Adaptation to illness and hospitalization. *American Journal of Orthopsychiatry,* 1961, *31,* 667-684.

Miller, W. B. Psychiatric consultation: A general systems approach. *Psychiatry and Medicine,* 1973, *4,* 135-142.

Monnelly, E. P., Ianzito, B. M., & Stewart, M. A. Psychiatric consultations in a children's hospital. *American Journal of Psychiatry,* 1973, *130,* 789-790.

Oremland, E. K., & Oremland, J. D. *The effects of hospitalization on children.* Springfield: C. C. Thomas, 1973.

Prugh, D. G., Staub, E. M., Sands, H. H., Kirschbaum, R. M., & Lenihan, E. A. A study of the emotional reactions of children and families to hospitalization and illness. *American Journal of Orthopsychiatry,* 1953, *23,* 70-106.

Rothenberg, M. B. Child psychiatry-pediatrics liaison: A history and commentary. *Journal of the American Academy of Child Psychiatry,* 1968, *7,* 492-509.

Rotmann, M. A model of an integrated psychosomatic consultation service. *Psychotherapy & Psychosomatics,* 1973, *22,* 189-191.

Schowalter, J. E. The utilization of child psychiatry in a pediatric adolescent ward. *Journal of the American Academy of Child Psychiatry,* 1971, *10,* 684-699.

4

The Final-Stage Conference
The Patient's Decision on Research Drugs in Pediatric Oncology

Ruprecht Nitschke, Shirley Wunder, Charles L. Sexauer, and George Bennett Humphrey
Oklahoma Children's Memorial Hospital

In recent years, numerous papers have been published in the lay and professional press, concerning the psychological needs of chronically ill and dying patients. The pediatric literature covers subjects ranging from maternal-child relationships (Freud, 1972; Natterson & Knudson, 1960) and parental response to the child's illness (Glaser, 1960; Gofman, Buckman, & Schade, 1957; Vander Veer, 1949) to the child's response to disease and treatment (Karon, 1973; Lansky, Lowman, Vats, & Gyulay, 1974) and altered life styles of the child and family (Heffron, Bommelaere, & Masters, 1973; Lansky, 1974).

This report will discuss a new approach developed in the last two years, toward the management of children who have cancer that fails to respond to conventional therapy. It will focus on the content of the final-stage conference and its effect on the child, the family, and professional staff. In this meeting, or meetings, the parents and the child are informed that the cancer has recurred and that death appears now inevitable. The future management is also outlined. The child and the parents may choose between the two options: treatment with a new research drug of unknown efficacy, or discontinuation of chemotherapy with continued supportive care.

The format of this report is as follows: first, the structure of the Hematology-Oncology Service of the Oklahoma Children's Memorial Hospital is briefly described. Next, the initial conference with the patients and their

Originally published in *Journal of Pediatric Psychology, 2*(2)(1977):58-64.

parents is outlined, in which the disease, prognosis, and treatment are discussed. A description of the final-stage conference follows, including a report on twenty patients who participated in the latter conference. Nine histories are presented in detail. Special emphasis is given to the relationship between the child, the family, and the physician.

STRUCTURE OF THE ONCOLOGY SERVICE

The Oklahoma Children's Memorial Hospital has a center for oncology patients under twenty years of age. They are cared for by a hematology-oncology service, the pediatric surgeons and their colleagues in the sub-specialties, the radiation therapists, and the specialists for diagnostic procedures. The Hematology-Oncology Service consists of three pediatric hematologists, a fellow, a physician's assistant, three nurses, social worker, and ancillary personnel. A psychologist and a psychiatrist are available on request. The chaplain of the hospital, with his staff, works closely with many of our patients. Patients admitted to the hospital are cared for by the house officers under the direct supervision of one of the oncologists.

Members of the oncology team are investigators in the Pediatric Division of the Southwest Oncology Group. All of the treatment plans, therefore, are carefully structured, and all treatment protocols are reviewed nationally. In addition, new drugs not available to the general public are evaluated. These research drugs (Phase II drugs) are anticancer agents for which the tolerated dosage and possible side effects are known. However, their effectiveness against the various types of malignancies is not established.

INITIAL CONFERENCE

It is the policy of the Hematology-Oncology Service that the parents are thoroughly informed about the diagnosis and the treatment of the child. The children, older than three years, and sometimes younger, are informed by one of the physicians about their disease, the name of the disease, and the treatment plan, usually in the presence of the parents. The details of the information given vary according to the age of the child. The conversation with a four-year-old child has the following content: the name of the disease, its progression to death without treatment, the treatment plan and possible side effects, and the need for continuous treatment, as well as the possible recurrence of the disease. Older children are informed in more detail about the disease process and the side effects, according to their intellectual capacity. Thus, all of our patients newly diagnosed with cancer are informed about their disease and their prognosis, but there is an emphasis on the fact that the disease will most likely be controlled by the treatment.

FINAL-STAGE CONFERENCE

The final-stage conference with the parents is arranged by the physician and the nurse. The previous response of the child to chemotherapy, radiation therapy, and surgery is reviewed. The parents are informed that all conventional means of controlling the cancer have been exhausted and the death of their child now seems inevitable.

In the conference the options of further chemotherapy with a research drug or no chemotherapy are given. The parents are told that research drugs are available and that while they might temporarily retard or control the child's cancer, it is highly unlikely, based on past experience, that a new drug even if efficacious would result in a cure. The treatment would involve hospitalization and frequent clinic visits, painful procedures such as venipuncture and bone marrow aspirations, and side effects such as vomiting and nausea. It is also emphasized that the professional team will continue to care for the patient and the family even if they choose to have no further chemotherapy. The physician has a similar talk with the child, usually after he or she has discussed the matter with the parents. The parents may be included in this talk if they wish. For a patient who has already had one or more research drugs, this type of conference is repeated each time a new Phase II drug is proposed.

The final-stage conference with the child has not been used consistently over the past two years, because it evolved gradually as a response to the needs of one group of patients, most of them ten years old or older. For another group of patients, the final-stage conference involved only the parents. The child, although told about the recurrence of the disease, was not completely informed about the consequences and was not confronted with the decision: chemotherapy vs. cessation of chemotherapy.

PATIENT REPORTS

Table 1 shows the number of patients who died in 1973-1974 and in 1974-1976. The number of patients receiving Phase II drugs is noted for both groups. Included in the second group are the 20 patients who par-

Table 1. Number of Patients Who Died after 1973 Having Received Either Phase II Drugs or No Chemotherapy

Group	Years	Final-Stage Decision Made by	Phase II Drugs One or More	None
I	1973-74	Parents Only	24	7
II	1974-76	Parents Only	15	6
		Parents and Child	15	5

Table 2. Final-Stage Decision of Child and Parents

Patient Number	Decision Made Parents	Child	Age of Child in Years
1	No Chemotherapy	No Chemotherapy	15
2	No Chemotherapy	No Chemotherapy	16
3	Phase II Drugs	Phase II Drugs	10
4	Phase II Drugs	Phase II Drugs*	14
5	No Chemotherapy	No Chemotherapy	14
6	Phase II Drugs	No Chemotherapy	20
7	Phase II Drugs	No Chemotherapy	15
8	Phase II Drugs	No Chemotherapy	7
9	No Chemotherapy	No Chemotherapy	6
10	Undetermined	Undetermined	18
11	No Chemotherapy	No Chemotherapy	18
12	Undetermined	Phase II Drugs	14
13	Undetermined	No Chemotherapy	6
14	Phase II Drugs	Phase II Drugs	13
15	No Chemotherapy	No Chemotherapy	13
16	Phase II Drugs	Phase II Drugs	14
17	Phase II Drugs	Phase II Drugs	18
18	No Chemotherapy	No Chemotherapy	11
19	Phase II Drugs	Phase II Drugs	14
20	Phase II Drugs	Phase II Drugs	14

*Later asked for cessation of chemotherapy.

ticipated in the final stage conference. Among these patients no increased tendency to discontinue chemotherapy occurred.

Table 2 indicates the ages of these 20 patients and the decisions made by patients and their parents in regard to further treatment.

The following paragraphs will give the histories of 9 of the patients who were confronted with the fact that modes of conventional therapy were exhausted. The patients are grouped together according to (a) their independence in making the decision on further therapy, (b) the similarity between their decisions and the parents' and physicians' views, and (c) age.

AUTONOMOUS PATIENT DECISION: CONCURRING WITH PARENTS' AND PHYSICIANS' VIEW

Patient #1. A 15-year-old boy known to have acute lymphocytic leukemia (ALL) for four years was admitted because of high fever, headaches, and a sore throat. Four days prior to admission, we informed him that his bone marrow showed many leukemic cells. At that time, treatment with prednisone and adriamycin was started. While he was in the hospital, his condition worsened. Skin lesions occurred. The progression of the disease was discussed with his stepmother, who stayed with him in the hospital, but the possibility of stopping treatment was not yet mentioned. On the fifth day after admission, our physician's assistant expressed her concern about the boy's progressively worsening condition. As the father had just arrived, a conference with the parents was arranged. The seriousness of their son's condition and the grave prognosis were outlined. Further treatment with chemotherapy, blood transfusions, and antibiotics was discussed, as well as the alternative of discontinuing all treatment for the leukemia while continuing supportive care. The parents did not want any further treatment. In their presence, we talked to the boy and he agreed, saying, "I know I will go to Heaven. I want to be close to home." Chemotherapy and blood transfusions were discontinued, and his transfer to a small hospital close to his home was arranged for the earliest possible date. The boy died before he could be moved.

Patient #2. A 17-year-old girl with chronic myelogenous leukemia diagnosed six months earlier was in the blastic phase of the disease, partially controlled by 5-azacytidine, prednisone, and vincristine. She was readmitted because of high fever and severe neutropenia. Her bone marrow showed blastic cells again. The findings were discussed with her parents, who felt that no further treatment should be initiated. The progression of the disease and the possibility of treatment with a Phase II drug or the discontinuation of the treatment were discussed with the girl. She, like her parents, did not want further treatment. Her question was, "Can I go home?" Because of high fever and bleeding episodes, she was transferred to a hospital close to her home. She died four days after discharge.

While the reports on these two patients show that patients may have the same opinion about further treatment as their family members and the professional staff, the following case histories demonstrate that individuals involved in caring for the child may have differing opinions about further treatment.

AUTONOMOUS PATIENT DECISION: DIFFERING FROM PHYSICIAN'S EXPECTATION

Patient #3. A 10-year-old boy, with neuroblastoma diagnosed two years earlier, relapsed. No effective conventional therapy was available. We talked to the parents about a Phase II drug known to have some effect against the disease. The parents said the treatment should be tried, but they agreed that we should talk to the boy. They insisted that we meet with him alone and stated, "If we are with him, he will do what he thinks we want." The boy was informed about the progression of his disease. He was asked if he wanted to be treated with a new drug which would have to be given intravenously in the hospital for five days and might produce many side effects. The alternative was to have treatment against his cancer discontinued so he could go home. He cried, but there was no question in his mind: he wanted to be treated.

This decision surprised the physician, who thought he would prefer to go home. A tape which the boy had prepared several months earlier, which was later made available to the team, explained his determined attitude: he was truly convinced that he would be cured in a few months.

The boy died in the hospital three weeks later. Right before his death, he said to the nurse, "If I keep this up [vomiting], I am going to die." She answered, "That's right, you will, but we will stay with you." He stated, "But I am afraid." She replied, "We'll help you," and they talked of his God and his Heaven.

Patient #4. A 14-year-old boy with Ewing's Sarcoma of his right arm was successfully treated for 18 months with radiation therapy and chemotherapy. Two months after the discontinuation of chemotherapy, the disease recurred: the boy had arm, femur, and multiple lung metastases. He was unable to walk, to use his right arm, and he was in pain. He and his parents were informed about the progression of the disease. They agreed to go ahead with a new drug combination which had to be given every week intravenously. The boy became very depressed. The medical staff had the impression that he did not want any further treatment. With his parents' permission, we discussed his prognosis with him without the parents present. We emphasized that treatment could be discontinued. "I want to live, and I want the treatment continued," he insisted. We expressed our disbelief at his statement because he acted like somebody who had given up. He shouted at us, "What would you do if you knew you had to die!" We stated, "We would hope to live until the time of death and not waste time mourning." We made it clear that if he really wanted to live he had to show the will to live; for example, to see his friends and to be active as much as his disease allowed him. After this discussion, he enjoyed his friends, went to football games, and insisted on going hunting. He used his left hand for shooting at first with a shotgun; later when he became weaker, he continued hunting with a pistol. Two months later his father came to the outpatient clinic and informed us that the boy refused to return to the clinic. An arrangement with a local physician was made to continue treatment if desired, but the boy refused. The parents of the boy, at this point, agreed to his decision. He died at home six weeks after discontinuation of chemotherapy.

In these two instances, the physician felt that further treatment with a Phase II drug would only increase the misery of the two boys. The patients and their families felt strongly, however, that treatment should be continued. In the next reports, the patient's decision differed from that of the parents.

AUTONOMOUS PATIENT DECISION: DIFFERING FROM PARENTS' WISHES

Patient #5. A 20-year-old patient diagnosed as having ALL for two years experienced a relapse for two months without responding to chemotherapy. He was admitted several times because of fever and chills, controlled by systematic antibiotics. The last bone marrow showed further deterioration. The findings and the poor prognosis were discussed. Because of his generally good condition, a new Phase II drug was suggested, but the possibility of discontinuation of treatment was raised. The parents felt that he should try another drug, but the young man decided to go home, celebrate his birthday and Thanksgiving, and then to "come back when he felt bad." On his return, when he had high fever and his leukemia had progressed further, he decided against treatment. He said, "I want to be treated against infection and be made comfortable." He died 10 days later. He related well to his family, friends, and the professional staff until three hours before his death, when he became dyspneic and unconscious.

Patient #6. A 14-year-old boy who had testicular embryonal carcinoma with lung metastases at the time of diagnosis responded well to radiation therapy, chemotherapy, and surgery. The disease was under control for one year, and then the recurrence became evident. New chemotherapeutic combinations did not control the disease any more. Because of further deterioration, the prognosis and the outcome were discussed with the boy. The choice between a Phase II drug and no further treatment was proposed. He asked, "How long do I have to live with treatment and how long without?" We replied, "We do not know. Without treatment, most likely a few months; with the new drug possibly longer if you respond to it, but you may have severe side effects." He asked for time to think about it. The parents were ambivalent about treatment and resented the physician at first, because he talked so openly to their boy and presented him with such a difficult decision. A week later the boy agreed to further treatment, but he wanted to start the following week. This decision surprised us because we knew how much he hated intravenous medications. In a conversation with a nurse, he stated that he had agreed to the treatment because the physicians were interested in the new compound and that he did not want to disappoint them by refusing this treatment. After we heard this fact, we explained to him that he should decide what he wanted for himself, not for his physician. If he did not want therapy, we would not abandon him, but would support him.

He chose to remain at home without chemotherapy. He talked openly with his friends about his dying. They visited him after the baseball games which were his main interest. He made several short trips with his parents to some of his favorite places with the aid of a wheelchair. He asked his father to see the psychologist, because he thought his father was having difficulty with the decision to discontinue chemotherapy. The boy died six weeks later at home.

All of the patients described up to this point made their decisions on their own. The next patient arrived at her decision after conferring with her family.

COOPERATIVE PATIENT-PARENT DECISION

Patient #7. A 14-year-old girl was diagnosed as having osteogenic sarcoma of the left femur, which was amputated. Intensive chemotherapy was initiated. A half year later multiple metastases of the lungs occurred. The patient was in generally good condition and felt well. The findings were discussed with the patient and the parents. A new drug combination was suggested. The patient and her family asked for time to discuss this treatment. A few days later they came back to the clinic. The older brother and the parents and the patient expressed their conviction that no further chemotherapy should be initiated. Their decision was based on a strong religious belief. The girl continued to be active in school and visited friends until the day of her death. She was hospitalized for the last few hours of her life.

AUTONOMOUS DECISIONS IN YOUNG PATIENTS

The previous paragraphs mentioned children older than ten years of age. Should younger children be involved in the final-stage conference? Generally, the younger a child is, the greater the likelihood that the parents will decide his or her treatment. A patient history may elucidate this statement: A 7-year-old relapsed three years after diagnosis. She was resistant to conventional therapy. The parents were given the option of a Phase II drug trial or discontinuation of therapy. Chemotherapy was continued for 10 months without success. In fact, the child had to be readmitted several times because of severe side effects. After four different Phase II drugs had been tried, the parents agreed to keep the child at home, where she died. The prognosis and possible treatment were never discussed with the child.

The next patient expressed his own wishes with regard to further chemotherapy. Since that time we have included young children in the final-stage conference.

Patient #8. A 7-year-old boy diagnosed as having rhabdomyosarcoma of the lungs and mediastinum was treated with radiation therapy and chemotherapy. The disease was brought under control for five months, when the tumor recurred. The boy was the only child. His father was very close to him. "No other father can have so close a relationship to his boy as I have with my boy," he told us. During the treatment, the father was extremely apprehensive and difficult to handle, and he was unable to accept the fact that his son's health was failing rapidly. Although the medical team seriously questioned the continuation of treatment, he insisted on it, and his wife agreed with him.

After we heard from a student that the boy expressed to him his fears of being "stuck" for a blood transfusion, we received the permission of the parents to talk to the boy about the progression of the disease, and whether or not chemotherapy should be initiated. The boy understood that he was in the final stage. He did not want any further treatment. The father agreed. A couple of weeks later the boy died at home.

Patient #9. A 6-year-old boy was treated with conventional and Phase II drugs for four years when his disease, including central nervous system leukemia, recurred. A Phase II drug or no further treatment was the choice. The parents decided on no further treatment. They did not want the boy to suffer any longer than necessary. We encouraged them to discuss the matter with him and brought him into the room. He sat in his chair sucking on the ice cubes in his cup with a straw. While we told him what we had discussed with his parents, he listened, but did not speak to us. We encouraged him to talk to the parents and tell them what he wanted. We were puzzled. Was it right to explain his status so openly to him? An unexpected answer came. While we talked to the parents, he was sitting in our clerk's room. Suddenly he asked, "Do I have to die?" Her answer was, "Yes, but we will be here to help you." The boy told his parents that he wanted only therapy to stop his severe headaches. He asked for intrathecal treatment and rejected the physician's recommendation of radiation therapy. Two weeks after the conversation, the boy began discussing death openly with both parents. No further treatment was initiated, except for oral dexamethasone and intrathecal therapy to allay severe headaches.

DISCUSSION

An open and frank talk about the problems associated with cancer, among the physician, the patient, and the family, is strongly advocated (Karon, 1973). With the exception of one report, there is no information available on how to approach children, if their disease is far advanced and death is inevitable (Karon, 1973). In this paper the authors report on their experience with a new approach: the final-stage conference. By this technique parents and children are informed about the advanced state of the child's disease, and both are included in the future treatment plan: chemotherapy vs. no chemotherapy. It is not the intent of the authors to analyze the grief reactions of the patients to the final-stage conference, according to the stage schema of Kubler-Ross (1969). Instead, the authors are concerned with the following questions: (1) Can we predict in advance how children will respond emotionally to the information given? (2) Will we be able to predict in advance their choice between further treatment and no treatment? (3) What motivates the patients' decisions? (4) What is the role of the parents? (5) What approach and techniques does the professional team use in this situation? (6) Did the participation of the patients in the final stage decision alter the percentage of patients who chose Phase II drugs? (7) Does the final-stage conference and decision make unjustified demands on the patient and the family?

THE CHILD'S REACTION

The first three questions given above are concerned with the child. The reaction to the final-stage conference varies from child to child. To predict how each child will react is impossible. Some will accept the grave news stoically, some will turn off, and others will cry bitterly. In our small sample, most of the parents came to the same final decision as their children. However, four of 20 children decided differently as shown in Table 2. The professional staff had difficulty in predicting the final decisions of the child, as demonstrated by patients #3, 4, 5, 6, and 7. It is also difficult to evaluate the patients' motives, but few patterns could be detected. Some patients with very advanced disease, for example, who realize they are succumbing, have one wish, namely, to be home or as close as possible to their home (patients #1, 2). The patients' thinking was greatly influenced by their families, and their own philosophical or religious background, as impressively demonstrated by the girl with osteogenic sarcoma (patient #7). Whereas this girl made her decision together with all family members, other children decide by themselves with or without the help of the parents (patients #1, 2, 3, 4, 5, 6, 8, and 9). Fear of side effects, intravenous injections, and long stays in the hospital might dictate the final decision, but all these fears can be overcome if the patient has the impression he or she should not disappoint someone, or should help other persons by agreeing to further treatment (patient #6). Finally, there is a group who have the will to fight this disease as long as possible (patient #3).

THE PARENTS' ROLE

The parents have a very difficult task in this grave situation. They have their own feelings and opinions about further treatment, and yet they must listen to and respect the child's desire. They have to face the fact that the time for their child is running out. If they have not talked to each other before about their child's worsening condition or about his or her imminent death they must now discuss the facts.

No one wants to lose his or her child. Some parents will try everything to prevent death (patient #8), while others come to understand that the child will not live much longer and want most of all to alleviate the child's suffering (patient #9).

Some parents may participate actively in the decision-making process because of their common religious belief (patient #7). Some may feel that their child should spend life according to his or her own will and they should not impose their wishes on the child (patients #1, 2, 3, 5, 6, 8, and 9). Still another group is so dominated by their own feelings that they cannot consider their child's best interest (patient #8).

THE PHYSICIANS' APPROACH

The physician in our hospital who discusses the future of the patient with the family is a part of the professional team. The physician relies on the observations and opinions of the team as much as his or her own (patients #1, 8). The physician has a double role. As a clinical researcher, the physician is searching for new therapeutic approaches for the treatment of the disease. As a physician and patient advocate, his or her interest lies in helping the patient and the family through this most difficult period. Therefore, the conference with the family will reflect the physician's philosophical background. There are physicians who are convinced that it is most important to explore new therapeutic approaches, not only for the benefit of future patients but because of the satisfaction of humanitarian contribution that it gives to the patient involved. They will, therefore, influence the parents and the children to go ahead with Phase II studies if the patient is able to tolerate the treatment. For example, the boy who wanted to go ahead with the treatment in spite of his fears could have easily been convinced to be treated with a new drug for the sake of other patients (patient #6). Other physicians believe in human self-determination and fulfillment within the bounds of one's existence. A physician with this philosophical view does not seek to impose a specific religious belief upon the patient and the family, nor to stress the importance of testing new research drugs. Such a physician feels that the most important thing is that these children spend the time they have left in the way in which they decide is best for themselves. To accomplish this goal, the physician and the professional team must present both alternatives, Phase II treatment or no treatment, as impartially as possible. The physician will observe and listen to the patients, their families, and their feelings, and will help them make their decision if necessary, whether this decision is in his or her own interest or not (patient #6).

ACCEPTANCE OF PHASE II DRUGS

The participation of patients in the final-stage conference did not change the incidence of those on Phase II drugs (see Table 1). This fact is not surprising if one considers that most of the children have the same attitude toward further therapy as their parents (see Table 2). However, more patients should be evaluated to verify this finding.

THE EFFECT OF THE FINAL-STAGE CONFERENCE

Each final-stage conference will vary in content and outcome. Any routine presentation by the physician is dangerous and destroys the intent of the meeting. Each conference is a new challenge for the professional staff, to lead the family through this grave situation and encourage them to make the decision which is right for them. However, one has to be aware that there is always a chance that the discussion could be harmful; for example, the physician who talked to the boy with ALL (patient #9) had the impression that the boy was alienated by the discussion. Fortunately, we learned later that this discussion proved to be a great help to the parents and the child.

One may ask if it is important or right to talk to the patients so openly. Studies in the last 10 years indicate that children with cancer are aware of the severity of their disease, and are disturbed if they feel that essential information is withheld from them or they are not told the truth (Bluebond-Langner, 1974; Karon, 1973; Spinetta, Rigler, & Karon, 1973; Vernick & Karon, 1965; Waechter, 1971). When the team first discusses the diagnosis of cancer with the family and the patient, they promise them that information will not be hidden from them. For that reason the team must continue to be open with them, even in the final stage. At this point, the staff no longer talks about the possibility of death, but tells the child outright that he or she will die from the disease. If the child asks about his or her death, "Do I have to die?," the answer is "Yes," but assurance is given that the child will not be left alone, "We will be there to help you" (patients #3, 9).

Two related questions emerge: Can we ask parents to make such a difficult decision for their child as the choice between research drugs vs. no chemotherapy? Schowalter, Ferholt, and Mann (1973) discussed these questions in reference to a 16-year-old girl with renal failure. They concluded that the child and her family made a rationally based decision in refusing further treatment. The patients' histories given above show that parents are able to make this decision (Table 2). Other parents not included in this report, cannot decide at first, but do so later, often with the help of their child or the professional team. A third group of parents is never able to make the choice. As for the child, no simple answer can be given. But it is apparent that the psychological maturity of many children who are experiencing terminal illness far exceeds their biological age. Even young children are able to grasp the alternatives and share in making the decisions.

In no instance was there evidence of prolonged anger or resentment at the professional team for discussing the final-stage condition so openly. The children and families accepted the fact that no cure was available and decided what they wanted to be done. The decision, whether for or against further chemotherapy, resulted in a feeling of relief. The family and the patient were able to discuss freely their personal feelings and concerns as evident in the child with ALL and the boy with testicular embryonal carcinoma (patients #6, 9). All patients continued to participate in their normal daily activities as much as their disease permitted.

In reviewing the histories in which a final-stage conference was employed, the staff feels that this technique was not detrimental to the families. On the contrary, it was helpful to them as well as to the medical staff. The authors submit that to date it is the method which is most consistent with their commitment to deal openly with the patient. Therefore the team will continue to use it.

This report may encourage other investigators who have a similar understanding about communicating with children and families to use a similar approach in the final stage, and to report their techniques and experiences.

CONCLUSION

The Oncology Service of Oklahoma Children's Memorial Hospital has developed an atmosphere of openness and honesty with its patients, which is considered essential for a system of supportive psychological care (Karon, 1973). In a series of histories we have focused on the turning point in the treatment of terminal illness, when conventional chemotherapy has failed to control the disease, and the patient is faced with the options of no further treatment or Phase II drugs. The emotional impact of the final-stage conference and the decision-making process require a perceptive approach on the part of the professional team.

The histories of nine out of the 20 patients who experienced the final-stage conference were reported in detail. In this small series the use of the final-stage conference did not alter the percentage of patients choosing Phase II drugs. Sixteen children had the same view as their parents in regard to further treatment. However, four decided differently. Of nine patients presented in more detail, eight made their decision independently of their parents. In not one instance did the child or the parents regret being told the truth about the status of the disease. In fact, the parents and children were enabled to express their feelings and concerns freely.

The patient's reaction and decision could not be predicted by the physician. The decision depended on various factors: the will to live, the fears of a long stay in the hospital and painful procedures, and the relationship to the family and the medical staff. One of the most important factors in making the decision was the religious or philosophical background of the patient and the family, and the approach of the professional team.

REFERENCES

Bluebond-Langner, M. M. I know, do you? A study of awareness, communication and coping in terminally ill children. In B. Schoenberg, A. C. Carr, A. H. Kutscher, D. Peretz, & I. Goldberg (Eds.), *Anticipatory grief.* New York: Columbia University Press, 1974.

Freud, A. The role of bodily illness in the mental life of children. In R. S. Eissler (Ed.), *Psychoanalytic study of the child.* New York: International Universities Press, 1972.

Glaser, K. Group discussion with mothers of hospitalized children. *Pediatrics,* 1960, *26,* 132-145.

Gofman, H., Buckman, W., & Schade, G. H. Parents' emotional response to child's hospitalization. *American Journal of Disease of Children,* 1957, *93,* 629-637.

Heffron, W. A., Bommelaere, K., & Masters, R. Group discussion with parents of leukemic children. *Pediatrics,* 1973, *52,* 831-840.

Karon, M. The physician and the adolescent with cancer. *Pediatrics Clinics of North America,* 1973, *20,* 965-973.

Kubler-Ross, E. *On death and dying.* New York: Macmillan, 1969.

Lansky, S. B. Childhood leukemia: The child psychiatrist as a member of the oncology team. *Journal of the American Academy of Child Psychiatry,* 1974, *13,* 499-508.

Lansky, S. B., Lowman, J. T., Vats, T., & Gyulay, J. School phobia in children with malignant neoplasms. *American Journal of Disease of Children,* 1975, *129,* 42-46.

Natterson, J. M., & Knudson, A. G., Jr. Observations concerning fear of death in fatally ill children and their mothers. *Psychosomatic Medicine,* 1960, *22,* 456-465.

Schowalter, J. E., Ferholt, J. B., & Mann, N. M. The adolescent patient's decision to die. *Pediatrics,* 1973, *51,* 97-103.

Spinetta, J. J., Rigler, D., & Karon, M. Anxiety in dying children. *Pediatrics,* 1973, *52,* 841-845.

Vander Veer, A. H. The psychopathology of physical illness and hospital residence. *Quarterly Journal of Child Behavior,* 1949, *1,* 55-71.

Vernick, J., & Karon, M. Who's afraid of death on a leukemia ward? *American Journal of Diseases of Children,* 1965, *109,* 393-397.

Waechter, E. H. Children's awareness of fatal illness. *American Journal of Nursing,* 1971, *71,* 1168-1172.

5

Homosexual Outcome of Discordant Gender Identity/Role in Childhood
Longitudinal Follow-Up

John Money and Anthony J. Russo

Department of Psychiatry and Behavioral Sciences, and Department of Pediatrics, The Johns Hopkins University and Hospital

Prospective, longitudinal studies of childhood sexuality are rare. Few people are able to commit themselves to a longitudinal study and remain budgeted long enough to complete it. In addition, the sexual taboo of our society is particularly antithetical to the recognition of sexuality in childhood, let alone the study of it. Until recently, if a problem of gender identity showed up in a boy's development, the usual medical tradition was to prophesy that he would grow out of it at puberty. This tradition is completely contradicted by the evidence of retrospective studies of the developmental antecedents of homosexuality, bisexuality, transvestism, and transsexualism, all of which typically have a history dating back to prepuberty.

The purpose of this paper is to report the findings of the outcome in adulthood of discordant gender identity/role differentiation relative to the criterion of gross morphologic sex in five boyhood cases, with specific reference to occupational status, psychosexual status, and mental health status.

The follow-up period is from 15 to 22 years. The size of the sample, five, is small in absolute terms, but large in terms of the availability of such long-term follow-up.

Supported by U.S. Public Health Service grant #HD-00325.
Originally published in *Journal of Pediatric Psychology*, 4(1)(1979):29-41.

METHOD

Subjects

In the middle 1950s, and as an extension of psychologic studies in hermaphroditism, a request went out from the psychohormonal research unit of The Johns Hopkins University and Hospital for referral of pre-pubertal boys with discordant gender identity/role. In the period from 1955 to 1962, 12 referrals were made by pediatricians and/or school social workers.

The criteria for referral were: exceptional interest in dressing in girls' clothing; avoiding play activities typical of boys and preferring those of girls; walking and talking more like girls than boys; and stating overtly the wish to be a girl. The presence of overt homosexual erotic behavior was not specified as a requirement for referral and, indeed, was not a presenting symptom for any of these boys.

The patients referred did not represent a random or probability sampling from the general population of boys manifesting discordant gender identity/role. The exact biasing factors are not known. There was no selective bias in favor of psychopathology or delinquency as usually defined, for the primary concern was gender identity/role. There was also no consistent bias with respect to IQ, socioeconomic status, physique, or somatic status.

Of the 12 patients, 11 qualified for inclusion in the present follow-up study on the criterion of being now older than 23, the oldest being 29; 2 of the 11 were earlier lost to follow-up and remained lost. Of the nine remaining candidates for follow-up, two were reluctant to be seen in current psychosexual follow-up but are not lost; and the two remaining are presently untraced, though not written off as permanently lost, as they were seen for teen-aged follow-up within the past 7 years. The remaining five gave the data tabulated in this report.

Procedure

Initially the patients were all followed annually, with intervening visits on a self-demand, no-charge basis until puberty was established. Subsequent visits were on self-demand until 1977, when the present follow-up was instituted. A longitudinal file has been kept on each patient. The files included: test data; transcribed, taped interviews based on a systematic schedule of inquiry; and notes of physical examinations and measurements from the pediatric endocrine clinic. In addition the files also included interviews with parents and/or other guardians, as appropriate.

Patients were called in for follow-up interviews, which were based on a systematic schedule of inquiry. The Cornell Medical Index, among other tests, was also administered to each patient as a source of inquiry regarding his general health.

The schedule of inquiry was drawn up specifically for this follow-up study. It consisted of 27 typed pages with space for the interviewer to record the responses. In the case of extended answers, a tape recorder was used and answers were transcribed. The topics of inquiry fell into categories dealing with education, indoor and outdoor recreational activities, hobbies, dress, make-up, jewelry and perfume, teasing, dreams, enuresis, sleep, self-image, parental relationships, employment and career, living arrangements, religion, nonromantic friendships and acquaintances, romantic friendships, aggressive/passive behavior, sexual activity, and any other special behavior. The follow-up evaluation required an average of 6 hours.

FINDINGS

Occupational Status

The educational and occupational information in Table I shows that none of the nine individuals for whom the information is available was a vocational failure. Except for two who were completing a college education when last contacted, all were, at a minimum, economically self-supporting at the middle-class level or higher. Among the seven who were already employed, six were professionally trained and were working at a level consistent with their training and intelligence. The seventh had irregular work in his chosen theatrical career, and took a second job in order to augment his salary in the meantime.

In view of the association between stage-acting and childhood effeminacy reported by Green and Money (1966) for the same group of individuals in childhood, it is noteworthy that two of them have pursued their interests professionally, one of them to a high degree of recognition.

Psychosexual Status

Inspection of Table II shows that the stated request to be a girl during childhood did not persist into a stated request to be a woman in adulthood.

Table I. Age, Education, and Occupation of Five Men with a History
of Discordant Gender Identity/Role in Childhood[a]

Patient no.	Age in years at follow-up	Education completed	Occupation
564988	29	B.A.	Small business entrepreneur
076559	23	College 3 semesters	Paramedical
141178	29	H.S.	Professional theater
868999	24	B.A.	Pedagogy and small business entrepreneur
6900501	24	A few college credits	Waiter; nonprofessional theater

[a] Among the six persons not seen in current follow-up and not included in Table I, educational data are known about four persons. Of the four, one had attended college for a year when last interviewed; one received a bachelor's degree as an art student; one is a fine arts director; and one is a graduate in American literature.

The current absence of a request to be a woman is paralleled by an absence of seeing the self as a woman during current dreams. Since the dreams of childhood as formerly reported did not include seeing the self as a girl, it is possible that the dream content in childhood may be utilized as a prognosticator of the status of gender identity/role in adulthood. This childhood dream content correlates in four cases with consistent absence of the possibility of the self as transsexual. In the fifth case the boy did, between the ages of 17 and 19, contemplate the possibility of sex reassignment as a solution to what he perceived as his life's dilemma. He went so far at the age of 19 as to embark on the real-life test of cross-dressing and presenting himself socially as a woman. After 6 weeks he gave up, having learned from the real-life test that sex reassignment was not for him.

By contrast with the cross-dressing interest as juveniles (see Table III), the current interest is zero in four cases and in the fifth case is restricted to costume parties.

With respect to the use of make-up and the wearing of jewelry, the change from childhood to adulthood follows in the same direction as the change in cross-dressing. That is to say, in daily life, none of the five men exhibit themselves as being feminine by reason of what they wear. The only signs, if any, that an observer might construe as being feminine would be subtle ones of body movements. In four of the five, such signs were minimal at most, and in the fifth a little more obvious to those educated in what to look for.

Table II. Gender Orientation: Reported Statements, Dreams, and Thoughts of Five Men with a History of Discordant Gender Identity/Role in Childhood

Patient no.	Stated request to be a girl during childhood	Stated request to be a woman, currently	Self seen as a woman in dreams, currently	Self seen as a girl in dreams in childhood	Thought of being transsexual
564988	Yes	No	No	No	Never
076559	Yes	No	No	No	Never
141178	Yes	No	No	No	Never
868999	Yes	No	No	No	Never
6900501	Yes	No	No	No	Yes (see text)

Table III. Preferences in Clothing, Make-up, and Jewelry of Five Men with a History of Discordant Gender Identity/Role in Childhood

Patient no.	As a child dressed up as a female	Currently dresses up as a female	Wore make-up in childhood	Wore make-up at time of follow-up	Wore jewelry in childhood	Wore jewelry occasionally at time of follow-up
564988	Yes	Costume parties only	No	Costume parties only	Yes	No
076559	Yes	No	Yes	No	Yes	No
141178	Yes	No	Yes	No	Yes	No
868999	Yes	No	No	No	Yes	No
6900501	Yes	No	Yes	Minimal	Yes	No

Table IV. Romantic and Erotic Status of Five Men with a History of Discordant Gender Identity/Role in Childhood[a]

Patient no.	Had a coitus with a female	Erotic status	Romantic	Involvement with females
564988	No	Homosexual	Yes	Yes
076559	No	Homosexual	No	Yes
141178	Yes	Predominantly homosexual	No	Yes
868999	Yes	Predominantly homosexual	No	Yes
6900501	No	Homosexual	No	Yes

[a] Among the six persons not seen in current follow-up and not included in Table IV, four are known to be homosexual in erotic status, and two are lost to follow-up.

With respect to current romantic and erotic status, Table IV shows that all five men considered themselves homosexual or predominantly so, as confirmed in their actual erotic behavior. Two have had the experience of copulating with females, but in a more perfunctory way than in their corresponding experience with males. One of these two appears to be in a phase of transition to a less perfunctory continued relationship with a girl friend. One man who had not had sexual intercourse with a female described what he called a dating relationship with a girl friend during his high-school years, subsequently totally discontinued. All five of the men have had romantic involvements or love affairs with males and two of them are in long-term living arrangements with their lovers. The other three men are living independently away from their parents. In all five cases, contact with the parents was maintained in the usual adult way when sons live away from their parents.

Mental Health

As stated in the section on Procedure, self-demand counseling was offered to all of the individuals in this study from childhood onward. Each of the five seen personally for current follow-up expressed his approval of this arrangement, and particularly of the nonjudgmental attitudes they encountered in their visits. They volunteered that they had strongly benefited from their counseling sessions and believed that they were better able to accept themselves as healthy individuals because of them. None of the five men was evaluated as being in the need of more frequent psychotherapy and none showed psychopathological symptoms requiring it.

DISCUSSION

Etiology

The starting date of the ideal longitudinal study of the outcome of psychosexual differentiation would be the day of conception; and the ideal prenatal methodology would be one in which the prenatal fetal hormonal history could be measured with greater precision than is today possible. Fetal sex hormones are known to influence brain pathways which in turn will subsequently mediate behavior that is to some degree sexually dimorphic: the relevant animal-experimental and human-clinical evidence is reviewed in Money and Ehrhardt (1972). This fetal-hormonal influence does not preordain masculine versus feminine behavior, but simply creates a threshold that will either help or hinder the manifestation of the one or the other, respectively. An excess of fetal androgenization of a genetic and gonadal female, for example, may induce a high degree of anatomical masculinization of the genitals. In extreme cases, there is instead of a clitoris a penis. In less extreme cases, the phallus looks like either a hypospadiac penis or a maximally hypertrophied clitoris. In some cases the baby is assigned, reared, and rehabilitated hormonally and surgically as a boy, especially when the phallus looks like a normal penis. Psychosexual differentiation then proceeds as masculine so that, in adulthood, the individual shows no signs of having a 46,XX chromosomal complement, nor of having been born with two ovaries (Money & Daléry, 1976). Conversely, when the postnatal medical biography is aimed at feminization, then the psychosexual differentiation, while not masculine, has a tomboyish underpinning, and it is easy for the girl to grow up to become bisexual or, in some instances, exclusively homosexual in young adulthood (Money & Schwartz, 1977).

In the present series of cases, there was no way of retrospectively retrieving information about the prenatal hormonal status of the individuals concerned. It is, therefore, purely speculative as to whether or not they were born with a prenatal hormonal disposition favoring the differentiation of a homosexual gender identity/role. Nonetheless, such a possibility cannot be rejected. If one allows this possibility, one must equally allow also that the possibility does not automatically dictate the outcome. As in the case of native language, the outcome of psychosexual differentiation is, in nature's economy of things, heavily dependent on postnatal input from the social environment. The two principles involved are identification with people of one's own assigned sex, and complementation to those of the other sex. The most important models of identification and complementation are typically the parents.

In the present group of cases, there was no consistency of evidence as to whether the child encountered an exogenous difficulty in identification and complementation as compared with one that emanated from within the child himself. In some cases, the relationship between the parents was blatantly pathological, in others not. When the parents were caught in a pathological relationship, the nature of the pathology was not consistent among families. In some instances the mother was the power broker, in some the father, and in some neither dominated the other. The variability of family relationships was not noticeably different from that found in families who bring their children to the clinic with other diagnoses; and the same kind of variability could have been found in nonclinic families sampled at random. In brief, we did not recognize any consistent postnatal developmental formula to account for the fact that it was in psychosexual differentiation and not in some other aspect of behavioral development, that the child encountered developmental difficulty. Different pathways led to the same destination.

In popular superstition, there is a commonly held dogma that boys are recruited to homosexuality by older homosexual boys or men. In the present sample, this was definitely not the case, for all the boys manifested the signs of gender identity/role discordance which led to their hospital referral in the absence of known homosexual play. In all 11 cases, there was only one known instance of homosexual involvement in childhood. It happened at age 10 when the boy concerned woke up from sleep to discover his 16-year-old baby sitter having interfemoral intercourse with him. One of the reasons why the parents asked their pediatrician for a psychological referral following this incident was that they had some apprehension that their son, an adopted child, might have unwittingly invited the incident because of what they construed as signs of effeminacy. An interview with the teenager showed this not to have been the case. The younger boy is the one in the present series who, more than the others, grew up to achieve a high degree of explicit bisexuality, partly with the help of continued therapy, self-initiated from age 16 onward.

There is another popular superstition that links the onset of homosexuality with the onset of hormonal puberty and, specifically, with a hormonal imbalance. The boys of the present series negate this superstition, for they all showed the developmental signs of what would later manifest itself as homosexuality well before puberty. The timing of the onset of puberty was within normal limits in all cases, and the degree of adolescent virilization of the body was evaluated as normal in the physical examination done by a clinical endocrinologist. The techniques of hormonal measurement were still relatively crude in those days, and were not expected to add significantly to the evidence of hormonal virilization as recorded in the physical examination. Hence there are no hormonal levels to report.

Diagnosis

In the present era of equal rights for both sexes and of the destereotyping of occupational, recreational, and legal sex roles, one may be called upon to justify the legitimacy of labeling a boy's behavior as girlish and then classifying it as pathological. In the present group of cases, it was not simply girlish or androgenous behavior that brought the boys to medical attention. Rather it was the pervasive discordance between the sex of the genitalia and the sex of the mind, so pervasive that each boy had developed a conviction that he should change into a girl, and that he should be able to do so by somehow or other losing his penis, for example, by praying to God to perform the miracle of having it wither and drop off. Other evidence of identification with girls and of adopting their socially coded roles, including their dress, was secondary to this rejection of the male anatomy. The manifestation of such discordance between genital anatomy and gender identity/role eventually provoked concern in the parents, even in those cases in which either one or both of the parents were in covert collusion with the child. The concern at home was matched by concern at school, and was exceeded by peer abuse. Other children persecuted the boy as a sissy and excluded him from their companionship, usually quite cruelly.

At the time they were first seen, these boys were unable to widen their repertory of behavior to encompass that which in our society is stereotypically coded as male as well as that which is coded as female. They had no option of moving back and forth between both sets of stereotypes, which is the true mark of sexual liberation and of behavioral androgyny. They were trapped in one of the two stereotypes, the one in which they were victimized as freakish, and in which they suffered too much at the hands of a disapproving society.

There is no traditionally accepted diagnostic term for boys with a discordant gender identity/role, the terminology utilized in this paper. It is incorrect to use the terms juvenile homosexual, transsexual, or transvestite (see Prognosis, below).

Prognosis

When the men of the present study were first seen in childhood, the strategy of longitudinal follow-up had already been decided upon. In those days, as now, funding for projects on sexuality in childhood was impossible to come by, the taboo on sexuality in our society being what it is. Economic necessity thus joined with a basic policy decision to be as helpful as possible, with minimal intrusion into the lives of the boys and their families. They were offered follow-up on a self-demand basis without charge, on the understanding that an appointment would be sent out from time to time for the purpose of a check-up and progress report. One boy, with his mother's collusion, soon insisted on never coming to the hospital again, though his parents did not. Only two families became permanently lost to follow-up.

Apart from the two early drop-outs, enough is known of the remaining nine men to permit the statement that they did not develop as transsexuals in adulthood. Since transvestites usually are rather theatrical about cross-dressing and not particularly secretive except with people who might punish or chastise them, it is probably correct to say that none of the nine is a transvestite, the evidence being quite definite in seven cases. The evidence is quite conclusive that in eight cases, including the one bisexual case, the boys grew up to be practicing homosexuals. The ninth might well be a case of erotic apathy and inertia, the details remaining undisclosed, except that he is not overtly heterosexual, and has exclusively gay friends.

There is no way of knowing to what degree, if any, the prognosis may have been altered by the minimal form of treatment given. Nonetheless, the follow-up does show that a syndrome that included cross-dressing in boyhood and appeared likely to be a precursor of transsexualism, and possibly of transvestism, did not in fact turn out to be either. Presently there is no known way of establishing a differential prognosis regarding transsexualism, transvestism, and homosexuality (or bisexuality) on the basis of discordance of gender identity/role in childhood. If one judges by the retrospective biographies of adulthood, then the childhood precursor of all three outcomes in adulthood could be indistinguishable from one another.

As adults, none of the men is known to have complained about inadequacy of genital functioning—no impotence, premature ejaculation, anorgasmia, or other erotic disability. To use a newly emerging terminology, they had no difficulty with the second, the acceptive phase of functioning with a sexual partner. This is the phase in which the couple accept one another bodily, the sex organs included. It is preceded by the proceptive phase, the phase of courtship and solicitation, of attracting and being attractive. This is the phase of establishing a pair-bond, otherwise known as falling in love. It is the phase in which the phenomenon of homosexuality essentially resides, for homosexuality is not, in fact, a sexual phenomenon at all, but a love phenomenon—an inability to fall in love with a person of the other sex, and an ability to fall in love with a person of the same sex as one's own. In consequence, the acceptive phase, when it follows the proceptive, does not lead on to the conceptive phase. Nonetheless, the conceptive phase of parenthood is not impaired. The men of the present sample all had a positive attitude toward children, and not a negative one, on the criterion of being able to be parental toward young children. They were able to develop a special avuncular relationship with their nieces and nephews, if they had them.

Treatment

In the present era of the ethics of informed consent and the rights of patients in medicine, some critics have questioned the morality of considering the problems of discordant gender identity/role in childhood as symptoms requiring treatment. Thus, it is not possible to find out what might happen to psychosexual differentiation should a group of boys with discordance of gender identity/role be transferred from the home of origin to, say, a children's recovery center or to foster homes for a period of time, as happens in the case of child-abuse dwarfism (Money, 1977), with ensuing catch-up growth, both statural and mental. At the present time it is also doubtful that one will be able to compare the effects of different forms of attempted intervention while the child stays living with the parents.

What can be said on the basis of the present findings is that the minimal form of treatment offered did no obvious harm. On the contrary, the verdict of those men interviewed in person during late adolescence or young adulthood was, without exception, that they had benefited from having someone, especially in the juvenile years, whom they could expect to be totally nonjudgmental and willing to help in time of need, when they disclosed intimate and confidential information that brought scorn, disapproval, and stigmatization from many other authorities. It is quite possible that they were assisted to maintain self-esteem and self-respect, and to become successful human beings, unencumbered by secondary psychopathology, because of this early experience of nonjudgmentalism. They certainly do not fit the common and faulty stereotype of homosexuality as a form of sickness, degeneracy, or abomination.

Addendum

Three of the five adults here reported were among those previously reported as children (Green & Money, 1960, 1961).

REFERENCES

Green, R., & Money, J. *Journal of Nervous and Mental Disease,* 1960, *130,* 160-168.

Green, R., & Money, J. *Pediatrics,* 1961, *27,* 286-291.

Green, R., & Money, J. Stage-acting, role-taking, and effeminate impersonation during boyhood. *Archives of General Psychiatry,* 1966, *15,* 535-538.

Money, J. The syndrome of abuse dwarfism (psychosocial dwarfism or reversible hyposomatotropism): Behavioral data and case report. *American Journal of Diseases of Children,* 1977, *131,* 508-513.

Money, J., & Daléry, J. Iatrogenic homosexuality: Gender identity in seven 46,XX chromosomal females with hyperadrenocortical hermaphroditism born with a penis, three reared as boys, four reared as girls. *Journal of Homosexuality,* 1976, *1,* 357-371.

Money, J., & Ehrhardt, A. A. *Man and woman, boy and girl: The differentiation and dimorphism of gender identity from conception to maturity.* Baltimore: Johns Hopkins University Press, 1972.

Money, J., & Schwartz, M. Dating, romantic and nonromantic friendships, and sexuality in 17 early-treated adrenogenital females, aged 16-25. In P. A. Lee, L. P. Plotnick, A. A. Kowarski, & C. J. Migeon (Eds.), *Congenital adrenal hyperplasia.* Baltimore: University Park Press, 1977.

6

Psychological Perspectives in Chronic Childhood Illness

Dennis Drotar

Departments of Psychiatry and Pediatrics, Case Western Reserve University, School of Medicine

Chronic physical illness is a major life stressor for increasing numbers of children and their families (Pless & Douglas, 1971; Pless & Roghmann, 1971). Owing to advances in medical treatment, children with such chronic conditions as cancer, cystic fibrosis, myelodysplasia, and endstage renal failure are now living longer than ever before and facing unforeseen problems as adolescents and adults (Dorner, 1976; Gogan, Koocher, Fine, Foster, & O'Malley, 1979; Grushkin, Korsch, & Fine, 1973; Rosenlund & Lustig, 1973). In concert with these developments, growing numbers of pediatric psychologists are engaged in clinical work with chronically ill children and their families, chronic illness-related research, and consultation with medical and nursing staff. To facilitate their work, psychologists must grapple with a complex and unfamiliar body of knowledge, including the physical aspects of disease as well as the psychological assessment, clinical intervention, and research methods uniquely suited to chronic illness populations.

This special section of the *Journal of Pediatric Psychology* extends our understanding of psychological practice and research with this important pediatric population with contributions from experienced practitioners and researchers. Brantley, Stabler, and Whitt describe the unique consultation, training, and research needs of a chronic illness program. The physicians' perspective is represented in Heisler and Friedman's thoughtful and empathic description of the comprehensive care of children with seizures. Finally, Spinetta, Swarner, and Sheposh's study of parental adjustment following the death of leukemic children illustrates an interesting family-centered approach to research. The present paper introduces these contri-

Originally published in *Journal of Pediatric Psychology,* 6(3)(1981):211-228.

butions with an overview of perspectives concerning the psychology of childhood chronic illness.

CLINICAL WORK WITH CHRONICALLY ILL CHILDREN

Chronically ill children are commonly referred to pediatric psychologists for assessment and treatment recommendations concerning a bewildering range of problems such as disruptive or disturbed behavior on hospital wards; poor compliance with treatment regimens; severe anxiety or depression; problematic adaptation to school, peers, or family; and preparation for hospitalization and/or surgery (Drotar, 1977a; Johnson, 1979; Magrab, 1978; Wright, 1979). Although these presenting problems overlap with those seen among physically healthy children, clinical assessment of chronically ill children involves a unique, comprehensive appraisal of the quality of the child's coping with disease-related stresses including pain, physical limitations, or treatment regimens, as well as psychosocial functioning in school, hospital, or family. Brantley and her co-workers' caveat for the clinician to consider the unique stresses posed by each individual disease and its treatment regimens, and to distinguish carefully between maladaptive versus adaptive coping illustrates the complexity of diagnostic assessments in this population. The fact that children's intellectual understanding of their disease (Campbell, 1975; Simeonsson, Buckley, & Monson, 1979), salient emotional concerns (Freud, 1952; Nagera, 1978; Schowalter, 1977), and expectations for management of physical treatment regimens varies with age and level of emotional maturity requires a special understanding of child development. The wise clinician also construes the child and family's coping as a *process* which unfolds over time rather than as a static attribute (Cohen & Lazarus, 1979; Mechanic, 1974). Since the onset of a chronic illness (Geist, 1979), assumption of a physical treatment regimen, or change in physical status present different stresses, chronically ill children's coping must always be evaluated against the backdrop of the stage and severity of disease. For this reason, evaluations of the chronically ill child's psychological progress over time are much more useful in treatment planning than any single evaluation. Many chronically ill children who are severely stressed by the onset of the disease, a lengthy hospitalization, or physical deterioration show surprising resilience and regain a level of adaptive coping without intensive psychological intervention. On the other hand, a protracted retreat from age-appropriate developmental tasks, particularly in a child with mild physical disease, can signal a more ominous disturbance requiring more intensive intervention (Drotar, 1975a; 1978). In contrast to similar work with physically healthy children, the goals of clinical intervention are highly dependent on the expectations for life functioning afforded by the child's physical status. For example, confrontation of family attitudes and relationships that maintain a child's perceived vulnerability within the family (Green & Solnit, 1964) may be needed to counter the psychological debilitation associated with relatively mild physical disease. On the other hand, families of children whose life functioning is realistically impeded by severe disease may require support to adjust to the painful implications of a diminished quality of life.

Setting priorities for psychological intervention is made difficult by the many potential problems, such as personality disturbance, family difficulties, acute psychological crises, etc., that can accompany a chronic illness (Drotar, 1977a; 1978). In addition, the weighty burdens of a chronic illness can tax the emotional and financial resources of child and family, limit options for intervention, and complicate the family's acceptance of psychological treatment. Since a recommendation for psychological intervention can be experienced as an added insult by children or parents who already feel singled out by their disease, intervention must be planned and timed so as not to undermine further the child's autonomy. An understandable wish to help a highly stressed child can sometimes lead to premature application of psychological "treatment" at a time when the child's needs for the continued and reliable presence of family and/or hospital staff are much more compelling (Drotar & Chwast, Note 1).

Assessing the Family Context

Since the chronically ill children's relationships with other family members are a critical source of emotional support (Anthony, 1970; Caplan & Killea, 1976; Litman, 1974; Sourkes, 1977), the quality of family coping with the financial, organizational, and relationship stresses incurred by a chronic illness should be a primary focus of assessment. Unfortunately, the emphasis on the child's physical condition tends to deflect total family participation from comprehensive care. For example, in many chronic illness centers, mothers often assume total responsibility for contacts with the medical staff, and other important family members such as fathers or siblings are rarely seen. For this reason, a family-centered approach, as exemplified by Ablin, Binger, Stein, Kushner, Roger, and Mikkelsen's (1971) use of a family conference to establish a relationship between physician and family, can be an important ingredient of comprehensive care. Moreover, clinical observation of family problem-solving, communication, and coping concerning the child's disease (Lewis, Beavers, Gosett, & Phillips, 1976; Power & Dell Orto, 1980) can reveal potentially maladaptive family alignments, such as overly close relationships between parent and child, and suggest psychological treatments that address the family context of children's adjustment problems (Jaffee, 1978). A family-oriented approach to treatment can also minimize the counterproductive labeling of the ill child as the sole focus of disturbance and provide support to fathers or physically healthy siblings, who may be highly stressed but silent participants in the child's care (Boyle, di Sant' Agnese, Sack, Millican, & Kulczycki, 1976; Cairns, Clark, Smith, & Lansky, 1979). Family therapy is a primary treatment modality for those emotional disturbances that are rooted in dysfunctional family transactions culminating in overprotection or scapegoating of the ill child (Minuchin, Rosman, & Baker, 1978). Finally, in cases of severe, life-threatening illness, family-oriented supportive intervention can be a highly productive means of encouraging family members' support and contact with their dying child or adolescent (Drotar, 1977b).

The Psychologist and Comprehensive Care

The interpersonal context of physical treatment, including such variables as openness of communication between staff and family (Spinetta & Maloney, 1978) or continuity of care (Breslau, Note 2) may play a critical role in family stress management. Recognizing that a chronic illness poses stresses to *all* children and their families, not only those who experience severe adjustment problems, physicians have established comprehensive care programs to provide ongoing psychosocial support to children and families. Comprehensive care can be defined as the systematic inclusion of psychosocial issues in the child's medical care within a family and community context (Rothenberg, 1976). In this section, Heisler and Friedman present an exemplary approach to the comprehensive care of children with seizures. However, it should be noted that the *content* and *structure* of comprehensive care programs in various centers differ widely in (a) frequency, continuity, and nature of contact between physicians, health care professionals, and family; (b) the focus of care, e.g., disease-related vs. family-centered; (c) the structure of leadership and decision-making; and (d) the nature of interdisciplinary communication and planning. In some settings, physicians and nurses provide the sole ongoing contact with most families, while mental health professionals work only with those children judged as having severe adjustment problems. Other programs feature shared professional contact with children and families over the entire course of the illness. Disease-related issues such as the child's physical status or compliance with regimens are the primary focus of many comprehensive care programs. In others, the impact of disease on the family, academic, and social adjustment are considered in close conjunction with physical care. Some comprehensive care teams meet and communicate regularly; while others meet only in response to crises. Finally, responsibilities for leadership and decision-making in comprehensive care may reside solely with physicians or be shared with other professional disciplines.

Our clinical experience suggests that the mere inclusion of a psychologist or mental health professional in a comprehensive care team without a well-defined salient role in clinical decision-making does not necessarily facilitate psychosocial support to children and families. The psychologist's ability to engage in the kind of dialogues with medical and nursing staff described by Brantley and her co-workers in this section and by others (Drotar, 1976; Koocher, Sourkes, & Keane, 1979; Stabler, 1979; Hollon, Note 3) assumes particular importance in chronic illness-related consultation. Further, the development of supportive-educational interventions (Drotar & Ganofsky, 1976; Heffron, Boomelaere, & Masters, 1973; Korsch, Fine, Grushkin, & Negrete, 1971; Pless & Satterwhite, 1972) for *all* chronically ill children and their families, not only those who undergo psychological crises, is a major goal of any comprehensive care program. Unfortunately, the close interdisciplinary problem-solving and communication which appears to be necessary for sound comprehensive care is very much affected by the structural and organizational problems of hospital settings (Mechanic, 1972; Tefft & Simeonsson, 1979). For example, the subspecialized efforts of many professionals leading to medical advances which have prolonged the lives of chronically ill children can disrupt the level of interdisciplinary communication and planning necessary to maintain the quality of life (Mechanic, 1972). In the hospital context, it is not uncommon for a single professional discipline to have access to only a small part of the total information concerning a chronically ill child and family. Finally, other features of hospital culture, such as time pressures, emphasis on action, and the absence of privacy can severely constrain care-givers' transactions with children and families (Drotar, Benjamin, Chwast, Litt, & Vajner, in press).

The physical care of the chronically ill child also takes place in a highly charged interpersonal arena. Physicians and family are locked into an ambivalent partnership in which "treatment" does not mean "cure" and from which neither can exit. Moreover, physical treatments for conditions such as cancer and renal failure have been developed without a thorough understanding of the psychosocial supports needed to enhance the quality of life and raise profound ethical questions for care-givers and families (Fox & Swazey, 1978; Illich, 1976; Katz & Capron, 1975); As a consequence, decisions concerning the provision of emotional support to chronically ill children are often made in an atmosphere of palpable uncertainty (Fox,

1979). Moreover, relating to chronically ill patients frustrates many physicians (Artiss & Levine, 1973; Ford, Liske, & Ort, 1962), partially because this work requires the kind of communication skills which are not usually emphasized in pediatric training (Haggerty, Roghmann, & Pless, 1975). In many training programs, physicians have much more experience with the hospital-based management of chronically ill children's acute physical problems than they do with the care of the chronically ill in their home settings.

The considerable stresses engendered by the care of the chronically ill child can also affect the medical and nursing staff's appraisal of psychosocial problems and trigger unrealistic requests for psychological consultation. In the stress-laden hospital context, severely ill children and their parents, especially those who demand extra support from the staff, can at times be erroneously construed as emotionally disturbed (Meyer & Mendelson, 1961). For example, in our setting, critically ill adolescents have been referred for psychological treatment of behaviors which the staff perceived as pathological which were better viewed as understandable reactions to painful illness-related stress (Drotar, 1975b; 1978). In such cases, helping medical and nursing staff begin to recognize how their personal reactions may color their appraisal of chronically ill children so that they provide more effective support can often be more useful than direct psychological treatment of the child (Drotar, 1977b; Drotar & Doershuk, 1979).

In their work with the chronically ill, psychologists are also asked to grapple with difficult ethical questions. For example, in our own setting, we were initially asked to evaluate the adjustment of children with end-stage renal failure to determine who would be a "good" psychosocial risk for transplant. These requests were especially troubling because we felt that the use of psychological assessments to make such predictions was neither realistic nor ethically desirable (Fox & Swazey, 1978; Sachs, 1978), Yet, not wanting to dismiss prematurely the prospects of collaborating with our pediatric colleagues, we answered these initial requests as best we could and helped to restructure the program to include ongoing support for all families, not just for those who were severely distressed (Drotar & Ganofsky, 1976; Drotar, Ganofsky, Makker, & DeMaio, 1981).

Like their physician colleagues, psychologists who work with the chronically ill witness human suffering that cannot be erased, even by the most humane interventions (Drotar, Note 4). For this reason, professionals who work closely with chronically ill children cannot help but be touched and, at times, severely distressed, by their poignant struggles (Axelrod, 1979; Cartwright, 1979). The capacity to remain open and available to the chronically ill child and family, while somehow not unduly stressing one's self is an inherent dilemma of work with the chronically ill. The ability to recognize and accept one's own limitations and develop respect for the individuality and strength of chronically ill childrens' coping can be a sustaining force for the care-giver. Moreover, the consistent interpersonal support of colleagues, and a varied, well-organized work routine, including activities which complement direct service, can serve to alleviate the considerable personal burdens of this work (Koocher, 1980).

RESEARCH STRATEGY IN CHILDHOOD CHRONIC ILLNESS

Clinical observations have long underscored the potential impact of chronic illness on areas of personality functioning such as body image and separation/individuation (Becker, 1977; Bergmann, 1965; Eissler, Freud, Kris, & Solnit, 1977; Freud, 1952), and patterns of coping associated with various diseases (Korsch et al., 1971; Mattsson, 1972; McCollum & Gibson, 1970). Following a clinical paradigm, initial research focused on personality adjustment and was characterized almost entirely by clinical descriptive methods and uncontrolled single-group designs with small samples (Gayton & Friedman, 1973; Shontz, 1970). Lacking a coherent conceptual framework, research in the psychology of chronic illness has also been quite fragmented. For example, consider the variety of overlapping definitions of "adjustment" which have included (a) acceptance of disease, including understanding and compliance; (b) freedom from severe psychopathology; (c) "normal" or age-appropriate personality functioning; (d) age-appropriate functioning in school, with family, and/or peers (Pless & Pinkerton, 1975). Unfortunately, personality-focused research in childhood chronic illness has been beset with the same problems involving unwarranted assumptions of cross-situational generality (Mischel, 1973) and inconsistent reliability and validity which have plagued the scientific study of child psychopathology (Achenbach, 1978; Achenbach & Edelbrock, 1978). Chronic illness research has concentrated on the identification of differences or deficits between chronically ill children and their physically healthy peers to the exclusion of factors that relate to competent adjustment *within* various chronic illness populations. Investigators who study group differences sometimes assume that what is adaptive behavior for a healthy child is also adaptive for a chronically ill child who faces very different life circumstances. As a consequence, adjustment patterns that are functionally related to the unique stresses posed by a chronic illness may be prematurely judged as indicative of psychopathology (Mohr, Note 5). For example, it is very possible that chronically ill children's discrepant (from age-matched peers) portrayals of human figures may reflect an accurate appraisal of their compromised physical state rather than a "disturbed" body image, as has been inferred by some (Boyle et al., 1976). Since measures of psychological adjustment have been standardized on physically healthy rather than chronically ill children, inferences concerning the meaning of obtained differences between physically healthy versus chronically ill populations must be made cautiously. Even so, recent research employing objective measures and controlled designs suggests that (a) no one personality pattern is associated with a given illness (Tavormina, Kastner, Slater, & Watt, 1976), (b) the personality strengths of chronically ill children outweigh their deficits (Drotar, Owens, & Gotthold, 1980; Gayton, Friedman, Tavormina, & Tucker, 1977; Tavormina et al., 1976), and (c) chronic illness is a life stressor which, in interaction with other variables, may contribute to increased risk but is *not* the sole cause of adjustment problems (Pless & Roghmann, 1971; Pless, Rhoghmann, & Haggerty, 1972).

Future Directions for Research: Coping and Life Outcomes

In recent years, a competence or coping based model which emphasizes the coping tasks and strategies involved in living with a chronic illness (Cohen & Lazarus, 1979; Lazarus, Averill, & Opton, 1974; Lazarus, 1980) has emerged as a cogent alternative to a psychopathology-based model. However, coping is a vague, all-inclusive concept which subsumes behaviors across a wide range of adaptive contexts (Lazarus & Launier, 1978) and is not easily operationalized. Explicit operational definitions of coping should differentiate the *modes* (e.g., information-seeking or action), *functions* (e.g., altering a stressful situation), and *outcomes* of coping (Lazarus & Launier, 1978). Koski's (1969) study of juvenile diabetes represents an early attempt to distinguish coping style or mode (external vs. internal) from function (constructive vs. nonconstructive). Developing objective procedures to assess disease-related coping tasks such as compliance with treatment regimens; management of anxiety; and adapting to peers, school, or family remains an important goal for future chronic-illness research. Recent approaches to the assessment of childhood coping strategies which merit further application include Zeitlin's (1980) rating of behavioral coping strategies in preschoolers, Yamamato's (1979) study of children's perceptions of stressfulness of experience, Spinetta and Maloney's (1978) classification of coping strategy in childhood cancer, and Siegel's (Note 6) study of children's coping with hospitalization.

Coping is best studied from an ipsative and/or developmental perspective (Lazarus, 1980) in which children or families from a chronic illness population are studied over time, ideally with measures which link coping processes to adaptive outcome in life situations. Covergent group designs involving prospective study of patient groups at different points of postillness contact (Mechanic, 1974; Turk, Note 7) can provide much-needed data concerning how chronically ill children and their families negotiate key developmental transitions such as the onset of adolescence or the entry into adulthood. Moreover, the study of coping should be linked to the development of children's social and emotional competencies as suggested by Murphy and Moriarity's (1976) work with physically healthy children and more recently in Harter's study of children's perceptions of their own cognitive, social, and physical competence (Harter, 1978; in press).

Most psychological researchers have not studied the potential influence of disease-related variables such as severity, recurrent hospitalizations, and physical deterioration on psychosocial variables, including response to psychosocial intervention (Gordon, Freidenbergs, Diller, Hibbard, Wolf, Levine, Lipkins, Ezrach, & Lucido, 1980). However, as more and more survivors of childhood chronic illness reach adulthood, the systematic follow-up of their adult life adjustment assumes special priority. Preliminary outcome studies suggest that adult survivors of childhood chronic illness cope surprisingly well with many life demands, but have a higher than average incidence of adjustment problems (O'Malley, Koocher, Foster, & Slavin, 1979), particularly in social adaptation (Boyle et al., 1976; Gogan et al., 1979; Korsch, Negrete, Gardner, Weinstock, Mercer, Grushkin, & Fine, 1973). Finally, the identification of factors associated with survivors' psychosocial competence or "invulnerability" (Rutter, 1979) might suggest interventions to enhance competent coping with illness-related stress.

ADJUSTMENT IN LIFE CONTEXTS

The Family

Research concerning the psychosocial aspects of chronic illness has generally focused on children's individual adjustment, to the exclusion of their adjustment in various life situations. For this reason, future research might be profitably directed to a greater understanding of chronically ill children's transactions "with significant persons in their lives, in particular settings and at particular times" (Hobbs, 1975, p. 80). The family appears to be an influential mediator of the chronically ill child's adjustment (Caplan & Killea, 1976; Litman, 1974; Litman & Venters, 1979), which deserves a primary place in future research efforts. Preliminary studies indicate that variables such as parents' perceptions of family functioning (Pless et al., 1972), flexibility of family problem-solving (Kucia, Drotar, Doershuk, Stern, Boat, & Matthews, 1979), perceived family cohesion (Moise, Note 8), and ratings of openness of communication (Spinetta & Maloney, 1978) are associated with children's adjustment to chronic illness. Although the impact of chronic illness on siblings, fathers, or on family functioning and organization has received some attention (Cairns et al., 1979; Crain, Sussman, & Weil, 1966; Gayton et al., 1977), the generalized effects of a chronic illness on intrafamilial transactions and family functioning are not well understood. In an interesting example of family-oriented research, Ritchie (1981) found that in contrast to families with a physically healthy child, families with an epileptic child had an autocratic matriarchal structure which was more efficient in problem-solving. Moreover, epileptic children tended to withdraw from family interaction. In addition, Venters (Note 9) found that families which attributed a positive meaning to cystic fibrosis had a higher level of participation in activities outside the home than families with alternative coping strategies.

The validation of family-functioning measures with applicability to chronic illness populations remains a priority for future research. Family or parent-centered measures developed on other populations which might be applicable to childhood chronic illness include perceived family environment (Moos & Moos, 1976), family concept (Van der Veen, Huebner, Jorgens, & Neja, 1964), family cohesion and adaptability (Olson, Sprenkle, & Russell, 1979), clinical ratings of family structure, expression of affect, etc. (Lewis et al., 1976), and parental coping with marriage and child-rearing (Pearlin & Schooler, 1978).

The School

Although school assumes great importance in the lives of chronically ill children, their school adjustment has not been well studied. Despite the fact that chronically ill children can have intermittent school absences and/or limitations requiring special tutoring or limitations in activity, teachers' ratings of the school adjustment of some chronic illness populations (e.g., cystic fibrosis) are surprisingly positive (Drotar, Doershuk, Boat, Stern, Matthews, & Boyer, 1981). However, school adjustment appears to vary considerably as a function of the type of condition. For example, Spinetta and Spinetta (1980) reported that children with cancer adjusted relatively well but were perceived by teachers as more inhibited, less active, and more cautious than a matched group of physically healthy children. Harper, Richman, and Snider (1980) found that type of physical disability and degree of physical impairment were related to different modes of behavioral adjustment in school in a population of children with cerebral palsy and cleft palate. Unfortunately, with few exceptions (Katz, Kellerman, Rigler, Williams, & Siegel, 1977), school-related interventions with chronically ill children have not been described, let alone systematically evaluated.

Chronically ill children are educated by teachers who generally are unfamiliar with their disease and may not have specific information from health professionals to aid their transactions with chronically ill children. For this reason, the attitudes and behaviors of teachers toward the chronically ill child also merit further study. Faust and Campbell (Note 10) found that increased personal familiarity with patients did not appear to affect teachers' knowledge and attitudes about childhood cancer. On the other hand, teachers' concern with children's vulnerability may contribute to unnecessary restrictions or contradictory attitudes toward children with conditions such as spina bifida (Glaser, Drotar, Jaffee, Nulsen, & Gosky, Note 11).

Peer Socialization

A chronic illness presents special problems for a child's socialization which are not well understood. Some chronically ill children are stigmatized by their appearance, limitations in activity owing to their disease, and having to take medications in school. Further, hospitalization and physical treatments limit time and opportunities for socialization with physically healthy peers, and can contribute to social stress and/or isolation. For example, Drotar (Note 12) found that young adults with cystic fibrosis perceived others as having a great many misapprehensions about their disease and perhaps as a consequence, preferred to share little information about their disease with them. One might also expect chronic physical disease to affect the development of intimate personal relationships in later life. Preliminary evidence based on long-term clinical observations suggests that socialization may be an area of special vulnerability for the survivors of chronic illness (Korsch et al., 1973; O'Malley et al., 1979).

On the other hand, contact with peers has been shown to enhance the socialization of physically impaired children in important ways, particularly in the school setting (Guralnick, 1976; Rapier, Adelson, Carey, & Croke, 1972). In an intriguing study that bears replication with children, Zahn (1973) reported that adults with more severe physical impairments had more effective interpersonal relationships than those with mild chronic conditions.

The Hospital

Despite the prevalence of comprehensive care programs for chronically ill children, objective evidence linking frequency, continuity, or nature of professional contact on chronically ill children's adjustment is lacking. However, preliminary evidence suggests that physician-family communication may be less than optimal. Many primary physicians do not play a major role in the management of children with chronic illness with respect to counseling and preventive mental health services (Pless, Satterwhite, & Van Vechten, 1976). Further, social-emotional issues appear to be neglected in communicating with parents about well-child care) (Francis, Korsch, & Morris, 1969) and evaded in the care of adolescents with some chronic conditions (Raimbault, Cachin, Limal, Elincheff, & Rappaport, 1975).

Since psychologists have generally not opened up their transactions with chronically ill children to scientific scrutiny, precious little information documents how psychologists actually function in comprehensive care settings and how their work is perceived by other professionals and/or families. Although the potential utility of psychological interventions with children with chronic illnesses has been eloquently described in a variety of case reports (Becker, 1972; Bergmann, 1965), the efficacy of psychological interventions has not been systematically evaluated in experimental designs (Johnson, 1979; Olbrisch, 1977), with the exception of controlled studies of preparation of nonchronically ill children for surgery (Melamed & Siegel, 1975; Peterson, Hartman, & Gelfand, 1980). Moreover, descriptions of clinical interventions with chronically ill children have generally focused on severe or exceptional disturbances rather than the adjustment difficulties experienced by the majority of chronically ill children. The evaluation of psychosocial interventions designed to enhance children's coping skills and management of disease-related stress, remains a priority for future research (Roskies & Lazarus, 1980). Such applied intervention research might best be directed toward measurable "target" outcomes (Turk, Note 7), such as interpersonal problem-solving (Spivack & Shure, 1974), perceived competence (Harter, in press), or compliance with treatment regimens rather than on global measures such as personality adjustment. Although ethical considerations generally preclude the use of true "no treatment" control groups with children presumed to be at risk, the efficacy of psychosocial treatments differing along potentially important dimensions such as frequency of contact, modality (individual vs. group), or context (home vs. school) can be assessed. The effects of new but untried intervention programs can also be compared against the base-line support provided by the customary level of comprehensive care.

FINAL NOTE

As Brantley and her co-workers attest, there is a strong need for psychologists who work with the chronically ill to develop ongoing research programs which are integrated with the clinical components of comprehensive care. Those who pursue such commitments face the extraordinary practical obstacles of energy-draining demands of patient care, teaching, and clinical responsibilities in other areas, and problems with funding. In many pediatric settings, there is an unfortunate trend for comprehensive care programs to spring up without concerted planning for the special intervention, research, and consultation needs of a particular chronic illness population. As a consequence, few programs have been able to generate new knowledge consistently concerning patient–professional transactions or the nature of chronically ill children's psychosocial outcome. The resources to anticipate needed services, organize psychosocial research, and build liaison with community resources must come from collaborative funding ventures shared by psychologists, physicians, and other health professionals. Moreover, to discourage fragmented, idiosyncratic approaches to research and clinical work, psychologists and other health professionals who work with the chronically ill should begin to share their methods of research, consultation, and clinical interventions in collaborations that transcend individual settings.

Research and clinical work with chronically ill children has much to contribute to our understanding of the impact of long-term stress on child and family coping and development as well as interventions designed to buffer the effects of such stress. It is my hope that the ideas presented in this special section will challenge psychologists to extend their research and clinical endeavors with chronically ill children and their families; to describe their transactions with children, families, and medical staff with greater precision; and to open up their work to scientific scrutiny.

REFERENCE NOTES

1. Drotar, D., & Chwast, R. *Family oriented intervention in chronic illness.* Paper presented at the meeting of the Ohio Psychological Association, Cleveland, 1978.
2. Breslau, N. Personal communication. Cleveland, Ohio, August 21, 1980.
3. Hollon, T. H. *The interaction model of consultation in the general hospital.* Paper presented at the meeting of the American Psychological Association, Montreal, September 1973.
4. Drotar, D. *Shared dilemmas of modern medical care.* Paper presented at the meeting of the American Psychological Association, Washington, D.C., September 1976.
5. Mohr, R. *Paradigms in the clinical psychology of a chronic illness.* Paper presented at the meeting of the American Psychological Association, Washington, D.C., September 1977.

6. Siegel, L. *Preparation of children for hospitalization.* Paper presented at the meeting of the American Psychological Association, New York, September 1979.
7. Turk, D. C. *Factors influencing the adaptive process with chronic illness.* Paper presented at the meeting of the American Psychological Association, New York, September 1979.
8. Moise, J. R. *Psychosocial adjustment of children and adolescents with sickle cell anemia.* Unpublished master's thesis, Case Western Reserve University, 1979.
9. Venters, M. *Chronic childhood illness/disability and familial coping.* Unpublished doctoral dissertation, University of Minnesota, 1980.
10. Faust, D. S., & Caldwell, H. S. *Community attitudes toward the child with a life threatening illness.* Paper presented at the meeting of the American Psychological Association, New York, September 1979.
11. Glaser, N., Drotar, D., Jaffee, M., Nulsen, F. E., & Gosky, G. *Educational and vocational attainments of adolescent and young adult survivors of spina bifida.* Unpublished manuscript, Case Western Reserve University Medical School, 1980.
12. Drotar, D. *Coping patterns of adolescents and young adults with cystic fibrosis.* Unpublished manuscript, Case Western Reserve University School of Medicine, 1980.

REFERENCES

Ablin, A. R., Binger, C. M., Stein, R. C., Kushner, T. H., Roger, S., & Mikkelsen, C. A. A conference with the family of a leukemic child. *American Journal of Disease of Children,* 1971, *122,* 362-366.

Achenbach, T. M. Psychopathology of childhood: Research problems and issues. *Journal of Consulting and Clinical Psychology,* 1978, *46,* 759-776.

Achenbach, T. M., & Edelbrock, C. S. The classification of child psychopathology: A review and analysis of empirical efforts. *Psychological Bulletin,* 1978, *85,* 1275-1301.

Anthony, E. F. The impact of mental and physical illness on family life. *American Journal of Psychiatry,* 1970, *127,* 138-145.

Artiss, K. L., & Levine, A. S. Doctor-patient relation in severe illness. *New England Journal of Medicine,* 1973, *288,* 1210-1214.

Axelrod, B. H. The chronic care specialist "but who supports us". In O. J. Sahler (Ed.), *The child and death.* New York: Mosby, 1979.

Becker, R. D. Therapeutic approaches to psychopathological reactions to hospitalization. *International Journal of Child Psychotherapy,* 1977, *1,* 65-96.

Bergmann, T. *Children in the hospital.* New York: International Universities Press, 1965.

Boyle, I. R., di Sant' Agnese, P. A., Sack, S., Millican, F., & Kulczycki, L. L. Emotional adjustment of adolescents and young adults with cystic fibrosis. *Journal of Pediatrics,* 1976, *88,* 313-326.

Cairns, N. U., Clark, G. M., Smith, S. P., & Lansky, S. B. Adaptation of siblings to childhood malignancy. *Journal of Pediatrics,* 1979, *95,* 484-487.

Campbell, J. D. Illness is a point of view: The development of children's concept of illness. *Child Development,* 1975, *46,* 92-100.

Caplan, G., & Killea, M. *Support systems and mutual help: Multidisciplinary explorations.* New York: Grune & Stratton, 1976.

Cartwright, L. K. Sources and effects of stress in health careers. In G. C. Stone, F. Cohen, & N. E. Adler (Eds.), *Health psychology.* San Francisco: Jossey-Bass, 1979.

Cohen, F., & Lazarus, R. Coping with the stress of illness. In G. C. Stone, F. Cohen, & N. E. Adler (Eds.), *Health psychology.* San Francisco: Jossey-Bass, 1979.

Crain, A. R., Sussman, M. B., & Weil, W. B. Effects of a diabetic child on marital integration and related measures of family functioning. *Journal of Health and Human Behavior,* 1966, *7,* 122-127.

Dorner, S. Adolescents with spina bifida: How they see their situation. *Archives of Disease in Childhood,* 1976, *51,* 439-444.

Drotar, D. The treatment of severe anxiety reaction in an adolescent boy following renal transplantation. *Journal of the American Academy of Child Psychiatry,* 1975, *14,* 451-462. (a)

Drotar, D. Death in the pediatric hospital: Psychological consultation with medical and nursing staff. *Journal of Clinical Child Psychology,* 1975, *4,* 33-35. (b)

Drotar, D. Psychological consultation in the pediatric hospital. *Professional Psychology,* 1976, *7,* 77-83.

Drotar, D. Clinical practice in the pediatric hospital. *Professional Psychology,* 1977, *8,* 72-80. (a)

Drotar, D. Family oriented intervention with the dying adolescent. *Journal of Pediatric Psychology,* 1977, *2,* 68-71. (b)

Drotar, D. Adaptational problems of children and adolescents with cystic fibrosis. *Journal of Pediatric Psychology,* 1978, *3,* 45-50.

Drotar, D., Benjamin, P., Chwast, R., Litt, C., & Vajner, P. The role of the psychologist in the pediatric outpatient and inpatient settings. In J. Tuma (Ed.), *The practice of pediatric psychology,* New York: Wiley, in press.

Drotar, D., & Doershuk, C. F. The interdisciplinary case conference: An aid to pediatric intervention with the dying adolescent. *Archives of the Foundation of Thanatology,* 1979, *7,* 79-96.

Drotar, D., Doershuk, C. F., Boat, T. F., Stern, R. C., Matthews, L., & Boyer, W. Psychosocial functioning of children with cystic fibrosis. *Pediatrics,* 1981, *67,* 338-343.

Drotar, D., Ganofsky, M. A. Mental health intervention with children and adolescents with end-stage renal failure. *International Journal of Psychiatry in Medicine,* 1976, *7,* 181-194.

Drotar, D., Ganofsky, M. A., Makker, S., & DeMaio, D. A family oriented supportive approach to renal transplantation in children. In N. Levy (Ed.), *Psychological factors in hemodialysis and transplantation.* New York: Plenum, 1981.

Drotar, D., Owens, R., & Gotthold, J. Personality adjustment of children and adolescents with hypopituitarism. *Child Psychiatry and Human Development,* 1980, *11,* 59-66.

Eissler, R. S., Freud, A., Kris, M., & Solnit, A. *Physical illness and handicap in childhood.* New Haven: Yale University Press, 1977.

Ford, A. B., Liske, R. E., & Ort, R. S. Reactions of physicians and medical students to chronic illness. *Journal of Chronic Diseases,* 1962, *15,* 785-794.

Fox, R. *Essays in medical sociology.* New York: Wiley, 1979.

Fox, R. C., & Swazey, J. P. *The courage to fail: A social view of organ transplants and dialysis* (2nd ed.). Chicago: University of Chicago Press, 1978.

Francis, V, Korsch, B. M., & Morris, M. J. Gaps in doctor-patient communication: Patients' response to medical advice. *New England Journal of Medicine,* 1969, *280,* 235-540.

Freud, A. The role of bodily illness in the mental life of children. *Psychoanalytic Study of the Child,* 1952, *7,* 69-81.

Gayton, W. F., & Friedman, S. B. Psychosocial aspects of cystic fibrosis: A review of the literature. *American Journal of Diseases of Children,* 1973, *126,* 856-859.

Gayton, W. F., Friedman, S. B., Tavormina, J. B., & Tucker, F. Children with cystic fibrosis: Psychological test findings of patients, siblings and parents. *Pediatrics,* 1977, *59,* 888-894.

Geist, R. A. Onset of chronic illness in children and adolescents: Psychotherapeutic and consultative intervention. *American Journal of Orthopsychiatry,* 1979, *49,* 4-22.

Gogan, J., Koocher, G. P., Fine, W. E., Foster, D. T., & O'Malley, J. E. Pediatric cancer survival and marriage: Issues affecting adult adjustment. *American Journal of Orthopsychiatry,* 1979, *49,* 423-430.

Gordon, W. A., Freidenbergs, I., Diller, L., Hibbard, M., Wolf, C., Levine, L., Lipkins, R., Ezrach, O., & Lucido, D. Efficacy of psychosocial intervention with cancer patients. *Journal of Consulting and Clinical Psychology,* 1980, *48,* 743-759.

Green, M., & Solnit, A. F. Reactions to the threatened loss of a child: A vulnerable child syndrome. *Pediatrics,* 1964, *34,* 58-66.

Grushkin, G. M., Korsch, B. M., & Fine, R. N. The outlook for adolescents with chronic renal failure. *Pediatric Clinics of North America,* 1973, *20,* 953-963.

Guralnick, M. The value of integrating handicapped and non-handicapped preschool children. *American Journal of Orthopsychiatry,* 1976, *46,* 236-245.

Haggerty, R., Roghmann, K. J., & Pless, I. B. *Child health and the community.* New York: Wiley, 1975.

Harper, D. C., Richman, L. C., & Snider, B. C. School adjustment and degree of physical impairment. *Journal of Pediatric Psychology,* 1980, *5,* 377-383.

Harter, S. Effectance motivation reconsidered: Toward a developmental model. *Human Development,* 1978, *1,* 34-64.

Harter, S. The perceived competence scale for children. *Child Development,* in press.

Heffron, W. A., Boomelaere, K., & Masters, R. Group discussion with the parents of leukemic children. *Pediatrics,* 1973, *52,* 831-837.

Hobbs, N. *The futures of children.* San Francisco: Jossey-Bass, 1975.

Illich, I. *Medical nemesis: The expropriation of health.* New York: Random House, 1976.

Jaffee, D. T. The role of family therapy in treating physical illness. *Hospital and Community Psychiatry,* 1978, *29,* 169-174.

Johnson, M. R. Mental health interventions with medically ill children: A review of the literature 1970-1977. *Journal of Pediatric Psychology,* 1979, *4,* 147-163.

Katz, E. R., Kellerman, J., Rigler, D., Williams, V. O., & Siegel, S. F. School intervention with pediatric cancer patients. *Journal of Pediatric Psychology,* 1977, *2,* 72-76.

Katz, J., & Capron, A. M. *Catastrophic diseases: Who decides what?* New York: Russell Sage, 1975.

Koocher, G. P. Pediatric cancer: Psychosocial problems and the high costs of helping. *Journal of Clinical Child Psychology,* 1980, *8,* 2-5.

Koocher, G. P., Sourkes, B. M., & Keane, W. M. Pediatric oncology consultation: A generalizable model for medical settings. *Professional Psychology,* 1979, *10,* 467-474.

Korsch, B. M., Fine, R. N., Grushkin, C. M., & Negrete, V. R. Experiences with children and families during extended hemodialysis and kidney transplantation. *Pediatric Clinics of North America,* 1971, *118,* 625-637.

Korsch, B. M., Negrete, V. F., Gardner, J. E., Weinstock, C. L., Mercer, A. S., Grushkin, C. M., & Fine, R. N. Kidney transplantation in children: Psychosocial follow-up study on child and family. *Journal of Pediatrics,* 1973, *83,* 339-408.

Koski, M. L. The coping processes in childhood diabetes. *Acta Paediatrica Scandinavia* Supplement 1969, *198,* 7-56.

Kucia, C., Drotar, D., Doershuk, C., Stern, R. C., Boat, T. F., & Matthews, L. Home observation of family interaction and childhood adjustment to cystic fibrosis. *Journal of Pediatric Psychology,* 1979, *4,* 189-196.

Lazarus, R. The stress and coping paradigm. In A. Bond & J. C. Rosen (Eds.), *Competence and coping during adulthood.* Hanover, New Hampshire: University Press, 1980.

Lazarus, R. S., Averill, T. R., & Opton, E. M. The psychology of coping: Issues of research and assessment. In G. V. Coelho, D. A. Hamburg, & T. E. Adams (Eds.), *Coping and adaptation.* New York: Basic Books, 1974.

Lazarus, R., & Launier, R. Stress related transactions between person and environment. In L. W. Pervin and M. Lewis (Eds.). *Perspectives in interactional psychology.* New York: Plenum, 1978.

Lewis, J. M., Beavers, W. R., Gosett, J. T., & Phillips, V. A. *No single thread: Psychological health in family systems.* New York: Brunner/Mazel, 1976.

Litman, T. J. The family as a basic unit in health and medical care: A social-behavioral overview. *Social Science and Medicine,* 1974, *8,* 495-519.

Litman, T. J., & Venters, M. Research on health care and the family: A methodological overview. *Social Science and Medicine,* 1979, *13A,* 379-385.

Magrab, P. (Ed.). *Psychological management of pediatric problems* (Vol. 1). *Early life conditions and chronic diseases.* Baltimore: University Park Press, 1978.

Mattsson, A. Long-term physical illness in childhood: A challenge to psychosocial adaptation. *Pediatrics,* 1972, *50,* 801-811.

McCollum, A. T., & Gibson, L. E. Family adaptation to the child with cystic fibrosis. *Journal of Pediatrics,* 1970, *77,* 571-578.

Mechanic, D. *Public expectations and health care.* New York: Wiley, 1972.

Mechanic, D. Social structure and personal adaptation: Some neglected dimensions. In G. V. Coelho, D. A. Hamburg, & J. T. Adams (Eds.), *Coping and adaptation.* New York: Basic Books, 1974.

Melamed, B. G., & Siegel, L. J. Reduction of anxiety in children facing hospitalization and surgery. *Journal of Consulting and Clinical Psychology,* 1975, *43,* 511-521.

Meyer, E., & Mendelson, M. Psychiatric consultations with patients on medical and surgical wards: Patterns and processes. *Psychiatry,* 1961, *24,* 197-205.

Minuchin, S., Rosman, B., & Baker, L. *Psychosomatic families.* Cambridge, Massachusetts: Harvard University Press, 1978.

Mischel, W. Toward a cognitive social learning reconceptualization of personality. *Psychological Review,* 1973, *80,* 252-283.

Moos, R., & Moos, B. A typology of family social environments. *Family Process,* 1976, *15,* 357-371.

Murphy, L. B., & Moriarity, A. E. *Vulnerability, coping and growth from infancy to adolescence.* New Haven: Yale University Press, 1976.

Nagera, H. Children's reactions to hospitalization and illness. *Child Psychiatry and Human Development,* 1978, *9,* 3-19.

Olbrisch, M. E. Psychotherapeutic interventions in physical health: Effectiveness and economic efficiency. *American Psychologist,* 1977, *32,* 761-777.

Olson, D. H., Sprenkle, D., & Russell, C. A circumplex model of marital and family systems. I: Cohesion and adaptability dimensions, family types and clinical applications. *Family Process,* 1979, *14,* 1-35.

O'Malley, T. E., Koocher, G., Foster, D., & Slavin, L. Psychiatric sequelae of surviving childhood cancer. *American Journal of Orthopsychiatry,* 1979, *49,* 608-616.

Pearlin, L. J., & Schooler C. The structure of coping. *Journal of Health and Social Behavior,* 1978, *19,* 2-21.

Peterson, L., Hartman, D. P., & Gelfand, D. M. Prevention of child behavior disorders: A life style change for child psychologists. In P. O. Davidson & S. R. Davidson (Eds.), *Behavioral medicine: Changing health lifestyles.* New York: Brunner/Mazel, 1980.

Pless, I. B., & Douglas, I. W. B. Chronic illness in childhood: Part I. Epidemiological and clinical characteristics. *Pediatrics,* 1971, *47,* 405-414.

Pless, I. B., & Pinkerton, P. *Chronic childhood disorders: Promoting patterns of adjustment.* Chicago: Year Book Medical Publishers, 1975.

Pless, I. B., & Roghmann, K. J. Chronic illness and its consequences: Observations based on three epidemiological surveys. *Journal of Pediatrics,* 1971, *79,* 351-359.

Pless, I. B., Roghmann, K., & Haggerty, R. F. Chronic illness, family functioning, and psychological adjustment: A model for the allocation of preventive mental health services. *International Journal of Epidemiology,* 1972, *1,* 271-277.

Pless, I. B., & Satterwhite, B. Chronic illness in childhood: Selection activities and evaluation of non-professional family counselors. *Clinical Pediatrics,* 1972, *11,* 403-410.

Pless, I. B., Satterwhite, B., & Van Vechten, D. Chronic illness in childhood: A regional survey of care. *Pediatrics,* 1976, *58,* 37-46.

Power, P. W., & Dell Orto, A. E. (Eds.). *Role of the family in the rehabilitation of the physically disabled.* Baltimore: University Park Press, 1980.

Raimbault, G., Cachin, O., Limal, J. M., Elincheff, C., & Rappaport, L. Aspects of communication between patients and doctors: An analysis of the discourse in medical interviews. *Pediatrics,* 1975, *55,* 401-405.

Rapier, J., Adelson, R., Carey, R., & Croke, K. Changes in children's attitudes toward the physically disabled. *Exceptional Children,* 1972, *39,* 219-224.

Ritchie, K. Research note: Interaction in the families of epileptic children. *Journal of Child Psychology and Psychiatry,* 1981, *22,* 65-71.

Rosenlund, M. L., & Lustig, H. S. Young adults with cystic fibrosis: The problems of a new generation. *Annals of Internal Medicine,* 1973, *78,* 959-961.

Roskies, E., & Lazarus, R. S. Coping theory and the teaching of coping skills. In P. O. Davidson & S. M. Davidson (Eds.), *Behavioral medicine: Changing health life styles.* New York: Brunner/Mazel, 1980.

Rothenberg, M. Comprehensive care in pediatric practice. *Clinical Pediatrics,* 1976, *15,* 1097-1100.

Rutter, M. Invulnerability, or why some children are not damaged by stress. In S. J. Shamsie (Ed.), *New directions in children's mental health.* New York: Spectrum, 1979.

Sachs, M. Social psychological contributions to a legislative subcommittee to organ and tissue transplants. *American Psychologist,* 1978, *33,* 680-690.

Shontz, F. C. Physical disability and personality: Theory and recent research. *Psychological Aspects of Disability,* 1970, *17,* 51-69.

Schowalter, J. E. Psychological reactions to physical illness and hospitalization in adolescence. *Journal of the American Academy of Child Psychiatry,* 1977, *16,* 500-516.

Simeonsson, R., Buckley, L., & Monson, L. Conceptions of illness in hospitalized children. *Journal of Pediatric Psychology,* 1979, *4,* 77-81.

Sourkes, B. Facilitating family coping with childhood cancer. *Journal of Pediatric Psychology,* 1977, *2,* 65-68.

Spinetta, J., & Maloney, L. J. The child with cancer: Patterns of communication and denial. *Journal of Consulting and Clinical Psychology,* 1978, *46,* 1540-1541.

Spinetta, P. D., & Spinetta, J. J. The child with cancer in school: Teachers' appraisal. *American Journal of Hematology/Oncology,* 1980, *2,* 89-94.

Spivack, G., & Shure, M. B. *Social adjustment of young children: A cognitive approach to solving real life problems.* San Francisco: Jossey-Bass, 1974.

Stabler, B. Emerging models of psychologist-pediatrician liaison. *Journal of Pediatric Psychology,* 1979, *4,* 307-313.

Tavormina, J. B., Kastner, L. S., Slater, P. M., & Watt, S. L. Chronically ill children: A psychologically and emotionally deviant population? *Journal of Abnormal Child Psychology,* 1976, *4,* 99-110.

Tefft, B. M., & Simeonsson, R. J. Psychology and the creation of health care settings. *Professional Psychology,* 1979, *10,* 558-570.

Van der Veen, F., Huebner, B., Jorgens, B., & Neja, P. Relationships between the parents' concept of the family and family adjustment. *American Journal of Orthopsychiatry,* 1964, *34,* 45-55.

Wright, L. A comprehensive program for mental health and behavioral medicine in a large children's hospital. *Professional Psychology,* 1979, *10,* 458-466.

Yamamoto, K. Children's ratings of the stressfulness of experiences. *Developmental Psychology,* 1979, *15,* 581-582.

Zahn, M. A. Incapacity, impotence, and invisible impairment: Their effects upon interpersonal relations. *Journal of Health and Social Behavior,* 1973, *14,* 115-123.

Zeitlin, S. Assessing coping behavior. *American Journal of Orthopsychiatry,* 1980, *50,* 139-144.

7

Effective Parental Coping Following the Death of a Child from Cancer

John J. Spinetta
San Diego State University

Joyce A. Swarner
University of Arizona

John P. Sheposh
San Diego State University

One of the consistent suggestions given in the literature for helping the child with cancer deal with the anxieties relative to the illness is to have the family and physician respond as openly and honestly as possible to the child's questions, at the child's level of development and readiness (Adams, 1980; Futterman & Hoffman, 1973; Kagen-Goodheart, 1977; Kellerman, 1980; O'Malley & Koocher, 1980; Schulman & Kupst, 1980; Slavin, 1980; Sourkes, 1977; Spinetta, 1977, 1978; Spinetta & Deasy-Spinetta, 1980). With openness and honesty regarding the diagnosis and prognosis a more common policy in our present treatment of children with cancer, concern has shifted from the issue of telling or not telling, to the issue of maintaining an open pattern of communication at a level that is both consistent and supportive. If it is true that a child as young as 5 or 6 years of age becomes aware eventually of the serious nature of his or her illness (Bluebond-Langner, 1978; Spinetta, 1974), what does the child do with this

This study was supported in part by Public Health Service Grant CA 21254, National Cancer Institute. The authors wish to thank Donald Schwartz, MD, and Gary Hartman, MD, of Children's Hospital and Health Center, San Diego, and Faith Kung, MD, of the University of California, San Diego, School of Medicine, and their staffs for their support and assistance in this research.

Originally published in *Journal of Pediatric Psychology,* 6(3)(1981):251–263.

knowledge and awareness? Does the child talk openly and frequently with the family about the prognosis, or does the child live in silence with the knowledge? What role does the family play in the child's wishing to talk or not to talk about the illness? Does talking about the illness help the child adapt more effectively?

A partial answer to these questions was attempted in a study of family communication patterns regarding the issue of cancer in the child (Spinetta & Maloney, 1978). Results indicated a strong correlation between the level of family communication about the illness and coping strategies in the child. Families in which levels of communication about the illness were high were those families in which the independently measured children (a) exhibited an open, nondefensive personal posture, (b) expressed a consistently close relationship to the parents, and (c) expressed a basic satisfaction with self. Although no conclusions were drawn regarding cause–effect relationships, results indicated that the level of family communication about the illness is related to coping strategies in the child. The children who exhibited a higher level of adaptation with the illness were members of families in which open discussions were allowed and maintained regarding the illness.

Our research team is currently engaged in a longitudinal study of families, from the point of diagnosis through the disease course, to determine prospectively which coping strategies appear to be the most effective in helping children and their families deal successfully with the stresses imposed by the disease and treatment. Maintenance of open communication is one of the variables of concern. In a pilot study regarding the effect of communication patterns on coping, we interviewed 23 families whose children had died of cancer prior to the initiation of our formal interventions.

Our goals were twofold. First, we wished to see if families adapted relatively well to life without their child as suggested by Futterman and Hoffman (1973), or relatively poorly, as suggested by Binger, Ablin, Feuerstein, Kushner, Zoger, and Mikkelsen (1969). Second, we wished to test the suggestions of Hofer, Wolff, Friedman, and Mason (1972) and of Stehbens and Lascari (1974), that some of the differences shown by parents in levels of postdeath adjustment could be due to the ways in which the parents handled the diagnosis, illness, and treatment regimen prior to the child's death. We wished to study the issue of communication as well as other disease-related issues that might affect ultimate adaptation.

An interview schedule was devised tapping the following areas: (a) present family status, (b) major changes in job, health, and friends since the death of the child, (c) other kinds of past crises and methods of resolution, (d) differences in the grieving process between spouses, (e) support systems during the illness and after the child's death, (f) parents' memories of the child, the child's awareness of the illness, and his/her questions regarding the illness and treatment procedures, (g) similar questions regarding the siblings, (h) extrafamilial resources, (i) the parent's basic philosophy of the meaning of life and how the illness fits into this philosophy, and (j) the parents' views of their own adaptational process. In order to avoid having the parents give socially desirable responses, the questions were devised in an open-ended manner, allowing parents to talk at length about feelings and concerns on any particular issue. In this way, the problems inherent in the forced-choice types of self-report instruments were minimized. Judgments of independent experts were used in determining interpretation of tone and content so that a reliable measure of adaptation could be obtained.

The parents who were asked to participate in the interviews were those whose children had been treated in one of the two local institutional pediatric cancer facilities that have participated in our longitudinal studies. The parents of children treated at a third facility and who subsequently died were also interviewed, and the results for them will be reported separately.

METHOD

All of the parents whose children had died at each of the two centers not more than 3 years before the interviews were contacted by letter asking their participation in the interviews and explaining the voluntary and minimally obtrusive nature of participation. The parents were not apprised of the specific hypotheses, but were told of the general nature of the study. Several letters were returned because of change of address. Those families that had moved but remained within driving distance were recontacted. Of the families contacted, only two refused permission for the interview. The interviews were conducted by the same interviewer in the home of each family, and all interviews were tape-recorded and later transcribed. Throughout, the parents were reminded that they did not have to respond to any question that was too obtrusive or overly personal. With very few exceptions, the parents responded to every question asked. The average interview lasted about 1 hour. Parents typically expressed gratitude for having been allowed the opportunity to participate, to share their feelings and concerns, and to place their own sufferings in perspective after the passage of time.

Content Analysis

The taped interviews were transcribed and analyzed as follows: A scoring form was devised, with spaces to be completed by the interviewer and by independent scorers. All of the tapes were scored using this form, both from the typed transcripts and from the actual taped interviews. A flow chart was then devised, with columns listing specific details in each area covered by the interviews. In order to avoid the "halo" type of response interpretation that might take place if one were to score each family's responses in their entirety at the same time, each family was evaluated for its response in each category before the next category was scored. In this manner, a finer point of comparison was possible, and the scorers were able to avoid responding to any individual family in a set manner. All of the responses were ultimately translated into numerical form, in the most conservative manner possible. There were two areas scored from the interviews: (a) the parents' present adaptational level, and (b) the parents' memories of life with the child during the course of the illness.

Present Adaptational Level

Parental responses regarding their current adaptational level were analyzed and scored on 10 criterion measures. The 10 criterion measures, given in full in Table I, centered about a general malaise and inability to return to full functioning. Included were such areas as continued apathy, lack of zest for life, continued feelings of sadness, inability to confront reminders of the child or talk comfortably about the child, remorse over what was not done for the child, and inability to make plans for the future. The 10 items that were chosen were based on statements made in the literature by a variety of authors regarding healthy adaptation (Adams, 1980; Binger et al., 1969; Fischoff & O'Brien, 1976; Futterman & Hoffman, 1973; Hamovitch, 1964; Kaplan, Grobstein, & Smith, 1976; Schiff, 1977). The items were scored in such a manner that the high score in each category represented a higher level of adjustment. Scores were summed across cate-

---

Table I. Postdeath Adaptation Measure

---

1. Parents have returned to normal activities: friends, recreation, eating habits.
   a. All three normal: 4 points
   b. Any two normal: 3 points
   c. Any one normal: 2 points
   d. None: 1 point

(Continued)

Table I. (*Continued*)

2. Parents exhibit apathy and lack of zest for life.
   a. None: 4 points
   b. Some, at times: 3 points
   c. Moderate: 2 points
   d. Considerable: 1 point

3. Family members can talk comfortably with one another about the child, and have pictures of the child around the house without stress and tears.
   a. Yes, parents and sibs: 4 points
   b. Yes, parents; no, sibs: 3 points
   c. Can talk, but with stress: 2 points
   d. Can't talk about child: 1 point

4. Parents exhibit feelings of sadness and crying spells.
   a. Few or none: 4 points
   b. Occasional nondisruptive: 3 points
   c. Occasional disruptive: 2 points
   d. Many: 1 point

5. Parents can make plans for the future.
   a. Yes: 5 points
   b. Yes, but with feelings of urgency: 4 points
   c. Yes, but on a limited basis only: 3 points
   d. No, taking one day at a time: 2 points
   e. No, feelings of betrayal: 1 point

6. Parents can confront physical reminders of the child outside the home without distress.
   a. Yes: 2 points
   b. No: 1 point

7. Parents have used the crisis as an opportunity to learn skills in coping.
   a. Yes, explicitly expressed: 4 points
   b. Yes, in vague and general terms: 3 points
   c. No, do not view crisis this way: 2 points
   d. No, experience represents a negative in terms of confidence to cope with other problems: 1 point

8. Parents feel they did all they could for child, with acceptance of any failings in that regard
   a. Yes: 4 points
   b. Yes, but with some reservations: 3 points
   c. No: 2 points
   d. No, with unresolved guilt: 1 point

9. Parents remain filled with questions and are still searching.
   a. No: 3 points
   b. Yes, in general terms: 2 points
   c. Yes, in very specific terms: 1 point

10. Unresolved feelings and symptoms persist with siblings: crying, guilt, health fears, refusal to discuss.
    a. Absence of fears, sadness, or guilt, can discuss: 4 points
    b. Questions indicating some fears, sadness, or guilt: 3 points
    c. Don't discuss, some fears, sadness, or guilt: 2 points
    d. Fears, secret crying, can't or won't discuss: 1 point

Range of potential scores: 10–38

gories to form a single postdeath adaptation score. The range of scores for parents was from 11 to 36.

Disease-Course Variables

The parents' responses to questions about their family during the life of their child were also analyzed, and reduced to five variables which best summarized parental areas of response. The five variables, defined by positive valence, are as follows:

1. Life Meaning. The presence of a consistent philosophy/theology/cosmology of life present during the diagnosis, which helped the family accept the diagnosis and its consequences as part of an overall life scheme. Meaning was measured by parents' responses to questions about the disease course, how it fit into their life view, and whether their philosophy of life helped them sustain a positive attitude throughout. Scores were based on consistency and strength of the parents' philosophy over time in giving meaning to the illness, and in helping them cope with the disease course.

2. Support. The presence of a viable significant other, usually the spouse, who helped the parents cope during the course of the illness. Spouse-support was measured by whether and to what degree the parents had found the spouse or significant other supportive during the course of the disease and after the death.

3. Communication with the Child. A level of communication with the child during his/her life which included full factual explanations of the diagnosis, treatment, and prognosis, consistent with the child's age and level of development, and allowing the child to express feelings, both positive and negative, toward the disease, the treatment procedure, and/or the hospital. Initiation and maintenance of an open level of communication with the child was judged on a point system based on parental responses to the following: how aware the child was of the illness, whether the child continued speaking about the illness either directly or indirectly throughout the course of the illness, whether the child initiated the conversations or waited, whether parents felt enough had been said, types of questions asked relative to prognosis, and whether parents answered prognosis-related questions honestly.

4. Normal Functioning. The ability of the family, after a period of time postdiagnosis, to return eventually to a semblance of normal family functioning while the child was alive and in remission.

5. Communication with Siblings. This was defined the same as no. 3 above, but with siblings. The five variables were submitted to a multiple regression analysis, with the overall postdeath adaptation score as the criterion measure.

Table II. Itemized Responses of Families to Postdeath Adaptation Measure

Family	\multicolumn{10}{c}{Items}										Total
	1	2	3	4	5	6	7	8	9	10	
1	3	2	2	2	3	1	2	4	1	3	23
2	4	4	4	2	5	2	3	4	3	3	34
3	3	4	3	4	5	2	3	3	2	2	31
4	1	1	1	1	1	1	1	1	2	1	11
5	4	4	4	4	4	2	4	3	3	4	36
6	3	4	1	4	3	2	2	4	3	2	28
7	4	4	4	4	5	2	2	3	3	3	34
8	3	4	2	2	3	2	2	3	1	2	24
9	3	2	2	3	2	1	2	3	2	2	22
10	3	4	4	3	5	2	2	4	3	2	32
11	3	4	3	2	3	2	3	4	3	3	30
12	4	4	2	2	3	2	2	3	2	3	27
13	4	4	2	3	5	2	4	4	3	3	34
14	2	3	2	2	3	1	2	3	1	2	21
15	3	4	2	2	2	1	2	3	2	2	23
16	3	4	4	4	5	2	4	4	3	3^a	36
17	4	3	3	2	2	1	4	3	2	1	25
18	4	1	1	1	3	1	2	1	2	2	18
19	4	4	4	3	5	2	3	4	3	3	35
20	4	3	2	3	4	2	2	3	3	3^a	29
21	4	4	2	4	5	2	2	4	3	3	33
22	4	1	4	1	5	1	1	4	1	3	25
23	2	4	3	4	5	2	3	3	3	1	30
Means	3.30	3.26	2.65	2.69	3.73	1.65	2.47	3.26	2.34	2.38	

Percentage of families accomplishing task:

Well	.48	.65	.13	.13	.43	.65	.17	.43	.52	.05	
Adequately	.87	.78	.48	.52	.52	.65	.39	.91	.52	.48	

^{a} Two families did not have other children. The score of 3 is given so that the family's overall adaptation score is not penalized for lack of siblings. However, column summations for column 10 are based on an n of 21, with items 16 and 20 omitted.

RESULTS

Postdeath Level of Adaptation

Table II summarizes the scores of parents on each item of the Post-death Adaptation Measure. If one were to place an arbitrary dividing line for the minimal level of healthy adaptation between the higher and lower possible scores on each item, and compare actual responses to this hypothesized median, then the percentage of families accomplishing each task adequately falls as listed at the bottom of Table II. With regard to specific coping tasks, the families as a group have adequately mastered item 1 (returning to normal activities), item 2 (having life become zestful and fulfilling again), item 6 (being able to confront physical reminders of the child outside the home without distress), and item 8 (being able to look back without regret). The families were having a more difficult time with the remaining tasks: talking comfortably with other family members about the child, controlling occasional disruptive feelings of sadness, planning for the future, viewing the death as an opportunity to learn new coping skills, resolving questions as to why it had to happen, and dealing with sibling issues and concerns relative to the illness.

If one were to look beyond adequacy of coping to full and effective resolution of the tasks, then very few families can be judged as coping well. With a stricter definition of effective coping, four of the items (items 3, 4, 7, and 10) remain critical areas of concern for the families as a group.

Disease-Course Variables

As already indicated, five variables were derived from an analysis of parental memory of behaviors occurring during the course of the child's treatment. These five variables were submitted to a multiple regression analysis, with the overall postdeath adaptation score as the criterion measure. Results are summarized in Table III. The first three variables, taken collectively, were able to predict the postdeath level of adaptation of the family. A multiple R of .70 (adjusted R^2 of .41) was achieved. The analysis demonstrated that items could be isolated by independent judges from the parents' memories of life with their child, which would relate to parents' postdeath level of adaptation.

Table III. Multiple Regression Analysis Predicting to Postdeath Adjustment

Predictor	Multiple R	r
Life meaning	.55	.55
Support	.63	.43
Communication with the child	.70[a]	.31
Normal functioning	.71	.23
Communication with siblings	.71	.16

[a] Adjusted $R^2 = .41$

Several other possible sources of variance were tested to see if they were related to postdeath level of adaptation. The factors were (a) length of time from the death of the child until the interview, (b) duration of the illness, (c) age of the child, and (d) sex of the child.

An analysis was performed to test whether the parents for whom there was a longer time period between the death of the child and the interview would have a higher level of postdeath adaptation. There was no support for this. Each 6-month time segment contained parents at both high and low adaptation levels, and there was no trend in the means for each time period. Thus, length of grieving time alone does not seem to be related to the postdeath adaptation level.

In comparing the duration of the child's illness with the postdeath level of adaptation, one would expect that those parents whose children were ill for a longer period of time would have had more opportunity to prepare for the death of the child and would be coping better at the time of the interview. While there is a trend in this direction, the results were not statistically significant. Although more of the families whose child's illness was of short duration did poorly, the longer duration of illness did not affect postdeath level of adaptation. Among those whose duration was longer, postdeath adaptation scores were not significantly different.

The age of the child at death was not related to the long-term level of adaptation of the parents, nor was the sex of the child related to parental adaptation. One might think that parents would be more likely to be open with an older child, but within the age range studied we found parents as likely to tell a younger child as an older one about the prognosis.

DISCUSSION

The families in our study exhibited difficulties in certain of the behavioral tasks that formed our Postdeath Adaptation measure. While the majority of families were able to return to a semblance of normal activities, were able to reinvest in life with some zest and positive feeling, and were content that they had done all they could for the child when he or she was alive, parents had difficulties avoiding feelings of sadness and crying spells when thinking about the child and could not talk comfortably within the family about the child without stress and tears. Unresolved feelings or symptoms persisted with siblings in the majority of families, including crying spells, health fears, feelings of remorse and guilt, and refusal to discuss the deceased child, even 2 or 3 years after the death. The issue is certainly not one of expecting the family member not to be sad over the death, for sadness at the memory of the child may well last the parents' and siblings' lifetimes.

What is of concern is the extent to which such memories may interfere with daily functioning and commitment to the future, most notably in the siblings.

In 1969, Binger et al. reported that in 11 of 20 families of children who had died from leukemia, one or more members had emotional disturbances severe enough to interfere with adequate functioning and required psychiatric help. We did not find such severe disturbances in our sample. Along with Futterman and Hoffman (1973), we observed few instances of severe psychopathology, severe maladaptive behavior, or permanent family disruption. Divorce rates were relatively low, a finding in congruence with that of Lansky, Cairns, Hassanein, Wehr, and Lowman (1978). The 23 sets of parents interviewed in our study comprised all but two available parents from our two-hospital sample over a specified period of time. Of the 23 sets of parents, two sets had been divorced and a third set separated prior to the diagnosis. Only one set of parents divorced during the course of the child's disease. None divorced after the death of the child. The remaining sets of parents remained married throughout the course of the illness and after the death.

Discrepancies with Binger's findings may be due to differences in the definition of what constitutes pathology or in the nature of the samples, or may be due to the changes in medical and psychosocial care that have taken place in the past decade. Our families expressed the positive feelings mirrored in the Futterman and Hoffman (1973) sample, that the crisis often leads to family cohesiveness and a positive redefinition of values. However, lack of psychopathology and the presence of a renewed value system do not preclude ongoing difficulties in coping with the death of the child. While the families in our study did not exhibit psychopathology or severe maladaptive behavior, certain areas in their adjustment to life without their child remain a concern. Professional commitment to the psychological health of the families cannot stop at the point of the child's death.

That family coping efforts during the course of the illness can make a difference in postdeath adaptation was the finding from the second of the two goals we set for this study. From the content analysis of interviews of the parents of the 23 children who had died of cancer, factors occurring during the course of the life of the child were isolated and shown to relate to how well the surviving family members adapt after the death of the child. From the parents' responses to questions about life with their child, independent judges isolated five variables, three of which related to the postdeath adjustment level of the surviving family members. Those parents who were best adjusted after the death of their child were those who had had a consistent philosophy/theology/cosmology of life during the child's life, which helped the family accept the diagnosis and cope with its consequences (Life Meaning), who had a viable and ongoing "significant other" as a support to whom they could turn for help during the course of the illness (Support), and who gave their child the information and emotional support the child needed during the course of the illness at a level consistent with their child's questions, age, and level of development (Communication with the Child).

The parents have shown us that families can adjust to life without their child. Pathology and maladjustment are not inevitable. We have demonstrated the generally beneficial effects on the ultimate adjustment of the family members of such variables as a viable support system, open and responsive communication with the child during the course of the illness, and a commitment to one's basic life view. What is called for in the light of the present results is to help strengthen the adaptive capabilities and coping styles specific to each family and to each member of the family, to help the family members struggle forward as best they can in a commitment to the value of the remaining months or years of their child's life, and to give them access to the intrafamilial sources of support they most need to help them in that struggle. Strengthening the family's own adaptive resources along the lines of the variables shown to be effective in the present study cannot but lead to generally beneficial effects, both on the family as a unit and on each member.

For the long-term benefit of the parents as well as for alleviating a sense of isolation in the child, openness of communication is recommended. This is a difficult task for parents, and further research is needed into the specific ways in which to tell the child and when to tell the child (Spinetta, 1978; Spinetta & Deasy-Spinetta, 1980). The specific course and nature of emotional support which is most helpful to parents in effecting and maintaining openness of communication should also be investigated, so that medical and psychological support staffs might be maximally helpful to the parents.

Present efforts are underway to study families prospectively from the point of diagnosis through to the point of death and after death, to see if data from the series of studies to date can be replicated following the same families over time. When the predictor variables are demonstrated in a multisource longitudinal study to be consistent in a prospective manner throughout the course of treatment and postdeath, then a further structure will have been laid for intensive programs that can help strengthen the family's ultimate ability to adapt to life without the child.

REFERENCES

Adams, D. W. *Childhood malignancy: The psychosocial care of the child and his family.* Springfield, Ill.: C C Thomas, 1980.

Binger, C. M., Ablin, A. R., Feuerstein, R. C., Kushner, J. H., Zoger, S., & Mikkelsen, C. Childhood leukemia: Emotional impact on patient and family. *New England Journal of Medicine,* 1969, *280,* 414-418.

Bluebond-Lagner, M. *The private worlds of dying children.* Princeton: Princeton University Press, 1978.

Fischoff, J., & O'Brien, N. After the child dies. *Journal of Pediatrics,* 1976, *88,* 140-146.

Futterman E., & Hoffman, I. Crisis and adaptation in the families of fatally ill children. In E. J. Anthony & C. Koupernik (Eds.), *The child and his family: The impact of disease and death.* New York: Wiley, 1973. (Yearbook of the International Association for Child Psychiatry and Allied Professions, Vol. 2)

Hamovitch, M. B. *The parent and the fatally ill child.* Los Angeles: Delmar Publishing, 1964.

Hofer, M. A., Wolff, C. T., Friedman, S. B., & Mason, J. W. A psychoendocrine study of bereavement, Part I: 17-hydroxycorticosteroid excretion rates of parents following death of their children from leukemia. *Psychosomatic Medicine,* 1972, *34,* 481-507.

Kagen-Goodheart, L. Re-entry: Living with childhood cancer. *American Journal of Orthopsychiatry,* 1977, *47,* 651-658.

Kaplan, D., Grobstein R., & Smith, A. Severe illness in families. *Health and Social Work,* 1976, *1,* 72-81.

Kellerman, J. (Ed.). *Psychological aspects of childhood cancer.* Springfield, Ill.: C C Thomas, 1980.

Lansky, S. B. Cairns, N. U., Hassanein, R., Wehr, J., & Lowman, J. T. Childhood cancer: Parental discord and divorce. *Pediatrics,* 1978, *62,* 184-188.

O'Malley, J. E., & Koocher, G. P. Implications for patient care. In C. P. Koocher & J. E. O'Malley (Eds.), *The Damocles syndrome: Psychosocial consequences of surviving childhood cancer.* New York: McGraw-Hill, 1980.

Schiff, H. S. *The bereaved parent.* New York: Crown Publishers, 1977.

Schulman, J. L., & Kupst, M. (Eds.). *The child with cancer: Clinical approaches to psychosocial care, research in psychosocial aspects.* Springfield, Ill.: C C Thomas, 1980.

Slavin, L. S. Evolving psychosocial issues in the treatment of childhood cancer: A review. In G. P. Koocher & J. E. O'Malley (Eds.), *The Damocles syndrome: Psychosocial consequences of surviving childhood cancer.* New York: McGraw-Hill, 1980.

Sourkes, B. Facilitating family coping with childhood cancer. *Journal of Pediatric Psychology,* 1977, *2,* 65-67.

Spinetta, J. J. The dying child's awareness of death: A review. *Psychological Bulletin,* 1974, *81,* 256-260.

Spinetta, J. J. Adjustment in children with cancer. *Journal of Pediatric Psychology,* 1977, *2,* 49-51.

Spinetta, J. J. Communication patterns in families dealing with life-threatening illness. In O. J. Z. Sahler (Ed.), *The child and death.* St. Louis: C. V. Mosby, 1978.

Spinetta, J. J., & Deasy-Spinetta, P. M. Coping with childhood cancer: Professional and family communication patterns. In M. G. Eisenberg, J. Falconer, & L. C. Sutkin (Eds.), *Communications in a health care setting.* Springfield, Ill.: C C Thomas, 1980.

Spinetta, J. J., & Maloney, L. J. The child with cancer: Patterns of communication and denial. *Journal of Consulting and Clinical Psychology,* 1978, *46,* 1540-1541.

Stehbens, J. A., & Lascari, A. D. Psychological follow-up of families with childhood leukemia. *Journal of Clinical Psychology,* 1974, *30,* 394-397.

8

An Investigation of Grief and Adaptation in Parents Whose Children Have Died from Cancer

Therese A. Rando

North Scituate Medical Center

Although in recent years there has been a burgeoning of interest in the topics of dying, death, and bereavement, and there has been an astronomical increase in the number of studies and investigations of these topics, there has been a strange reluctance to address the issue of childhood terminal illness with the same vigor. There has been even less investigation of the reactions and experience of the parents of the terminally ill child. There is, however, no lack of agreement that such studies are warranted and it is far from uncommon to see such research advocated in the conclusions of other investigations.

Objective data concerning parental grief are particularly needed in view of the deleterious and malignant effects that can result from unresolved and inappropriate grief (Solnit & Green, 1959; Cain & Cain, 1964; Gorer, 1965; Wallace, 1967; Binger, Ablin, Feuerstein, Kushner, Zoger, & Mikkelsen, 1969; Alby & Alby, 1970; Kaplan, Smith, Grobstein, & Fishman, 1973; Kaplan, 1974; Townes, Wold, & Holmes, 1974; Heller & Schneider, 1978).

In reviewing the literature on the quasi-experimental and descriptive studies that have been undertaken to research the experience of parents of terminally ill children, there is consistent repetition of 11 investigations which form the backbone of the research on the topic (Solnit & Green, 1959; Binger

The author gratefully acknowledges the editorial suggestions of Dennis Drotar, Lawrence C. Grebstein, J. Eugene Knott, and Vanderlyn R. Pine in the preparation of this manuscript. She recognizes the invaluable contribution of Samuel Gross, formerly of the Pediatric Hematology-Oncology Department, Rainbow Babies and Childrens Hospital, Cleveland, Ohio, who provided the opportunity for the collection of the data in this investigation. Originally published in *Journal of Pediatric Psychology,* 8(1)(1983):3–20.

et al., 1969; Bozeman, Orbach, & Sutherland, 1955; Orbach, Sutherland, & Bozeman, 1955; Richmond & Waisman, 1955; Natterson & Knudson, 1960; Knudson & Natterson, 1960; Friedman, Chodoff, Mason, & Hamburg, 1963; Chodoff, Friedman, & Hamburg, 1964; Hamovich, 1964; Easson, 1970). However, these previous studies and writings have led to results that are often inconsistent in findings and emphasis, and often based upon subjective clinical observation without objective, valid, or reliable measures of adjustment. Moreover, these investigations were generally conducted prior to the advances in the treatment of cancer, which has become more of a chronic life-threatening illness in recent years. Recent developments in treatment are reflected in altered familial life-styles, treatment regimens, life expectancies, and disease process. In addition, these studies have tended to slight the investigation of the experiences of fathers. For these reasons, the results of the initial pioneering studies are less applicable to present clinical reality. Their neglect of research on parental bereavement subsequent to the death leaves a lack of information about the postdeath grief experiences and adaptations of parents. It has only been in the very recent past that there have been conducted relatively more comprehensive studies of parental experience during and after the child's terminal illness (in 1979: Kerner, Harvey, & Lewiston; and in 1981: Foster, O'Malley, & Koocher; Kemler; Spinetta, Swarner, & Sheposh; and Kreuger, Gyllensköld, Pehrsson, & Sjölin).

It was in response to the aforementioned deficits that the present investigation was conducted. It provides empirical data in a field which presently lacks empirical justification for the psychotherapeutic interventions proposed and utilized. Eight major hypotheses (generating 31 specific predictions) concerning parental bereavement were tested. Eight major variables were hypothesized to influence parental grief and adaptation subsequent to the death of a child. They included (a) the amount of support received during the terminal illness; (b) the amount of previous loss sustained prior to the death; (c) the duration of the child's illness; (d) the length of time since the death; (e) the sex of the parent; (f) the parental evaluation of the child's treatment experiences; (g) the parental anticipatory grief; and (h) the parental participation in the care of the child during hospitalization.

METHOD

Subjects

The subjects were 54 parents (27 married couples) whose children had died from cancer following treatment at Rainbow Babies and Childrens

Hospital in Cleveland, Ohio. Criteria for selection were that the parents were still married and living together; that they resided in a location within a 3-hour-drive of Cleveland; and that their child had died from a form of cancer from 2 months to 3 years previously. With the exception of three fathers, all the parents were the biological parents of the deceased children. The three stepfathers had been intimately involved with the children and the families prior to the diagnosis of the illness.

The age range for the parents was from 26 to 58 years with the mean parental age being 40 years old. Family income ranged from $11,000 to $70,333 a year. In 41% of the couples both parents were employed. Educationally, all save two of the parents had completed high school (or in one case, trade school), with 56% of the parents having gone on to training or education past the high school level. Sixty-one percent of the parents were of Protestant denomination, 30% were Catholic, and 9% reported they had no religion. Racial background was white, with the exception of one set of black parents. There was a mixture of ethnic backgrounds with Slovak and German nationalities predominant.

In total, there were 39 couples who were known for sure to have been definitely contacted to participate in the study. Of these 39 couples, 31 initially agreed to participate. Of these, 27 couples fully completed the study.

Clearly the main reason for the parents' participation in a study which was intensely painful at times was their desire to provide information that would be helpful to parents and children in similar situations in the future.

Setting

All interviews took place in the private homes of the subjects. The subjects corroborated the initial feeling of the investigator that participation in the study would be precluded for many parents if it was contingent upon their returning to the hospital where their deceased child had been treated. For many, the emotional feelings attached to the facility were too painful.

Procedure

The vast majority of the initial contacts were made by the pediatric oncology nurse who had worked with all the parents and children during the illness. She introduced the study and obtained consent for participation. At the interview both parents were initially seen together by the investigator in order to describe to them in more detail the nature and objectives of the study as well as to address any questions or concerns they may have had.

Parents were then separated. One parent was given a Structured Interview (Rando, 1980) while the other completed the Grief Experience Inventory (Sanders, Mauger, & Strong, 1978). When each had finished they reversed roles. After the Structured Interview was administered to each parent, the Parental Experience Assessment Form (Rando, 1979) was completed by each parent. (The first 10 parents in this study were administered an earlier version of this form. The differences are very slight, reflected only in several new ratings.) All interviews were audiotaped for future analysis.

Instruments

The state of the art in bereavement research is still relatively unsophisticated. The concept of grief has been so nebulous and unrefined that objective, valid, and reliable measures have been lacking and are only now in initial stages of development and standardization. In spite of some shortcomings the measurements utilized in this investigation were the best available at the time to collect and evaluate the specific information desired.

There were four sources of data in the investigation: The Grief Experience Inventory (GEI), the Structured Interview, the Parental Experience Assessment Form (PEAF), and hospital medical charts.

The GEI (Sanders et al., 1978) is a self-report, objective instrument to assess an individual's grief experience through a 12-scale profile of the subject's grief. It is the sole instrument of its kind in existence at the present time in the area of bereavement research. The instrument has received norming on various populations, including a sample of parents whose children died from various causes. For purposes of this investigation seven of the subscales were chosen as variables to be analyzed. They included Atypical Responses, Despair, Anger/Hostility, Loss of Control, Rumination, Depersonalization, and Somatization. Five GEI scales were not used in the direct testing of hypotheses due to lower alpha coefficients, but have been included in the discussion to offer possible explanations for several of the findings. These include Death Anxiety, Social Isolation, Guilt, Social Desirability, and Denial.

The topics addressed in the Structured Interview (Rando, 1980) were taken from prior research on grief with special emphasis on the parental loss of children. The format had been designed to assist the parents in describing their experiences from the time of their child's diagnosis to the period of readjustment subsequent to death. The questions were all open-ended.

There was a series of discrete questions in the areas that had been addressed in the Structured Interview for which the parents provided objective ratings. This comprised the PEAF (Rando, 1979) and provided more objective quantification of the parents' perceptions and judgments, and gave a formal comparative basis for such data. The PEAF contains parental reports and/or ratings of (a) source, quality, and frequency of support received during the illness; (b) prior loss experiences, with assessments of successfulness of coping with each prior loss and a comparison of the stress it generated compared to that of the child's terminal illness and death; (c) types and frequency of parental behaviors participated in during the child's hospitalizations; (d) extent of involvement with hospital staff around the child's care; (e) extent of involvement with the child during hospitalizations and satisfaction with this extent; (f) existence of important "last wish" of the child and whether parent was able to grant it; (g) satisfaction with the health care and treatment received by the child from specific health-care personnel; (h) anticipatory grief behaviors engaged in prior to the child's death; (i) seeking of professional treatment to help the parent cope with the illness or death; (j) preparation at the time of death; (k) coping abilities prior to the onset of the child's illness (premorbid coping ability); (l) present overall coping abilities; and (m) coping with the child's death specifically (Subsequent Adjustment). Three open-ended questions allowed delineation of (n) the most difficult aspects of the child's illness and death; (o) those things which assisted the parent in coping; and (p) areas of problems still to be resolved.

Hospital and outpatient medical charts were utilized to provide such information as dates of diagnosis, number of hospitalizations, treatment regimens, numbers of remissions and relapses, and other information relating to the course of the child's illness.

Statistical Procedures

There were three primary statistical analyses performed on the data. A chi-square analysis was performed wherever possible. When the expected frequency was less than five in any one of the cells in the fourfold tables, the Exact Probabilities method for calculating p directly was used. The third major statistical procedure involved Student's t test of significance of the difference between means.

DISCUSSION OF RESULTS

Personal Characteristics Influencing Parental Grief and Adaptation

Previous Loss. In analyzing the impact of previous loss this study found that high Subsequent Adjustment was associated almost twice as often with low previous loss as with high previous loss. In contrast, there was almost an equal split between low and high previous losses for parents who had low Subsequent Adjustment. This implies that previous loss experiences are associated with poorer bereavement outcomes. It had been anticipated that successful resolution of past losses would predict a more favorable outcome.

Related to this is the implication that previous loss may preclude more anticipatory grief behaviors; 50% of the parents in the low anticipatory grief group had high previous loss as compared to only 31% of the parents in the medium and high anticipatory grief groups. If anticipatory grief is taken as an important and necessary aspect of the parents' experiences during and after the child's illness, then previous loss experience is again related to poorer bereavement outcome.

Sex of Parent. Overall, mothers appeared to experience, or at least admitted to, more intense reactions to bereavement and poorer Subsequent Adjustment than fathers.

On the GEI, the sole subscale that statistically differentiated mothers and fathers was Somatization, on which mothers scored significantly higher, $t = 1.98, p < .05, df = 106$. Fathers were higher than mothers (although not to a statistically significant extent) on only one index of bereavement: the Anger/Hostility subscale of the GEI.

Sexual response differences were also analyzed on the PEAF variables of anticipatory grief behaviors, parental participation behaviors during the child's hospitalizations, and parental reports of Subsequent Adjustment following the death. There was a statistically significant difference among parents with regard to the amount of their participation during their child's hospitalizations. Mothers reported engaging in significantly more participation behaviors than did fathers, $t = 2.52, p < .02, df = 106$. There was no statistically significant difference among mothers and fathers in the amount of anticipatory grief behaviors engaged in, although mothers reported more. Neither was there a significant difference among parents with regard to their Subsequent Adjustment; however, fathers were clearly higher in their adjustment than were mothers.

These findings suggest several interesting thoughts. Previously researchers had postulated that the mothers' increased participation during the child's illness facilitated her anticipatory grief and her higher adjustment following the death (Hamovitch, 1964) and had asserted the crucial importance of parental anticipatory grief for successful adaptation following the death (Richmond & Waisman, 1955; Friedman et al., 1963; Chodoff et al., 1964; Friedman, 1967; Wiener, 1970). The implications from these writings are not supported with the data from this investigation. Although fathers were definitely inferior to mothers in the amount of behavioral participation during the child's hospitalizations, they were almost equal in their amount of anticipatory grief and even surpassed mothers in Subsequent Adjustment following the death. The mothers' higher participation was not coincided with and did not ensure higher anticipatory grief or Subsequent Adjustment. Therefore, contrary to the implications of previous theorists, these data indicate that fathers are actually as involved in the process of anticipatory grieving as are mothers. The social role of the male would not seem to preclude his emotional experience of anticipatory grief, and better coping after the death, although it may affect his ability to participate behaviorally in his child's care. The data also indicate that care must be taken not to insinuate emotional involvement, anticipatory grief, or future subsequent adjustment solely from participation behaviors (as many of the earlier writers in this field have done) since they appear not to be reliable solitary predictors of the levels of such experiences.

Time Factors Influencing Parental Experience and Adaptation

Length of Illness. The results suggested that there may be an optimum length of terminal illness as it is related to parental grief experience. There appeared to be an optimum duration of illness, above and below which (a) parental preparedness at the time of death and (b) Subsequent Adjustment after the death were inferior. The number of parents who were low on preparedness for their child's death and low on Subsequent Adjustment following the death was the highest for those groups with the least warning (length of illness less than 6 months) and with the most warning (length of illness 18 months or longer). Those whose child died in the interim ranges (length of illness from 6 to 18 months) appeared to be the most prepared for the death and had better Subsequent Adjustment afterwards.

When analyzing which condition seems to be worse for the parents in relation to their preparation at the time of death and Subsequent Adjustment it is clear that it is most difficult for those parents whose children had the longest illnesses. There was also clear evidence of a pattern suggesting that as the length of the illnesses increased the percentages of parents with high Anger/Hostility and Atypical Responses scores also increased. This suggests that the longer the illness continues the angrier and more disturbed are the parents after the death.

In summary, in its role as a determinant of parental preparation at the time of death and parental Subsequent Adjustment following the death, the length of the illness can be neither too short nor too long. When it is too short, parents appear to be unable to adequately prepare themselves as well as they might. Apparently when an illness is too long the experience and stress associated with it act to militate against adequate preparation when death finally comes following such a long course, one presumably filled with remissions as well as relapses. The possibility of parental denial of death arising since the child has survived so long with the disease may be important. Such a lengthy illness exacerbates disturbed reactions following the death, lessens coping ability, and increases the intensity of feelings of anger and hostility. It is possible that the long and arduous experience of such an illness saps the parents of their ability to cope as effectively as desired and thus their ability to be appropriately prepared at the time of death is compromised, as is their ability to subsequently adjust. The role of steadily increasing abnormal responses (Atypical Responses) and intensifying anger and hostility may also preclude better therapeutic readiness and subsequent adjustment.

Length of Time Since the Death. There were numerous suggestions derived from the present investigation with respect to the influence of the length of time since death and parental grief. All GEI subscales, as well as the PEAF ratings of Subsequent Adjustment and Discrepancy between premorbid and present coping, were analyzed within one of the three 1-year intervals between the occurrence of death and the interview. The range of time for the lengths of time since the death was from 2 months 10 days to 2 years 11 months 27 days. The major finding is that there was a configural pattern to which the PEAF rating of Subsequent Adjustment and all the GEI subscales except Atypical Responses conformed. Although not statistically significant the pattern is a "V" configuration in which there is a decrease in the intensity of the experience in the 2nd year of bereavement which is followed by an increase in intensity in the 3rd year; 78% of the variables tested evidenced this configuration.

This pattern suggests that the 3rd year of bereavement constitutes an experience which shifts the parents' responses from the positive to the negative direction. Exactly what the nature of this experience might be is unclear at the present time. The finding is quite surprising in light of the fact that traditionally theorists have posited that bereavement symptoms decrease over time. There are data from several other GEI scales which may shed some light on the phenomenon found in this investigation. Several GEI scales were administered to the parents but not included in the hypotheses due to insufficient alpha coefficients in the normative findings of the instrument. However, although they were not utilized in the statistical procedures, they are included here in the hope that they could provide some indication of what could contribute to this "V" configuration. These are Death Anxiety, Social Desirability, Social Isolation, Denial, and Guilt. The first two reflected the "V" configuration seen in the majority of the subscales. Social Isolation remained the same during the first 2 years prior to decreasing in the 3rd year. Denial steadily rose over each year. Guilt declined steadily during the 3 years.

A possibility immediately apparent is that the rising Denial allows for the decreasing Guilt, as the normal parental defensive process reconstitutes after the severe blow dealt to it by the death of a child. Herein a rise in Denial would be considered adaptive. What appears to be less adaptive is the increasing tendency of the parents towards an abnormal grief experience, as is evidenced by a steady increase in Atypical Responses over each of the 3 years and a steady decrease of the percentages of parents experiencing high Subsequent Adjustment each year. Taken together these suggest that bereavement and coping may actually worsen over time.

One possible explanation for the typical "V" configuration may be that the increasing rise of Atypical Responses and the increasing percentages of parents with lower Subsequent Adjustment reflects an increase in the intensity of bereavement experience and symptomatology which influences the other subscales towards intensification in the 3rd year subsequent to their normal course of diminution in the second year following the death. Possibly the steadily rising intensity is what shifts the other variables toward a more negative direction.

As mentioned previously, the rising GEI scale of Atypical Responses is coincided with by a similarly rising scale of Denial. This may reflect their both responding to a particular experience which would prompt them both to rise, i.e., an intensification of the grief process, or the Denial may elevate in response to the rise of Atypical Responses. In the first case the rising Denial may be construed to be more symptomatic, while in the second case it may be viewed as more defensive.

A phenomenon influencing the rise of both Denial and Atypical Responses may be the decrease of Social Isolation and the increase in Social Desirability in the 3rd year. There may be something in the experience of resumed social contact that warrants an increase in Denial, especially as parents are increasingly exposed to the world ongoing in spite of the loss of their child. If this "reentry" is too painful it could prompt a temporary intensification of bereavement, resulting in the 3rd year (at the precise time of the decreased Social Isolation) in a swing in the negative direction for the majority of GEI subscales (hence the "V" configuration) and the exacerbation of Atypical Responses, Denial, and poor Subsequent Adjustment. Guilt is relieved by both the increase in Denial as well as its not being a necessarily consequent emotion in the aforementioned conjectured situation.

The rising Denial and lowered Guilt may contribute to the parents' evaluations that the further they get from their child's death, the better they rate their present coping relative to their premorbid coping. In fact, as evidenced by their Discrepancy scores (between parental premorbid and present coping), they appear to have some definite need to assert that they are actually coping *better* than they were prior to their child's diagnosis and illness. In fact, there is a steady rise in the percentages of parents who report experiencing positive change as represented by these Discrepancy scores. This seems to indicate that with the passage of time comes the increasing ability to cope at levels superior to those existent prior to the child's death. Several possible implications may be derived from this. First, that the experience of losing a child and surviving that loss indicates to the parents that they can cope with anything and that this recognition becomes more salient as time progresses and they continue to live on without their child. An alternative explanation is that the parents who had recently lost a child were so stunned that their Discrepancy scores indicating negative or "no change" artificially lowered the positive discrepancy scores and that what is construed as an increase in positive coping may actually only be a decrease in negative or neutral coping. A third implication is that the apparent increase in positive change discrepancies actually reflects an increase in level of denial on the part of the parents. As was mentioned previously, Denial rose consistently each year.

Another pattern that was clearly apparent during the 3-year spectrum investigated was that the percentages of parents experiencing low and high levels of Anger/Hostility on the GEI remained almost consistent throughout each of the six 6-month periods. Thus, there appears to be little change in the way that anger and hostility were distributed over time. The mean scores of each time period differed slightly, but the percentages of parents experiencing them did not.

In summary, analysis of the relationships between time and bereavement experience indicates that it is clear that time does not provide full relief from symptomatology nor necessarily a diminution of experience. In fact, the collected evidence argues for a worsening of the experience in the 3rd year, independent of that indicating some lessening of intensity during the 2nd year. The findings suggest the opposite of the commonsense notion and widely held belief that time "heals" grief. In fact it may not, particularly with bereaved parents. Our expectations for parents in these situations may be entirely inappropriate and therefore needed therapeutic endeavors may be deficient or lacking.

Parental Experience During the Illness

Anticipatory Grief. For purposes of this investigation anticipatory grief was operationalized by eight elements. A parent's anticipatory grief score was determined by the numerical sum of the behaviors he/she had reported they engaged in during their child's terminal illness. These behaviors included (a) Discussing with someone the possibility that their child would die; (b) Grieving in anticipation of the loss of their child; (c) Thinking what the future would be without their child; (d) Acknowledging the fact that their child was going to die; (e) Discussing their child's dying with their child; (f) Planning the type of death they wanted for their child; (g) Making funeral preparations; and (h) Starting to partially disengage themselves emotionally from their child. Two associations were found to be statistically significant. First, anticipatory grief was positively associated with preparedness at death, $\chi^2 = 6.3180$, $p < .05$, $df = 2$. Parental preparation increased directly as the amount of anticipatory grief increased. This finding supports the contention that anticipatory grief leads to relatively more preparation than does the lack of it.

Second, a stronger level of statistical significance describes the association between anticipatory grief and Atypical Responses (abnormal grief), $\chi^2 = 9.8873$, $p < .01$, $df = 2$. The more there is anticipatory grief prior to the death, the less abnormal grief is present following the death.

Several other patterns imply the relative importance of anticipatory grief. Although not statistically significant there is a strong suggestion that support is related to the experience of anticipatory grief. Those parents who were low on support during the child's illness tended to have engaged in fewer anticipatory grief behaviors. This suggests that the engagement in anticipatory grief may be assisted by, or possibly requires, the support of other people.

Individuals who were low in their Subsequent Adjustment following the death tended to have engaged in fewer anticipatory grief behaviors before the death. As the amount of anticipatory grief behaviors increased the percentages of parents with high Subsequent Adjustment also increased. This finding provides more evidence for the assertion that anticipatory grief facilitates grief work and that the absence of it predisposes one to worse bereavement outcomes. It follows both theoretically and empirically the relationship between anticipatory grief and Atypical Responses.

Several findings argue for the therapeutic effects of avoiding too little or too much anticipatory grief. There appears to be an optimum amount of anticipatory grief as it is related to parental participation during the child's hospitalizations and the GEI subscales of Anger/Hostility and Loss of Control. Parents reporting low and high amounts of anticipatory grief behaviors were found to have engaged in fewer participation behaviors during their child's hospitalizations. The greatest number of low participators were found among those who were also low in anticipatory grief. Low participation is related to individuals obsessed with more external problems (Hamovitch, 1964) which would most probably preclude adaptive anticipatory grief. The medium amount of anticipatory grief appeared to be most therapeutic and therefore facilitative of participation or at least subject to the same process which allows expression of both. Too much anticipatory grief appeared to compromise the parents' ability to continue interacting with their child. The fears of Travis (1976) and Levitz (1977), who warn against premature detachment secondary to the parents' process of decathexis through their anticipatory grief, may be reflected in this finding. Additionally, the low and high anticipatory grief groups contained higher percentages of parents with high Anger/Hostility and Loss of Control scores on the GEI.

Parental Participation During Child's Hospitalizations. Seven behaviors were used to operationalize the concept of parental participation during the child's hospitalizations. These included (a) Rooming in; (b) Visiting; (c) Feeding/dining with child; (d) Clothing/dressing child; (e) Bathing child; (f) Helping hospital staff with procedures; and (g) Discussing illness with child. The number of behaviors participated in were totaled for each parent. Three findings of statistical significance were discovered in the investigation. The GEI subscale of Rumination was found to be significantly associated with participation during the child's hospitalizations, $\chi^2 = 4.6855, p < .05, df = 1$. As the amount of participatory behaviors increased, so did the amount of Rumination. This finding is directly contrary to theory. However it supports Hamovitch's (1964) data. He noted that "full" participation predisposed the parents to be more volatile and "so wrapped up" in the care of the child that there was neglect of other responsibilities. This being so wrapped up with the child appears to continue after the death according to the present data. With low levels of participation there is lower Rumination. What remain to be investigated are the delimitation points of appropriate participation. It is clear that there may very well be "too much of a good thing" with regard to participating in the care of the fatally ill child, especially as it is related to subsequent grief following the death. This notion is the same as that found with regard to anticipatory grief.

The second statistically significant finding is the difference between mothers and fathers. Mothers were found to be significantly higher in their participation scores, $t = 2.52, p < .02, df = 106$ (see discussion on "Sex of Parent").

Parents' evaluations of their child's treatment experiences were associated with participation behaviors to a statistically significant extent (exact probabilities analysis $= p = .05$). Virtually all parents who reported a low level of satisfaction with the treatment experience had engaged in a lower amount of participation behaviors. Those who reported high levels of satisfaction were more evenly split on both low and high amounts of participation behaviors. This suggests the trend that satisfaction with treatment increases as the number of participation behaviors increases.

There is an implication that participation behaviors have some kind of relationship with or effect upon Subsequent Adjustment. Although not statistically significant, low Subsequent Adjustors in general were associated with a greater percentage of low participators than were high Subsequent Adjustors. Although high participation by itself does not guarantee high Subsequent Adjustment (as seen in the analysis of the sex of parents and the findings related to their participation and Subsequent Adjustment), the fact that the low adjustors tended to include so many parents who were correspondingly low in participation implies that too few participation behaviors generally predisposes one toward poorer Subsequent Adjustment than it does toward high Subsequent Adjustment.

The relationship between participation behaviors and anticipatory grief has already been analyzed in a previous section (see discussion on "Anticipatory Grief"). Suffice it to say at this point that there appears to be a relationship between the two suggesting an optimum level of anticipatory grief which facilitates the greatest percentage of high participation behaviors. Of course, it must be remembered that in many instances participatory behaviors either are, or pave the ways for, experiences of anticipatory grief.

Parental Evaluation of the Child's Treatment Experiences. The effect of the parents' evaluations was studied with respect to their Anger/Hostility scores on the GEI. In the present sample, 92% of the subjects rated themselves as highly satisfied with their child's treatment experiences. This figure is quite impressive and had not been expected.

When the parents' Anger/Hostility scores and their evaluations of their child's treatment experience were analyzed, 50% of the population were high on both Anger/Hostility and satisfaction with treatment. This was contrary to the prediction that high satisfaction would be more closely associated with lower Anger/Hostility scores. The pattern that was suggested revealed that those who were low satisfied were three times more likely to have low Anger/Hostility scores, while those who were high satisfied were almost evenly split among low and high Anger/Hostility scores. This implies that there is an increase in Anger/Hostility as there is an increase in satisfaction. The reason for this is unclear from data or from theory.

There was a significant association between satisfaction and the number of parental participation behaviors (exact probabilities analysis $= p =$ .05) (see discussion on "Participation Behaviors"). Suffice it to say it appears that increasing levels of satisfaction are associated with increasing amounts of participation behaviors on the part of the parents.

Amount of Support Received During the Terminal Illness. This final aspect of parental experience was addressed to investigate the influence of the amount of support received during the terminal illness.

In the present study 20 discrete sources were rated by parents according to the quality of support received. Those providing some measure of support were summed to generate a support score and were then analyzed with respect to the parents' Subsequent Adjustment and anticipatory grief scores from the PEAF and the GEI Atypical Responses scores. It was found that there was a relative increase in the tendency for parents to have lower Atypical Responses scores (a positive sign) as they reported increasing amounts of support during the illness. It was also found that parents with low support tended to have engaged in fewer numbers of anticipatory grief behaviors. This suggests that the experience of support facilitated the parents' coping during the illness and probably enabled them to undertake some difficult but necessary tasks, e.g., anticipatory grief.

Contrary to this was an unexpected finding illustrating the association between support and subsequent adjustment after the death. It appears that as parents had more support during the terminal illness they reported less Subsequent Adjustment following the death. The explanation for this is unclear from the data. One possibility is that the amount or type of support received during the illness is relatively unrelated to that which would be required after the death to facilitate parental Subsequent Adjustment. What may have constituted support prior to the death may fail to do so afterwards. This could account for its pattern of positive association with anticipatory grief prior to the death, since both take place during the same time period, but would not explain its pattern of association with Atypical Responses. Another possibility is that in the case of parents of terminally ill children the illness may continue for so long that at the time of death and afterwards support is no longer forthcoming. This lack of support is most important in that it may not only impede mourning but also preclude desired Subsequent Adjustment following the death. This prompts the need for a future analysis of the association between support and Subsequent Adjustment with regard to the length of the illness, in addition to the length of time since the death.

SUMMARY AND IMPLICATIONS

The findings from this investigation generate profound treatment implications. These include:

1. The findings suggest that parental bereavement may not diminish over time, but may in fact intensify. This demands that current expectations about parental grief be reviewed. A well-defined course of therapeutic intervention is mandated to assuage the intensification of bereavement which appears to occur sadly when most social supports have been withdrawn (e.g., "It's been several years now, I'm sure they're over it by this time").

2. Those findings regarding the "optimum" amount of anticipatory grief and parental participation during the child's hospitalizations suggest the necessity of examining current treatment practices which may encourage or discourage more involvement in both these areas in order to facilitate the most therapeutic parental experience. Although traditionally we have been aware of the negative results of insufficient anticipatory grief and participation, we now need to expand this awareness to realize the potentially undesirable consequences which may result from "too much of a good thing." At the same time we also need to appreciate and recognize that appropriate amounts of anticipatory grief and participation are associated with numerous indices of more positive coping during the illness and adjustment subsequent to the death. Clearly further research is needed to clarify what constitutes "appropriate" and "optimum" amounts of these variables and to be able to identify, differentiate, and predict what will be most therapeutic for different parents in differing situations.

3. The data have provided us with some criteria that can be employed to assist in identifying parents who may be at high risk in terms of their grief and adaptation. Parents whose children have sustained longer illnesses (in this investigation, illnesses longer than 18 months in duration) and who have had high previous loss appear to fare poorer. This information, when integrated with that revealing the detrimental effects of insufficient amounts of anticipatory grief, participation with the child during hospitalizations, and social support during the illness, can generate a profile descriptive of the parents' risk. (As indicated by the data there are deleterious effects of an excessive amount of anticipatory grief and participation but the delimitation points of what constitutes "too much" are ambiguous at present. Therefore, until further research can clarify this, only the condition of an insufficient amount of these variables should serve as a factor indicating high risk. At this juncture, without further research, it would be imprudent to tell people not to engage in anticipatory grief or participation behaviors out of fear they would surpass the optimum amount.)

4. Support during the illness appears to facilitate the important process of anticipatory grief, which in turn seems to facilitate numerous other positive experiences. It also tends to be associated with less abnormal grief after the death. Therefore, it is evident that health care personnel have the potential to influence more positive parental grief since they are in a position to support parents during the illness.

5. The data from this investigation clearly illustrate that despite a few differences mothers and fathers are more similar in their grief than previously noted. Historically fathers have often received "bad press" about their involvement with the dying child and their experience of grief after the death. Although in general mothers appeared to sustain grief experiences reflective of higher degrees of intensity and poorer adjustment than fathers, this was not usually to a statistically significant extent. They were statistically higher than fathers on participation during the child's hospitalizations, but not on anticipatory grief or Subsequent Adjustment. This demands that we revise some of the older theories postulating that fathers grieve less intensely and that we rethink our notions regarding participation with the child being such a major predictor of anticipatory and subsequent grief experience.

6. All of the findings demand replication with a larger population in order to secure a statistical base on which to utilize more sensitive statistical procedures. This will provide the opportunities to cull out much of the important information that may have been missed in the gross statistical procedures employed in this investigation due to the sample size. Variables such as the child's specific diagnosis and treatment regimen, along with the age, sex, and birth order of the child, demand further analysis in relation to parental bereavement. Ideally future studies will include single and divorced parents; will be prospective in nature and examine more discriminately the experience of the parents during the child's illness; and will utilize more objective behavioral and statistically rigorous measurements within a repeated measures design geared to follow the parents longitudinally during the illness and after the death.

REFERENCES

Alby, M., & Alby, J. Le medecin face a la mort de l'enfant. *Medicine de l'Homme,* 1970, *30,* 30-34.

Binger, C. M., Ablin, A. R., Feuerstein, R. C., Kushner, J. H., Zoger, S., & Mikkelsen, C. Childhood leukemia: Emotional impact on patient and family. *New England Journal of Medicine,* 1969, *280*(8), 414-418.

Bozeman, M. F., Orbach, C. E., & Sutherland, A. M. Psychological impact of cancer and its treatment. III. The adaptation of mothers to the threatened loss of their children through leukemia. Part I. *Cancer,* 1955, *8,* 1-19.

Cain, A. C., & Cain, B. S. On replacing a child. *Journal of the American Academy of Child Psychiatrists,* 1964, *3,* 443-456.

Chodoff, P., Friedman, S. B., & Hamburg, D. A. Stress, defenses and coping behavior: Observations in parents of children with malignant disease. *American Journal of Psychiatry,* 1964, *120,* 743-749.

Easson, W. M. *The dying child.* Springfield, Ill.: Charles C Thomas, 1970.

Foster, D. J., O'Malley, J. E., & Koocher, G. P. The parent interviews. In G. P. Koocher & J. E. O'Malley (Eds.), *The Damocles syndrome: Psychosocial consequences of surviving childhood cancer.* New York: McGraw-Hill, 1981.

Friedman, S. B. Care of the family of the child with cancer. *Pediatrics,* 1967, *40,* 498-504.

Friedman, S. B., Chodoff, P., Mason, J. W., & Hamburg, D. A. Behavioral observations on parents anticipating the death of a child. *Pediatrics,* 1963, *32,* 610-625.

Gorer, G. *Death, grief, and mourning.* London: Cresset Press, 1965.

Hamovitch, M. *The parent and the fatally ill child.* Los Angeles: Delmar, 1964.

Heller, D. B., & Schneider, C. D. Interpersonal methods for coping with stress: Helping families of dying children. *Omega,* 1978, *8*(4), 319-331.

Kaplan, D. M. *The impact of childhood leukemia on patients and families.* Paper presented to the American Cancer Society Writers Seminar, Saint Augustine, Florida, March 30, 1974.

Kaplan, D. M., Smith, A., Grobstein, R., & Fishman, S., Family mediation of stress. *Social Work,* 1973, *18*(4), 60-69.

Kemler, B. Anticipatory grief and survival. In G. P. Koocher & J. E. O'Malley (Eds.), *The Damocles syndrome: Psychosocial consequences of surviving childhood cancer.* New York: McGraw-Hill, 1981.

Kerner, J., Harvey, B., & Lewiston, N. The impact of grief: A retrospective study of family function following the loss of a child with cystic fibrosis. *Journal of Chronic Diseases,* 1979, *32,* 221-225.

Knudson, A. G., & Natterson, J. M. Participation of parents in the hospital care of fatally ill children. *Pediatrics,* 1960, *26,* 482-490.

Kreuger, A., Gyllensköld, K., Pehrsson, G., & Sjölin, S. Parent reactions to childhood malignant diseases. *The American Journal of Pediatric Hematology/Oncology,* 1981, *3,* 233-238.

Levitz, I. N. Comment in section on "The Parents." In N. Linzer (Ed.), *Understanding bereavement and grief.* New York: Yeshiva University Press, 1977.

Natterson, J. M., & Knudson, A. G. Observations concerning fear of death in fatally ill children and their mothers. *Psychosomatic Medicine,* 1960, *22,* 456-465.

Orbach, C. E., Sutherland, A. M., & Bozeman, M. F. Psychological impact of cancer and its treatment. III. The adaptation of mothers to the threatened loss of their children through leukemia. Part II. *Cancer,* 1955, *8,* 20-33.

Rando, T. A. *Parental Experience Assessment Form,* U.S.A. Copyright, 1979.

Rando, T. A. Structured interview for parents of deceased children. In *An investigation of grief and adaptation in parents whose children have died from cancer.* Unpublished doctoral dissertation, University of Rhode Island, 1980.

Richmond, J. B., & Waisman, H. A. Psychological aspects of management of children with malignant diseases. *American Journal of Diseases in Children,* 1955, *89,* 42-47.

Sanders, C. M., Mauger, P. A., & Strong, P. N. *The Grief Experience Inventory,* U.S.A. Copyright, 1978.

Solnit, A. J., & Green, M. Psychological considerations in the management of deaths on pediatric hospital services. I. The doctor and the child's family. *Pediatrics,* 1959, *24,* 106-112.

Spinetta, J. J., Swarner, J. A., & Sheposh, J. P. Effective parental coping following the death of a child from cancer. *Journal of Pediatric Psychology,* 1981, *6,* 251-263.

Townes, B. D., Wold, D. A., & Holmes, T. H. Parental adjustment to childhood leukemia. *Journal of Psychosomatic Research,* 1974, *18,* 9-14.

Travis, G. *The experience of chronic illness in childhood.* California: Stanford University Press, 1976.

Wallace, J. Comment on "Family Functioning." In "Care of the child with cancer." *Pediatrics,* 1967, *40,* 515-517.

Wiener, J. M. Reaction of the family to the fatal illness of the child. In B. Schoenberg, A. C. Carr, D. Peretz, & A. H. Kutscher (Eds.), *Loss and grief: Psychological management in medical practice.* New York: Columbia University Press, 1970.

9

Adaptive Noncompliance in Pediatric Asthma
The Parent as Expert

Ann V. Deaton

Cumberland, A Hospital for Children and Adolescents

Physicians and psychologists have long been aware that noncompliance with medical regimens is a relatively common occurrence, with probably one-third to one-half of all medical recommendations not being adhered to (Kirscht & Rosenstock, 1979; Stone, 1979). Research aimed at identifying noncompliers has suggested that persons with chronic illnesses and persons at the age extremes are at even greater risk for noncompliance than most individuals (Blackwell, 1973; Haynes, Taylor, & Sackett, 1979). Awareness of the magnitude of noncompliance has resulted in extensive efforts to design interventions which increase compliance and, presumably, result in better illness control (Eney & Goldstein, 1976; Haynes et al., 1979). Recently, however, a number of researchers have begun to question the underlying assumption of a one-to-one correspondence between treatment adherence and medical outcome (e.g., Epstein & Cluss, 1982; Janis, 1983). These authors have proposed the somewhat novel notions of adequate and inadequate regimens and "adequate" levels of compliance. At the same time, investigators in the related area of patient–physician interactions have begun to consider the idea that decisions regarding whether to comply with treatment ought to be considered the patient's, and not the physician's, prerogative (Kassirer, 1983; Stimson, 1974). These converging areas of study have suggested that a gradual change is taking

This paper is based on a dissertation completed at The University of Texas at Austin under the supervision of Mary Ellen Olbrisch, PhD, Department of Psychology, in September 1983. The comments and support of Dr. Olbrisch are gratefully acknowledged. The study was supported in part by two research grants from The University of Texas to Ann V. Deaton. Originally published in *Journal of Pediatric Psychology, 10*(1)(1985):1–14.

place in the traditional view of the "physician as expert." In keeping with this change, it may also be necessary to refocus compliance research away from the issue of identifying noncompliers and persuading them to comply, attempting instead to understand the nature of patients' decision making and the relationship these compliance decisions may have to outcome variables.

Typically, patients and their physicians have held conflicting views on the issue of noncompliance. The physicians' perspective may be best captured in Janis and Rodin's (1979) explanation that "ill persons are supposed to put themselves into the hands of medical authorities and do whatever they say without complaining too much" (p. 488). Proponents of this view have emphasized the negative aspects of noncompliance, including poor illness control, wasted resources, increased rates of morbidity and mortality, inaccurate results from clinical drug trials, overdoses as medications are increased because of their presumed ineffectiveness at lower doses, and the spread of communicable diseases (Eney & Goldstein, 1976; Hulka, Cassel, Kupper, & Burdette, 1976; Kinsman, Dirks, & Schraa, 1981; Kirscht & Rosenstock, 1979; Roth & Caron, 1978). For obvious reasons, the result has been considerable frustration for the treating physician when patients fail to comply.

From the patient's perspective, the problem is not so simple: "A recommendation by a health professional becomes one possibility to be judged by its perceived value for dealing with the threat (of illness) and in light of barriers to acting" (Kirscht & Rosenstock, 1979). In contrast to the generally held view of noncompliance as problematic and maladaptive, several authors have suggested the possibility that the decision not to adhere may be a well-reasoned and, indeed, adaptive choice on the part of the patient. They point to the growing body of literature on iatrogenic (physician-caused) illness such as the study by Trunet and colleagues in which 12.6% of 325 ICU admissions were due to physician errors, nearly half of which were potentially avoidable (Trunet, LeGall, Lhoste, Regnier, Saillard, Carlet, & Rapin, 1980). The notion that physicians make mistakes may be a powerful impetus to noncompliance; however, it is also important to note that sources of knowledge other than the physician exist and that these may contribute greatly to the patient's decision regarding compliance. A number of authors have suggested that the patient be viewed as a decision-making individual who evaluates medical treatment in terms of its efficacy and also with regard to the physician's past performance, the patient's own health and illness experience, and the experience of others (Janis & Rodin, 1979; Stimson, 1974; Stone, 1979). Because medical recommendations are only one aspect of a patient's daily existence, their perceived value may need to be quite high relative to their negative characteristics if compliance is to be chosen (Strauss, 1975).

PEDIATRIC ASTHMA: A PROTOTYPICAL CASE

The complexity of compliance decisions depends in part on the nature of an illness and its treatment. In the present study, the participants were children who suffered from asthma and the primary parent who made treatment decisions for the child. Although asthma is not the only chronic illness which frequently affects children, it is the most commonly occurring chronic childhood illness and, as such, may serve as a prototype for other chronic illnesses. Asthma treatment presents some problems which are specific to asthma but resembles other chronic disorders in that the treatment regimen is most often complex, difficult to implement, and only partially efficacious. In order to adequately comprehend some of the difficulties faced by pediatric asthma patients, their parents, and physicians treating them, it is necessary first to have a general working knowledge of the illness and a typical treatment regimen.

Asthma is most often defined as "an intermittent, variable, and reversible airway obstruction" (Chai, 1975; Creer, 1979). This definition is a concise summary of an illness which, as the words suggest, is quite unpredictable. Exacerbation of asthma occurs on an irregular basis. The attacks themselves may range from mild to severe within the same individual. With treatment, or sometimes spontaneously, the condition can reverse to normality. Medical treatment for asthmatic patients has three primary goals: (a) to reduce chronic symptoms (e.g., coughing, wheezing); (b) to minimize the frequency of acute attacks; and (c) to control the symptoms of acute attacks as quickly as possible when they occur (Kinsman, Dirks, & Dahlem, 1980). A typical treatment regimen includes some medications to be taken on a regular basis prophylactically, some medications to be taken as the need arises, and some behavioral recommendations to be followed in conjunction with taking the prescribed medications (Reichman, 1977). In emergencies, injections of epinephrine (adrenaline) or aerosolized bronchodilators may become necessary (Ben-Zvi, Lam, Hoffman, Teets-Grimm, & Kattan, 1982). When the asthma is severe or life threatening, corticosteroid drugs, which reduce inflammatory and allergic reactions, frequently are used as well. Additionally, allergic asthma can often be improved through the process of hyposensitization injections taking place over a period of months or years to increase the patient's tolerance for specifiable allergens (Parish, 1980). Behavioral recommendations may include the avoidance of certain allergens (e.g. dog hairs, dust, pollens), use of moderate exercise, and avoidance of cigarette smoke and overexertion (American Lung Association, 1978; Murray & Ferguson, 1983; Nickerson, Bautista, Namey, Richards, & Keens, 1983; Reichman, 1977).

As a rule, medical regimens for asthma are designed for maximal efficacy and minimal side effects (Dirks & Kinsman, 1981; Miklich, 1979). However, treatment regimens for asthma are not always efficacious and are rarely without undesirable characteristics such as those noted in Table I. Obviously, these side effects may make noncompliance a more attractive choice. In addition to physical side effects, negative aspects of an asthma treatment regimen can include inconvenient scheduling of medications, bad taste of medications, embarrassment at being under treatment, lowered self-esteem, and frustrating limitations in the activities of daily living such as sports (due to recommendations against overexertion) and the enjoyment of pets or the outdoors (due to recommendations to avoid allergens) (Becker, Radius, Rosenstock, Drachman, Schuberth, & Teets, 1978; Miklich, 1979). Sometimes the degree to which these characteristics disrupt the pediatric patient's life are seen as reasons for noncompliance. This is especially true when the treatment regimen is of uncertain efficacy. And, as one paper has noted, "even the most compliant (asthmatic) patient can suffer further episodes" (Becker et al., 1978, p. 268).

In summary, parents' decisions about whether to adhere to their asthmatic child's prescribed treatment regimen must be made under conditions of substantial uncertainty about the effectiveness of the regimen and significant concerns about its potential adverse effects. In addition, these decisions may be based on acquired knowledge. For instance, parents may recognize the variability in attack-inducing triggers (e.g., weather changes, seasonal allergens, infections), and correctly infer that control may be quite good for periods of time without aggressive treatment. Under these circumstances, it is not surprising nor, perhaps, particularly maladaptive, that some parents choose noncompliance or partial compliance as a viable alternative to complete adherence to the regimen.

In asthma, as in many illnesses, there may be numerous reasons for noncompliance. Thus far, there appears to be no clear finding in the literature which would indicate that noncompliance is always associated with treatment failure and compliance with treatment success. Therefore, the present study was conducted to evaluate the nature of parents' decision making in an attempt to identify adaptive and maladaptive decision makers and to evaluate the degree to which adaptiveness may predict outcome, both in terms of quality of life and illness control.

Table I. Pediatric Asthma: Side Effects of the Treatment Regimen

Medications

1. Medications for continuous bronchodilation (preventive maintenance medications)
   A. Sympathomimetic drugs
      Side effects: disorders of heart rate and rhythm, insomnia, nervousness, excitement, nausea (in large doses), headaches
   B. Xanthine compounds
      Side effects: stomach irritation, nausea, rapid heart rate, restlessness, nervousness
2. Medications for acute attacks
   A. Aerosols
      Side effects: dependency, risk of fatality with overuse, shakiness
   B. Injections
      Side effects: anxiety, restlessness, palpitations, headaches, dizziness, nausea, rapid heart rate, changes in blood pressure
3. Corticosteroids
      Side effects: suppression of body's own production of corticosteroids, weight gain, reduced resistance to infection, edema, effects on bone growth and hardness, effects on metabolism of salt, sugar, and protein, "moon face," excessive hair growth, disorders of the nervous system, indigestion, peptic ulcers, insomnia, nervousness, behavior changes (inhaled steroids have fewer of these side effects)
4. Management of allergic asthma
   A. Cromolyn sodium
      Side effects: bronchi and throat irritation; withdrawal may trigger an attack
   B. Desensitization/hyposensitization
      Side effects: pain, local swelling, increased number of attacks. Other negative aspects: inconvenience, expense
   C. Antihistamines
      Side effects: vary, but may include drowsiness, worsening of asthma attack by drying up bronchial secretions, loss of appetite, numerous drug interactions possible, stomach irritation, stimulation

Nonmedication components of regimen

1. Purification of the house (e.g., no rugs, no stuffed animals, books, curtains, etc. in child's room, special air filters)
   Undesirable effects: decreased quality of environment for child and family, expense, inconvenience, reduction of normative experiences
2. Avoidance of allergens (e.g., dog dander, pollens)
   Undesirable effects: restriction of activities and accompanying emotional stresses on child and family
3. Avoidance of overexertion and extreme emotions
   Undesirable effects: restriction of activities, decreased ability to enjoy strong emotional reactions or experiences (e.g., birthday parties), overprotectiveness by parents
4. Use of moderate exercise
   Undesirable effects: ??perhaps increased incidence of exercise-induced asthma

METHOD

Participants

Participants in this study were thirty 6-to 14-year-old children (mean = 9.3 years) who had been given a diagnosis of asthma by a pediatric allergist and were under treatment for control of their illness. Seventeen boys and 13 girls participated. Most had received their diagnosis at a relatively young age (mean = 3.3 years) and a number of years had passed since their diagnosis (mean = 6.0 years). For the most part, the sample tended not to have extremely severe asthma: 24 of the children were rated by their physicians as having asthma of average or below average severity; 22 had never been hospitalized for respiratory difficulties (range of hospitalizations = 0 to 20; mean = 2.7; median = 0.2).

Half of the sample was referred by private practitioners in Texas and the other half by a medical center clinic in Virginia. The two geographical groups did not differ significantly with respect to age, asthma severity, or number of physician visits in the last year, and therefore these groups were combined for purposes of data analysis. Five families declined to participate in the study. An ANOVA followed by Tukey's HSD post hoc comparison test indicated that children from these families had significantly fewer physician visits over the 9-month period of the study than either the Texas or Virginia samples ($F = 3.90, p < .05$) but did not differ with regard to age or rated asthma severity.

Parents of the children ranged from 29 to 47 years (mother's mean age = 36.3; father's mean age = 38.1) and the majority had at least a high school education ($n = 29$ mothers; $n = 27$ fathers). The families tended to be relatively well off financially, with a mean annual income of $42,000.

Measures

Structured Interview. An audiotaped, structured interview was conducted with each parent-child dyad. This interview included questions requiring that parents give a description of the child's asthma and its impact on the child and the family. Parents were also asked to describe the prescribed treatment regimen including the purpose and side effects of each component and the extent and reasons for any noncompliance. They also described in some detail their attitudes about the medical regimen and their decisions regarding the child's asthma and its treatment. At the end of the interview, parents were asked to predict their children's performance on each of four tasks in comparison to the normative scores of same-age peers on these tasks (which were provided).

On the basis of the interview, ratings of the severity of the child's asthma from 1 (much less severe than most children with asthma) to 5 (much more severe) were made. Interrater reliability between the experimenter and an independent rater was obtained for a randomly selected 20% of the interviews and was quite acceptable ($r = .94$).

The Adaptiveness Rating Scale (Deaton & Olbrisch, 1983) was also completed on the basis of the interview. This scale was devised for this study and enables the patients' decisions about compliance to be rated, regardless of whether the decisions were to comply or not to comply. The eight 5-point dimensions of this scale include two relating to the activeness and clarity of the compliance choice; two regarding knowledge of the child and whether this has a role in making compliance decisions; two dimensions relating to knowledge of the regimen itself; and, finally, two which assess how compliance decisions are evaluated. The total score on these eight dimensions is subtracted from 40 to get an "adaptiveness rating." Interrater reliability using this scale was assessed using six randomly selected tapes (20%) and an independent rater. The correlation between the two raters was .94 for scores summed across the eight dimension and ranged from .70 to .97 for individual dimensions. With the exception of the dimension "knowledge of side effects," ($r = .70$), interrater reliability was at least .80. In addition, when the two raters disagreed on exact ratings, the difference in their ratings, in all cases but one, was a single point on the rating scale.

On the basis of the interview, the child's quality of life was also rated on a 5-point scale, with a rating of 5 considered excellent and 1 very poor. Factors on which the rating was based included restrictions imposed by the asthma on activities and environment (e.g., limited sports participation, no pets, sterile room, etc.); familial attitudes (e.g., parental overprotectiveness, sibling resentment); and interference with normal activities (e.g., school absences, frequent requirements for medical care, experiencing side effects which preclude normal activities).

Finally, the parent's reported level of compliance with medications (Comp1M) and with behavioral recommendations (Comp1B) were each rated on a 5-point scale with 1 indicating complete noncompliance and 5 complete compliance.

Breathing Self-Report Postcard. This postcard is a self-report form requiring that parents report breathing difficulties, asthma attacks, and medical regimen followed by their child each day during three 1-week periods of time during the 3 months following the interview. These cards were used to provide data on the severity of the child's asthma and the stability of the medical regimen over a period of time.

Tasks Performed by the Child. Each child was asked to complete four tasks: (a) the Wechsler Intelligence Scale for Children-Revised (WISC-R) Information subtest, which provided a measure of each child's general store of information; (b) WISC-R Digit Span, used to assess verbal memory, that is, how many digits the child could recall in forward and reverse order; (c) the Benton Test of Visual Retention, which required that the child reproduce each of 10 designs (age 6 and 7 copying; age 8 and above immediate recall); and (d) sit-ups, included here as a measure of overall physical condition. This last task required that each child do as many bent-knee situps as possible in a period of 30 seconds.

Medical Outcome Data. In addition to the parents' completion of follow-up postcards, the physician and medical chart were consulted for information on the number of phone calls and visits to the physician over a 9-month time span, the number and duration of hospitalizations during this period, the prescribed medical regimen, and ratings of asthma severity.

Procedure

Patients were referred by three pediatric allergists. Each patient was contacted with a letter describing the study and a phone call within 2 weeks after the letter to schedule an appointment. Forty-three families were contacted. Of these, eight agreed to participate but were unable to schedule a convenient time to do so; five families (12%) refused to participate because they felt the child's asthma was too mild ($n = 3$) or because they felt it would be harmful to the child to be "labeled" asthmatic by participating in the study ($n = 2$). The remaining 30 families (70%) participated in the study and make up its sample.

Collection of the data was structured as follows. Each parent was given a copy of an informed consent form describing the study procedures and requesting that the experimenter be allowed to tape the interview and to consult the physician and the medical record for specified information. Following this, the structured interview took place, with parents initially being given some latitude to describe their child's asthma and its treatment. The interviewer then requested additional information which had not been provided in this unstructured format. The total time necessary for the interview was approximately 45 to 75 minutes. Following the interview, children were asked to complete the four tasks described previously. After the completion of these, parents and children were allowed to ask questions about the study. Parents frequently voiced their relief and pleasure at finally talking to someone who understood some of their feelings about the child's asthma and its treatment.

Following the interview, each parent–child pair was asked to record breathing difficulties and medication usage over the next week's time on a stamped, addressed, Breathing Self-Report Postcard. At the end of the week they mailed this to the experimenter. Study participants were sent additional postcards to complete at 1 and 3 months postinterview. At the end of the 3-month period following the interview, physicians and medical charts were consulted for medical outcome data.

Although interviews took place over 11 months, data on medical outcome for the same 9-month period (Sept. 1, 1982–May 31, 1983) were collected for all subjects so that seasonal fluctuations in allergens would not affect the results.

RESULTS

Underlying Assumptions

This study was based in part on the assumption that participants would be highly variable in both their degree of compliance and the rated adaptiveness of their compliance choices. These expectations were borne out in the results of the study. Although only one of the 30 participants (3.3%) adhered completely to both medication and behavioral aspects of the regimen, the remaining 96.7% of the sample ranged from mostly noncompliant to mostly compliant in their decisions about the treatment regimen. Similarly, with a possible range on the Adaptiveness Rating Scale from 0 to 32, actual adaptiveness scores in this study were from 8 to 32, indicating that some parents could be viewed as extremely maladaptive and others as very adaptive based upon the eight dimensions considered.

Compliance

As has been found previously in much of the compliance research, in this study time since diagnosis was negatively correlated with degree of compliance with medications ($r = -.32$, $p < .05$). An examination of the raw data indicated that parents tended to underutilize medications increasingly with the passage of time since diagnosis.

A second finding was that compliance with medications was positively related to the physicians' ratings of asthma severity ($r = .42$, $p < .05$), such that when physicians viewed the asthma as less severe, medications were less likely to be given to the child as prescribed. No similar correlation was found between compliance with behavioral recommendations and physicians' ratings of asthma severity ($r = .13$, $p > .10$).

Compliance with medications (Comp1M) and with behavioral recommendations (Comp1B) were not significantly related to the medical outcome variables of amount of hospitalization (Comp1M $r = .03$, $p > .10$; Comp1B $r = .18$, $p > .10$) or number of physician contacts during the 9-month study period (Comp1M $r = .01$, $p > .10$; Comp1B $r = -.10$, $p > .10$). Compliance was similarly unrelated to rated quality of life of the asthmatic child (Comp1M $r = .06$, $p > .10$; Comp1B $r = -.12$, $p > .10$) and to number of school absences (Comp1M $r = -.16$, $p > .10$; Comp1B $r = .00$, $p > .10$).

Adaptiveness Ratings

Although compliance was not related to outcome variables in the present study, medication compliance (but not compliance with behavioral recommendations) was correlated with parents' rated adaptiveness ($r = .50$, $p < .01$). Although some parents who were rated as adaptive did not comply (adaptive noncompliers) and one who was maladaptive did comply (maladaptive complier), compliance with medications and rated adaptiveness were not independent of one another.

Adaptiveness was not significantly related to either the amount of time the child was hospitalized ($r = -.19$, $p > .10$) or the number of physician contacts during the 9-month study ($r = -.24$, $p = .10$). Both of these correlations were in the predicted direction, however, with greater adaptiveness being associated with fewer medical interventions.

In contrast to its somewhat disappointing relationship to medical outcome variables, rated adaptiveness was correlated with quality of life outcome variables. Its correlation with quality of life ratings was .42 ($p < .05$), indicating that the children of more adaptive parents tended to experience less disruption (i.e., fewer restrictions in activities and environment) and other negative effects due to the asthma. Similarly, degree of adaptiveness was negatively correlated with number of school absences in the last year ($r = -.38$, $p < .05$). However, when the scatterplot for this latter correlation was studied, a single outlying score (a very maladaptive parent whose child was frequently absent) appeared to account for much of the relationship. When the outlier was removed the correlation decreased to a nonsignificant $-.14$.

Accuracy of Parental Predictions

It was expected that the accuracy of parental predictions of the child's task performance would be correlated with both adaptiveness and the outcome measures used in this study. To compute accuracy, the absolute values of the differences between predicted and actual performance were summed across tasks, with zero representing perfect accuracy in prediction. The resulting correlation between inaccuracy of prediction and rated adaptiveness was −.36 ($p < .05$), supporting the hypothesis that the more accurate the parents are in their ratings (and hence, their knowledge of the child), the more adaptive their decisions regarding compliance tend to be. Parental inaccuracy was also correlated with both of the objective measures of medical outcome. Its correlation with the amount of time the child spent in the hospital during the 9-month data collection period was .52 ($p < .01$) and with the number of contacts (visits or phone calls) with the physician during this period a nonsignificant .21 ($p < .10$). The more accurate parents were in their prediction of the child's task performance, the less the children were hospitalized. There was also a tendency for them to require fewer visits to the physician ($r = .26$, $p < .10$) but not necessarily to make fewer phone calls ($r = .13$, $p > .10$). The correlation between parental inaccuracy and overall quality of life ratings was of borderline significance ($r = −.24$, $p < .10$) and the correlation between inaccuracy and school absences was nonsignificant ($r = .10$, $p > .10$). This suggests that in the present study there was a trend in the direction of the children of more accurate parents having a better quality of life overall but not necessarily fewer school absences.

DISCUSSION

Research on the compliance of pediatric patients with medical regimens has traditionally been based upon the assumptions that the physician is the expert, that compliance is essential to illness control, and, therefore, that all noncompliance with prescribed regimens is problematic and maladaptive. The present study was undertaken to evaluate these assumptions; specifically to explore the notions that (a) the parents of pediatric asthma patients might have some expertise of their own; (b) that compliance might not be the sole factor predicting good outcome; and (c) that noncompliance, therefore, might not be invariably maladaptive.

With regard to the first of these, the idea of parent as expert, it was clear from the present study that parents certainly viewed themselves as having some special expertise complementary to that of the physician. Parents frequently made comments such as: "A doctor sometimes is right but they better listen to a mother sometimes too because she's with these kids 24 hours a day" or "We (the family) have to balance it. He (the physician) is real good on the technical medical aspects."

In addition to their own perceptions of their contributions to treatment, it is significant that parental accuracy and rated adaptiveness were predictive of several of the outcome variables considered in this study. The children of more accurate parents tended to require fewer medical interventions while parental adaptiveness predicted quality of life outcomes and, to a lesser degree, tended to relate to medical outcomes. These findings suggest that the parent–physician relationship can perhaps be better conceptualized as a partnership of experts, each with his or her own area of expertise and respect for the other person's capabilities.

While parental adaptiveness and accuracy were related to several of the outcome variables utilized in this study, compliance with the regimen was unrelated to either the quality of life or illness control outcomes. This finding certainly raises the question of whether compliance should be the goal of so many treatment interventions. Unless complying with the regimen yields a better outcome than not complying, the effort devoted to increasing levels of compliance seems unwarranted. The issue that Epstein and Cluss (1982) raise of "adequate levels" of compliance may be relevant here: most of the parents in the present study did follow some of the physician's recommendations. However, they did so after weighing their positive effects on the child's asthma against negative aspects such as side effects, inconvenience, interference with normal developmental experiences, and so forth. It appeared as though parents considered the prescribed regimen a guideline and used it accordingly to shape their compliance decisions. One parent described the process of her decision making with regard to a child's acute symptoms: "You're damned if you do and damned if you don't. You hear this kid wheezing and congested and you give him the medication but at the same time you have to weigh what's going to happen to him (insomnia, hyperactivity) and how it's going to be on the rest of the family."

Given these findings, the notion that all noncompliance is maladaptive must be reconsidered. In this study, many parents obviously viewed modification of the treatment regimen as an option. The fact that they decided not to comply is an important point, one which contrasts with the more traditional perspective that noncompliance reflects forgetfulness, irresponsibility, or carelessness on the part of the patient. A conscious decision which is based on adequate information about the regimen and on intimate knowledge of the child may in fact be superior to passive compliance with the regimen. In the present study at least, the adaptiveness of the decision was a better predictor of outcome than was the actual degree of compliance.

If the notion of parents/patients as active, adaptive decision makers is accepted, what implications does this have for future clinical applications and research? Insofar as medical treatment is concerned, it seems apparent that this perspective would support the growing emphasis on patient education and patient–physician partnerships. These are consistent with the renegotiation of the respective roles of parents and physicians in the health care of children. Physicians may begin to see themselves as "expert consultants," educating parents about the illness and its treatment while acknowledging the parent's (or patient's) right to make the decisions. This approach is likely to facilitate more adaptive decision making, in part by enhancing the level of communication between physicians and their patients.

With regard to research in this area, the present exploratory study leaves a great deal to be done. Some of the questions which should be addressed in future research include: (a) How is illness severity related to adaptiveness, e.g., is adaptive decision making more important when the illness is severe? (b) In addition to the cognitive aspects of adaptiveness (i.e., parental knowledge of the child, the illness, and the regimen) emphasized in the present study, what are the behavioral and affective components of adaptiveness? (c) At what age can children begin to make their own adaptive decisions concerning treatment? How can they be prepared to do this?

In addition to these (and other) specific questions, further research in this area is needed to address the question of the relationship between compliance and outcome variables for various acute and chronic conditions to evaluate to what degree compliance should be emphasized. Moreover, the association between adaptiveness and outcome variables should be replicated in additional studies and strategies for assessing the adaptiveness of decision making and for teaching parents and children how to be more adaptive should be designed. If physicians and parents are to negotiate a partnership whose aim is to produce the best possible outcome, both need to recognize the other's special expertise.

REFERENCES

American Lung Association of Texas. (1978). *Family asthma program*. Austin: American Lung Association of Texas.

Becker, M. H., Radius, S. M., Rosenstock, I. M., Drachman, R. H., Schuberth, K. C., & Teets, K. (1978). Compliance with a medical regimen for asthma: A test of the health belief model. *Public Health Reports, 93,* 268-277.

Ben-Zvi, Z., Lam, C., Hoffman, J., Teets-Grimm, K. C., & Kattan, M. (1982). An evaluation of the initial treatment of acute asthma. *Pediatrics, 70,* 348-353.

Blackwell, B. (1973). Drug therapy: Patient compliance. *New England Journal of Medicine, 289,* 249-252.

Chai, H. (1975). Management of severe chronic perennial asthma in children. *Advances in Asthma and Allergy, 2,* 1-12.

Creer, T. L. (1979). *Asthma therapy: A behavioral health care system for the respiratory disorders.* New York: Springer.

Deaton, A. V., & Olbrisch, M. E. (1983). *Adaptiveness Rating Scale.* Unpublished manuscript.

Dirks, J. F., & Kinsman, R. A. (1981). *Medication compliance. Considerations relating to current scope, definitions, and methods of measurement* (Report No. 98). Denver: National Jewish Hospital/National Asthma Center.

Eney, R. D., & Goldstein, E. O. (1976). Compliance of chronic asthmatics with oral administration of theophylline as measured by serum and salivary levels. *Pediatrics, 57,* 513-517.

Epstein, H. H., & Cluss, P. A. (1982). A behavioral medicine perspective on adherence to long-term medical regimens. *Journal of Consulting and Clinical Psychology, 50,* 960-971.

Haynes, R. B., Taylor, D. W., & Sackett, D. L. (1979). *Compliance in health care.* Baltimore: Johns Hopkins.

Hulka, B. A., Cassel, J. C., Kupper, L. L., & Burdette, J. A. (1976). Communication, compliance, and concordance between physicians and patients with prescribed medicines. *American Journal of Public Health, 66,* 847-853.

Janis, I. L. (1983). The role of social support in adherence to stressful decisions. *American Psychologist, 38,* 143-160.

Janis, I. L., & Rodin, J. (1979). Attribution, control, and decision-making: Social psychology and health care. In G. C. Stone, F. Cohen, & N. E. Adler (Eds.), *Health psychology* (pp. 487-521). San Francisco: Jossey-Bass.

Kassirer, J. P. (1983). Adding insult to injury: Usurping patients' prerogatives. *New England Journal of Medicine, 308,* 898-901.

Kinsman, R. A., Dirks, J. F., & Dahlem, N. W. (1980). Noncompliance to prescribed-as-needed (prn) medication use in asthma: Usage patterns and patient characteristics. *Journal of Psychosomatic Research, 24,* 97-107.

Kinsman, R. A., Dirks, J., & Schraa, J. C (1981). Psychomaintenance in asthma: Personal styles affecting medical management. *Respiratory Therapy.* (Reprinted by Barrington Publications)

Kirscht, J. P., & Rosenstock, I. M. (1979). Patients' problems in following the recommendations of health experts. In G. C. Stone, F. Cohen, & N. E. Adler (Eds.), *Health psychology* (pp. 189-215). San Francisco, Jossey-Bass.

Miklich, D. R. (1979). Health psychology practice with asthmatics. *Professional Psychology, 10,* 580-588.

Murray, A. B., & Ferguson, A. C. (1983). Dust-free bedrooms in the treatment of asthmatic children with house dust or house dust mite allergy: A controlled trial. *Pediatrics, 71,* 418-422.

Nickerson, B. G., Bautista, D. B., Namey, M. A., Richards, W., & Keens, T. G. (1983). Distance running improves fitness in asthmatic children without pulmonary complications or changes in exercise-induced bronchospasm. *Pediatrics, 71,* 147-152.

Parish, P. (1980). *The doctors' and patients' handbook of medicines and drugs.* New York: Alfred A. Knopf.

Reichman, S. (1977). *Breathe easy: An asthmatic's guide to clear air.* New York: Thomas Y. Crowell.

Roth, H. P., & Caron, H. S. (1978). Accuracy of doctors' estimates and patients' statements on adherence to drug regimen. *Clinical Pharmacology Therapeutics, 23,* 361-370.

Stimson, G. V. (1974). Obeying doctor's orders: A view from the other side. *Social Science and Medicine, 8,* 97-104.

Stone, G. C. (1979). Patient compliance and the role of expert. *Journal of Social Issues, 35,* 34-59.

Strauss, A. L. (1975). *Chronic illness and the quality of life.* St. Louis: Mosby.

Trunet, P., LeGall, J. R., Lhoste, F., Regnier, B., Saillard, Y., Carlet, J., & Rapin, M. (1980). The role of iatrogenic disease in admissions to intensive care. *Journal of the American Medical Association, 244,* 2617-2620.

III

Children's Perceptions and Understanding of Pediatrics

Michael C. Roberts
University of Kansas

Psychologists have long attempted to gain an understanding of how children view the world and its components. A particular interest within pediatric psychology has been children's perceptions of such environmental components as medical events, personnel, and procedures; diseases; handicapping conditions; and hazardous situations and behaviors. Knowing how children perceive is important for the adults in their lives so that efforts can be made to change the environment to produce more positive perceptions or to change the perceptions per se directly. The burgeoning research has assessed what have been variously called children's knowledge, attitudes, attributions, understanding, conceptions, and perceptions of health-related events, issues, and concepts. All of these are subsumed in this chapter's topic, although certainly differences are present. Studies have been done about sick and well children's medical fears, their knowledge about medical events such as X rays and surgery, their coping strategies, and the effectiveness of interventions to modify fears and knowledge. Similarly, researchers have tried to understand children's perceptions of diseases such as diabetes or seizure disorders in order to design interventions and explanations for those with the conditions, and for those who do not have them but who may be around those who do (viz. siblings and peers) to enhance their acceptance. In another line, clinical investigators have assessed children's views of medication and the causes of disease in order to influence adherence to treatment regimens. The recent epidemic of AIDS has spurred a spate of research into the knowledge and attitudes of children, adolescents, and adults about the etiology, nature, and consequences of AIDS in order to devise more effective prevention interventions. In related aspects of pediatric psychology and public health, knowing how children view hazards in the environment is useful for determining risks for injury and when or how to allow child exposure to them as well as how to design effective interventions to prepare children to deal with hazards.

THEORIES OF CHILDREN'S PERCEPTIONS AND ATTITUDES

Several theoretical frameworks have been developed or adapted within which to conceptualize children's perceptions and understanding. The Health Belief Model (HBM) has been widely used to conceptualize adults' motivations to adopt health-enhancing behaviors (Rosenstock, 1974). Research has been generally supportive of the HBM with adults. Markedly less research has investigated the applicability of HBM with children. A similar theoretical model, Protection Motivation Theory (PMT), has been advanced as a more comprehensive and adaptable model. PMT postulates that preventive health behavior results from the cognitive mediational processes of threat appraisal and coping appraisal. As with HBM, PMT relies on cognitive perceptions and has been supported by considerable research with adults (Prentice-Dunn & Rogers, 1986). Only recently have PMT concepts been extended to children (e.g., Knapp, 1991) in a study which found little support for the extension. Thus, with both HBM and PMT frameworks, the downward extension of adult-oriented theories to children have not been sufficient, just as they have not been in other aspects of health and clinical psychology.

More developmentally oriented models have been advanced with regard to children's perceptions of phenomena in pediatrics (Maddux, Roberts, Sledden, & Wright, 1986; Roberts, Maddux, & Wright, 1984). Many of these formulations have relied upon Piaget's concepts in which increasing cognitive sophistication leads directly to changes in children's health conceptions (e.g., Bibace & Walsh, 1979, 1980; Perrin & Gerrity, 1981).

As an example of this line of research, in an article published in the *Journal of Pediatric Psychology* (*JPP*) and reprinted in this section, Simeonsson, Buckley, and Monson (1979) examined hospitalized children's conceptions of illness and health. These researchers determined that conceptions of illness causality follow developmental trends from global, undifferentiated beliefs to specific causative agents to relatively abstract conceptions. Burbach and Peterson (1986) reviewed the studies utilizing cognitive developmental principles and concluded that "children's concepts of illness do evolve in a systematic and predictable sequence consistent with Piaget's theory of cognitive development" (p. 307).

Many research studies reported in *JPP* and elsewhere have not been organized by a particular theoretical framework. These studies have been guided more by pragmatic considerations or questions of "what are children's beliefs and perceptions?" and "what influences children's conceptions?" These have been valuable for explicating children's beliefs and as heuristics. The following sections summarize the research studies into children's conceptions of various pediatric phenomena.

RESEARCH INTO CHILDREN'S CONCEPTS

The rich literature in psychology and pediatrics on children's conceptions contains research reports investigating a wide range of phenomena. These include (a) children's conceptions of illness and specific diseases, (b) their reactions to peers with illness or disorders, (c) their perceptions of other health-related phenomena, and (d) interventions to modify the beliefs, attitudes, and perceptions. These aspects will be examined with a brief discussion of adults' perceptions of children as they relate to pediatric situations before providing an overview to the articles reprinted in this section.

Children's Conceptions of Illness

Early work into children's concept of illness per se was conducted with healthy children. For example, Nagy (1951) determined that very young children (3–5 years) were rather unsophisticated in their causal explanations for illness, slightly older children explained illness as due to infections (6–7 years) and to germs (8–10 years), while children ages 11–12 years understood multiple causes of illness. This age-developmental relationship was further investigated by later researchers (Brodie, 1974) who found evidence that children might perceive illness as punishment for misbehavior. Potter and Roberts (1984), in an application of Piagetian constructs, determined that preoperational children perceived themselves as more vulnerable to contagion. Whitt, Dykstra, and Taylor (1979) also used Piagetian concepts to help pediatricians develop clearer explanations of disease and treatment for children of different ages.

Research into healthy children's disease conceptions has begun to investigate perceptions of AIDS in terms of contagion, vulnerability, attitudes toward persons with AIDS, etc. Researchers have determined that children and adolescents, for example, have limited understanding of AIDS and possess a variety of conceptions of the disease not commensurate with professional knowledge (but probably not unlike what adults know and believe) (e.g., Brown & Fritz, 1988; DiClemente, Boyer, & Morales, 1988). Eiser, Eiser, and Lang (1990) determined that healthy younger children believed in the personal responsibility of individuals for the onset of AIDS (and other diseases). Walsh and Bibace (1991) found that children's conceptions of AIDS followed developmental trends related to cognitive development and are similar to their understanding of other diseases. Mason, Olson, Myers, Huszti, and Kenning (1989) surveyed patients with hemophilia regarding their knowledge and need for information on AIDS. McElreath and Roberts (1992) recently assessed perceptions of AIDS by children and their parents. They found a moderately high degree of AIDS-related knowledge for both groups and mostly tolerant attitudes toward people with AIDS. Parents' knowledge statistically predicted their children's attitudes, but not the children's knowledge. Zimet et al. (1991) determined that knowing somebody with AIDS lowered adolescents' social anxiety about interacting with a person with AIDS, but had no effect on perceptions of personal vulnerability. Other research has been conducted with children in the hospital or who are ill into their conceptions about their situation.

Children's Reactions to Peers with Illness or Disorders

The pediatric psychology research previously noted considered children's perceptions of health and illness in general. Even when specific to a disease such as AIDS or diabetes, the interest has been relatively focused on their conceptions in the abstract. A large body of literature has developed into how children view, interact with, and hold attitudes about those individuals who may have an illness or disorder. Knowledge of children's understanding of handicapping conditions can assist all parties during integration of children with handicaps into the classroom. Several studies have found that children hold more negative attitudes about peers who are different, namely, who are mentally retarded, visually, hearing, or speech impaired, and physically handicapped. Across perceived conditions, younger children and girls tend to hold more positive attitudes than do older children and boys (e.g., Royal & Roberts, 1987; Wisely & Morgan, 1981).

Different research methodologies have been used to assess children's attitudes and perceptions. Rosenbaum, Armstrong, and King (1986), for example, developed a psychometrically based questionnaire to measure children's attitudes toward peers with disabilities. This questionnaire sampled children's endorsement of statements assessing affective, cognitive, and behavioral intent components. Potter and Roberts (1984) presented vignettes or stories about peers with chronic illnesses (diabetes, epilepsy) and varied information to children who were at two cognitive stages before assessing perceptions. Sigelman and Begley (1987) provided vignette descriptions of a child in a wheelchair, a child who was obese, a child who had a learning disability, or an aggressive child. The vignettes either included or did not include information about the child's personal responsibility for the disorder. These researchers found that low personal responsibility resulted in more positive evaluations. In another methodology, Harper, Wacker, and Seaborg Cobb (1986) presented line drawings of disabled or nondisabled children. They found that varying orders of preference for the disabilities depended on the questions asked, social context, type of children sampled, etc. In general, though, they supported earlier findings that nondisabled children preferred the nondisabled stimulus children. In a different approach, Perlman and Routh (1980) presented nondisabled boys with either a boy in a wheelchair or one in a desk chair. They found that children played more with the boy when presented as nonhandicapped, and they expressed a preference for this child more.

In general, regardless of methodology, these studies consistently show that perceptions about peers with physical, medical, or psychological disorders tend to be more negative than those about peers without disorders and show age or developmental relationships.

Conceptions of Other Health-Related Phenomena

Children's perceptions of a variety of other health-related phenomena have also been investigated in pediatric psychology. Some of these have studied relatively abstract concepts such as health locus of control. This is the belief that health is either under one's own control (internal) or determined by external elements such as chance or other people. Originally conceptualized for adults, children's beliefs in locus of control of health have been examined by a few reports (Knapp, 1991; Parcel & Meyer, 1978), with mixed findings of a relationship between perceived locus of control and health outcomes.

Researchers have studied other relatively abstract concepts such as the development of concepts about death and personal mortality. Reilly, Hasazi, and Bond (1983) found belief in personal mortality beginning in children about age 6 years. Death is a fairly abstract concept, but apparently death-related experiences facilitate acquisition and increased understanding of death concepts.

Research has also examined more concrete and specific conceptions of health-related phenomena than general concepts of illness or health and death. Of particular interest to pediatric psychologists, children's views of health care and medical personnel have been investigated. For example,

Rifkin, Wolf, Lewis, and Pantell (1988) reported on the development of two measures of children's perceptions of physicians and health care. Similarly, Bush and Holmbeck (1987) devised a questionnaire of children's attitudes about health care which found such attitudes follow complex trends and are general attitudes, rather than specific to particular health care entities. This study was followed up by Hackworth and McMahon (1991).

In studying perceptions of specific phenomena in pediatrics, the importance of knowing children's knowledge and attitudes about medication and treatment regimens has been demonstrated in several reports. Practitioners have asserted that attitudes and beliefs about treatment and its components influence the acceptance, the adherence, and the outcome of health care interventions. For example, Allen, Tenner, McGrade, Affleck, and Ratzan (1983) assessed parents' and children's perceptions of the management of diabetes. They found that educational and support services for children with diabetes should consider "age-related meaning of the diseases of the child" (p. 139). Insulin injections are seen as a primary indicant of management independence which is related to age. A similar study of diabetes knowledge in newly diagnosed children and their parents was conducted by Auslander, Haire-Joshu, Rogge, and Santiago (1991). In a study of children with hyperactivity, Baxley, Turner, and Greenwold (1978) found they had "generally mixed attitudes toward drug treatment" (p. 175) and that much of their information and attitudes about stimulant medication was gained from physicians with reinforcement by parents. However, about 80% of these children indicated they would continue on stimulant medication even given an opportunity to stop. Levenson, Copeland, Morrow, Pfefferbaum, and Silverberg (1983), working with parents and adolescent patients with cancer, assessed perceptions of treatment. They found significant discrepancies over such issues as need for information and participation in treatment; parents believed the adolescents should be more involved than the patients themselves did. Attitudes about treatment such as these influence communication, information seeking, and adherence.

Children's perceptions of hazards in their environment relate to their potential risk-taking behavior as well as to professionals' developing interventions for preventing harm. Two articles are reprinted in the present section of this volume (Coppens, 1986; Peterson, Mori, & Scissors, 1986) as examples of this research line into children's conceptions of health-related phenomena.

Interventions to Modify Children's Perceptions

Recognizing that children (as well as adults) generally perceive people with physical and behavior disorders as less acceptable than those without disorders (e.g., Roberts, Beidleman, & Wurtele, 1981), health care and educational professionals have attempted a variety of interventions to influence the perceptions and improve acceptance and understanding. These interventions were often envisioned to have positive effects for the child with a disorder (e.g., illness, physical handicap, or behavioral problems) to understand their own situation and improve regimen compliance, lessen anxiety, and enhance adjustment. In addition, children without problems could better understand their peers or siblings who may be different. For example, some cancer treatment programs developed explanation modules for children with cancer (e.g., Claflin & Barbarin, 1991).

Utilizing Piagetian constructs, Potter and Roberts (1984) provided verbal descriptions and explanations of epilepsy and diabetes to children at preoperational and concrete operational stages. This study found that children receiving explanations exhibited more comprehension than those receiving symptom description. Children in the concrete operational stage were better able to comprehend and retain the information provided than those in the less sophisticated cognitive stage. The authors concluded that information given a child should be adjusted to his or her cognitive development.

Other research has found that direct interactions between children with physical disabilities and those without offer opportunities to observe, ask questions, and learn. As a result, understanding and peer acceptance have been improved. Westervelt, Brantley, and Ware (1983) attempted to determine whether a film emphasizing similarity between a child with a physical handicap and peers would influence attraction. They found that the film improved children's attitudes toward the peer with the handicap, but did not support the theoretical postulations. This type of intervention indicated how interventions might influence conceptions, perceptions, and attitudes about health, illness, handicaps, and children who are different.

Investigators have found that dental health promotion programs can influence children's knowledge of dental hygiene and improve their toothbrushing and flossing skills (Blount, Baer, & Stokes, 1987; Knapp, 1991). Other professionals have implemented curricula to influence (a) adolescents' attitudes toward and behavior in the misuse of alcohol (e.g., Dielman, Shope, Butchart, & Campanelli, 1986), (b) preadolescents' and adolescents' knowledge, attitudes, intentions, and behavior on onset of smoking (e.g., Evans, 1988), and (c) adolescents' knowledge about tolerance of and intended behavior about AIDS (e.g., Brown & Fritz, 1988; DiClemente et al., 1988; Zimet et al., 1991). In many of these programs, the purpose has been to influence knowledge or attitudes. Behavior change also ultimately has been the purpose of the programs whether for improved adherence or adjustment of those with a disorder or for those around them to accept or behave more positively toward those with a disorder.

Adults' Perceptions of Children

Although this chapter and section ostensibly deal with *children's* conceptions, the research literature in pediatric psychology is developing on how adults view, understand, and hold attitudes about children within the pediatric setting. These are relevant for the adults' interaction with the children in the pediatric setting and the adults' actions on behalf of, for example, in arranging services and interactions with other children. In one study, Miller and Ottinger (1986) investigated a phenomena of adults' beliefs called the "prematurity stereotype." This line of research has found that merely labeling a newborn as a preterm infant, regardless of other characteristics about the child, resulted in adults' negative judgments and attitudes about the infant, such as being less healthy, less competent, less attentive, less sociable, less enjoyable to interact with, and less liked than infants labeled as full term (cf. Stern & Karraker, 1988). These preset attitudes or perceptions form biases toward these infants which are important because the adults might interact differently with the child, with the result of perpetuating the stereotype.

Another similar line of research has investigated adults' perceptions of children with cancer. Stern and Arenson (1989) discovered that college students and medical students rated children with leukemia as less sociable, less cognitively competent, and less likely to adjust well to the future than children given a healthy label. Stern, Ross, and Bielass (1991) conducted a follow-up study which found that cancer stereotypes in medical students could be modified by providing accurate information about cancer and remission. Thus, adults' interactions with these children may be influenced by these perceptions. Comparing adult and child perceptions of cancer and treatment similarly can shed light on how communication and interactions might be assisted (e.g., Levenson et al., 1983). Other studies have investigated child-rearing attitudes in adolescent mothers (e.g., Camp & Morgan, 1984) and maternal perceptions of medical severity about children with congenital heart disease (De Maso et al., 1991) with the potential for intervention—both preventively and remedially.

OVERVIEW TO ARTICLES

Each of the three papers reprinted here represents aspects of children's conceptions. The Simeonsson et al. (1979) article followed a cognitive developmental framework to investigate how hospitalized children viewed illness causality. The methodology relied on the interview approach developed by Piaget, and the categorization of responses followed Piagetian stages. Simeonsson et al. found that the children with illnesses moved from global conceptions to increasingly more abstract conceptions. Also, increasing sophistication in concepts of illness was related to physical causality tasks. The importance of this research comes in articulating and supporting the need to understand the child's view of the world. Other studies published in *JPP* followed and expanded the concepts from the article by Simeonsson et al. (e.g., Potter & Roberts, 1984; Redpath & Rogers, 1984).

The reprinted articles by Coppens (1986) and Peterson et al. (1986) were first published in a special issue of the *Journal* on "Health Promotion and Problem Prevention in Pediatric Psychology." The overview article by Roberts (1986) is reprinted later in this volume. The articles by Coppens and Peterson et al. clarify the contributions of psychology to understanding the major threat to children's health and welfare—nonintentional injuries. These researchers demonstrate the value of examining how children perceive the world—its hazards and its safety rules. Prevention interventions can then be devised in light of such knowledge.

Coppens (1986) determined that children exhibit age-related changes in conceptions of safety and prevention. Consequently, safety education and behavioral change programs need to capitalize on the cognitive–developmental relationship. Peterson et al. (1986) investigated the correspondence between children's and their parents' awareness of rules about home safety when the children were left unsupervised. Through interviews and questionnaires, these researchers determined that children recalled very few parent rules. Parents and children disagreed in their perceptions of suggested rules for safety. However, both parents and children perceived the children as well prepared for staying home alone. The results of this study about children's and adults' perceptions of safety rules relate to the need for preventive interventions not solely to shape the perceptions, but more importantly, to increase children's safety behavior.

Research into children's conceptions of illness, their perceptions of peers with disorders, their comprehension of medical treatments, and their understanding of hazards, is useful for understanding children's development and their views of the world. Interventions to improve each of these aspects often follow from this understanding. Pediatric psychology, having the qualities of both basic and applied research, has given important attention to both in studying children's perceptions and understanding of pediatrics.

REFERENCES

Allen, D. A., Tenner, H., McGrade, B. J., Affleck, G., & Ratzan, S. (1983). Parent and child perceptions of the management of diabetes. *Journal of Pediatric Psychology, 8,* 129–141.

Auslander, W. F., Haire-Joshu, D., Rogge, M., & Santiago, J. V. (1991). Predictors of diabetes knowledge in newly diagnosed children and parents. *Journal of Pediatric Psychology, 16,* 213–228.

Baxley, G. B., Turner, P. F., & Greenwold, W. E. (1978). Hyperactive children's knowledge and attitudes concerning drug treatment. *Journal of Pediatric Psychology, 3,* 172–176.

Bibace, R., & Walsh, M. E. (1979). Developmental stages in children's conceptions of illness. In G. C. Stone, F. Cohen, & N. E. Adler (Eds.), *Health psychology* (pp. 285–301). San Francisco: Jossey-Bass.

Bibace, R., & Walsh, M. E. (1980). Development of children's concepts of illness. *Pediatrics, 66,* 912–917.

Blount, R. L., Baer, R. A., & Stokes, T. F. (1987). An analysis of long-term maintenance of effective toothbrushing by Headstart school children. *Journal of Pediatric Psychology, 12,* 363–377.

Brodie, B. (1974). Views of healthy children toward illness. *American Journal of Public Health, 64,* 1156–1159.

Brown, L. K., & Fritz, G. K. (1988). Children's knowledge and attitudes about AIDS. *Journal of the American Academy of Child and Adolescent Psychiatry, 27,* 504–508.

Burbach, D. J., & Peterson, L. (1986). Children's concepts of physical illness: A review and critique of the cognitive-developmental literature. *Health Psychology, 5,* 307–325.

Bush, J. P., & Holmbeck, G. N. (1987). Children's attitudes about health care: Initial development of a questionnaire. *Journal of Pediatric Psychology, 12,* 429–443.

Camp, B. W., & Morgan, L. J. (1984). Child-rearing attitudes and personality characteristics in adolescent mothers: Attitudes toward the infant. *Journal of Pediatric Psychology, 9,* 57–63.

Claflin, C. J., & Barbarin, O. A. (1991). Does "telling" less protect more? Relationships among age, information disclosure, and what children with cancer see and feel. *Journal of Pediatric Psychology, 16,* 169–191.

Coppens, N. M. (1986). Cognitive characteristics as predictors of children's understanding of safety and prevention. *Journal of Pediatric Psychology, 11,* 189–202.

DeMaso, D. R., Campis, L. K., Wypij, D., Bertram, S., Lipshitz, M., & Freed, M. (1991). The impact of maternal perceptions and medical severity on the adjustment of children with congenital heart disease. *Journal of Pediatric Psychology, 16,* 137–149.

DiClemente, R. J., Boyer, C. B., & Morales, E. S. (1988). Minorities and AIDS: Knowledge, attitudes, and misconceptions among Black and Latino adolescents. *American Journal of Public Health, 78,* 55–57.

Dielman, T. E., Shope, J. T., Butchart, A. T., & Campanelli, P.C. (1986). Prevention of adolescent alcohol misuse: An elementary school program. *Journal of Pediatric Psychology, 11,* 259–282.

Eiser, C., Eiser, J. R., & Lang, J. (1990). How adolescents compare AIDS with other diseases: Implications for prevention. *Journal of Pediatric Psychology, 15,* 97–103.

Evans, R. I. (1988). How can health life-styles in adolescents be modified? Some implications from a smoking prevention program. In D. K. Routh (Ed.), *Handbook of pediatric psychology* (pp. 321–331). New York: Guilford.

Hackworth, S. R., & McMahon, R. J. (1991). Factors mediating children's health care attitudes. *Journal of Pediatric Psychology, 16,* 69–85.

Harper, D. C., Wacker, D. P., & Seaborg Cobb, L. (1986). Children's social preferences toward peers with visible physical differences. *Journal of Pediatric Psychology, 11,* 323–342.

Knapp, L. (1991). Effects of type of value appealed to and valence of appeal on children's dental health behavior. *Journal of Pediatric Psychology, 16,* 675–686.

Levenson, P. M., Copeland, D. R., Morrow, J. R., Pfefferbaum, B., & Silverberg, Y. (1983). Disparities in disease-relation perceptions of adolescent cancer patients and their parents. *Journal of Pediatric Psychology, 8,* 33–45.

Maddux, J. E., Roberts, M. C., Sledden, E. A., & Wright, L. (1986). Developmental issues in child health psychology. *American Psychologist, 41,* 25–34.

Mason, P. J., Olson, R. A., Myers, J. G., Huszti, H. C., & Kenning, M. (1989). AIDS and hemophilia: Implications for interventions with families. *Journal of Pediatric Psychology, 14,* 341–355.

McElreath, L. H., & Roberts, M. C. (1992). Perceptions of acquired immune deficiency syndrome by children and their parents. *Journal of Pediatric Psychology, 17,* 477–489.

Miller, M. D., & Ottinger, D. R. (1986). Influence of labeling on ratings of infant behavior: A prematurity prejudice. *Journal of Pediatric Psychology, 11,* 561–572.

Nagy, M. H. (1951). Children's ideas of the origin of illness. *Health Education Journal, 9,* 6–12.

Parcel, G. S., & Meyer, M. P. (1978). Development of an instrument to measure children's health locus of control. *Health Education Monographs, 6,* 149–159.

Perlman, J. L., & Routh, D. K. (1980). Stigmatizing effects of a child's wheelchair in successive and simultaneous interactions. *Journal of Pediatric Psychology, 5,* 43–55.

Perrin, E., & Gerrity, P. S. (1981). There's a demon in your belly: Children's understanding of illness. *Pediatrics, 67,* 841–849.

Peterson, L., Mori, L., & Scissors, C. (1986). Mom or dad says I shouldn't: Supervised and unsupervised children's knowledge of their parents' rules for home safety. *Journal of Pediatric Psychology, 11,* 177–188.

Potter, P. C., & Roberts, M. C. (1984). Children's perceptions of chronic illness: The roles of disease symptoms, cognitive development, and information. *Journal of Pediatric Psychology, 9,* 13–27.

Prentice-Dunn, S., & Rogers, R. (1986). Protection motivation theory and preventive health: Beyond the health belief model. *Health Education Research, 1,* 153–161.

Redpath, C. C., & Rogers, C. S. (1984). Healthy young children's concepts of hospitals, medical personnel, operations, and illness. *Journal of Pediatric Psychology, 9,* 29–40.

Reilly, T. P., Hasazi, J. E., & Bond, L. A. (1983). Children's conceptions of death and personal mortality. *Journal of Pediatric Psychology, 8,* 21–31.

Rifkin, L., Wolf, M. H., Lewis, C. C., & Pantell, R. H. (1988). Children's perceptions of physicians and medical care: Two measures. *Journal of Pediatric Psychology, 13,* 247–254.

Roberts, M. C. (1986). Health promotion and problem prevention in pediatric psychology: An overview. *Journal of Pediatric Psychology, 11,* 147–161.

Roberts, M. C., Beidleman, W. B., & Wurtele, S. K. (1981). Children's perceptions of medical and psychological disorders in their peers. *Journal of Clinical Child Psychology, 10,* 76–78.

Roberts, M. C., Maddux, J. E., & Wright, L. (1984). The developmental perspective in behavioral health. In J. D. Matarazzo, N. E. Miller, S. M. Weiss, J. A. Herd, & S. M. Weiss (Eds.), *Behavioral health: A handbook of health enhancement and disease prevention* (pp. 56–68). New York: Wiley.

Rosenbaum, P. L., Armstrong, R. W., & King, S. M. (1986). Children's attitudes toward disabled peers: A self-report measure. *Journal of Pediatric Psychology, 11,* 517–530.

Rosenstock, I. M. (1974). The health belief model and preventive health behavior. *Health Education Monographs, 2,* 354–386.

Royal, G. P., & Roberts, M. C. (1987). Students' perceptions of and attitudes toward disabilities: A comparison of twenty handicapping conditions. *Journal of Clinical Child Psychology, 16,* 122–132.

Sigelman, C. K., & Begley, N. L. (1987). The early development of reactions to peers with controllable and uncontrollable problems. *Journal of Pediatric Psychology, 12,* 99–115.

Simeonsson, R. J., Buckley, L., & Monson, L. (1979). Conceptions of illness causality in hospitalized children. *Journal of Pediatric Psychology, 4,* 77–84.

Stern, M., & Arenson, E. (1989). Childhood cancer stereotype: Impact on adult perceptions of children. *Journal of Pediatric Psychology, 14,* 593–605.

Stern, M., & Karraker, K. (1988). Prematurity stereotyping by mothers of premature infants. *Journal of Pediatric Psychology, 13,* 255–263.

Stern, M., Ross, S., & Bielass, M. (1991). Medical students' perceptions of children: Modifying a childhood cancer stereotype. *Journal of Pediatric Psychology, 16,* 27–38.

Walsh, M. E., & Bibace, R. (1991). Children's conceptions of AIDS: A developmental analysis. *Journal of Pediatric Psychology, 16,* 273–285.

Westervelt, V. D., Brantley, J., & Ware, W. (1983). Changing children's attitudes toward physically handicapped peers: Effects of a film and teacher-led discussion. *Journal of Pediatric Psychology, 8,* 327–343.

Whitt, J. K., Dykstra, W., & Taylor, C. A. (1979). Children's conceptions of illness and cognitive development. *Clinical Pediatrics, 18,* 327–339.

Wisely, D., & Morgan, S. (1981). Children's ratings of peers presented as mentally retarded and physically handicapped. *American Journal of Mental Deficiency, 86,* 281–286.

Zimet, G. D., Hillier, S. A., Anglin, T. M., Ellick, E. M., Krowchuk, D. P., & Williams, P. (1991). Knowing someone with AIDS: The impact on adolescents. *Journal of Pediatric Psychology, 16,* 287–294.

10

Conceptions of Illness Causality in Hospitalized Children

Rune J. Simeonsson
Frank Porter Graham Child Development Center, University of North Carolina at Chapel Hill

Lenore Buckley
University of Rochester School of Medicine

Lynne Monson
University of North Carolina at Chapel Hill

Charting the developmental characteristics of children's understanding of illness and health might make important contributions to the applied context of pediatric care. Earlier work has provided anecdotal descriptive information on children's hospital experiences (Adams & Berman, 1965), examined correlates of child health attitudes and beliefs (Goochman, 1971; Mechanic, 1964), and compared mother–child conceptions of illness (Campbell, 1975), but little has been done to explore the stage-related development of illness concepts, paralleling earlier investigations of such concepts as life and consciousness (Piaget, 1929), prayer and religious identity (Elkind, 1962; 1967), and death (Childers & Wimmer, 1971; Koocher, 1973). The aim of the present study was to document the development of illness and health causality concepts in young hospitalized children (ages 4-9 years) whose stage of cognitive development may limit understanding

This research was conducted while the first author was a faculty member of the Department of Pediatrics, University of Rochester School of Medicine and Dentistry, Rochester, New York. Appreciation is expressed to the Department of Pediatrics and the nursing staff for their cooperation in the conduct of this study. An earlier version of this paper was presented at the meeting of the Society for Research in Child Development, Denver, 1975.
Originally published in *Journal of Pediatric Psychology,* 4(1)(1979):77–84.

of illness and treatment. It was hypothesized that developmental transitions would characterize children's conceptions of illness and that these transitions would parallel other indices of cognitive growth such as conservation and decentration.

METHOD

Subjects

Subjects were 30 boys and 30 girls (4 through 9 years of age) admitted to a university teaching hospital. All of the children included were judged to be capable of responding to task demands and were not in acute distress or terminally ill at the time of the interview. An analysis of the bases for hospitalization for 57 of the subjects indicated approximately similar percentages of patients in four broad categories (elective admissions, 25%; accidents, 23%; chronic conditions, 23%; and acute conditions, 30%). Subjects were selected to constitute approximately equal numbers of boys and girls in three age groups (4-0 to 5-11 years; 6-0 to 7-11 years; and 8-0 to 9-11 years).

Materials and Procedure

The Concept Assessment Kit (CAK: Goldschmid & Bentler, 1968), Form A, was administered to assess conservation. The role-taking skills of children were assessed by administering a set of five cartoon drawings developed by Chandler (Note 1) and described in detail by Blacher-Dixon and Simeonsson (1978). Cards are scored from 0 to 3, with a high score (maximum 15) indicating egocentrism. Seven questions were administered to elicit the child's response to questions of causality. The first utilized Piaget's (1930) questions: (a) "What makes clouds move?" to probe notions of physical causality. Six additional questions tapping causality of illness were constructed as follows: (b) "How can children keep from getting sick?" (c) "What does medicine do?" (d) "How do children get sick?" (e) "How do children get stomachaches?" (f) "How do children get bumps or spots?" (g) "When children are sick, how do they get better again?" Half of the children were presented only verbal questions, whereas for the other half, verbal questions were accompanied by appropriate illustrations (e.g., pictures of medicine, child in a hospital bed, etc.) to determine if mode of presentation would influence response quality. The scoring criteria involved the assignment of responses to one of three defined stages (Elkind, 1967): Stage I (global or undifferentiated responses including "don't know"), Stage II (concrete, specific responses reflecting rule breaking, rule keeping, and/or specific acts and events), Stage III (abstract verbalizations or expressions of principle).

Each child was first administered a receptive language test (Peabody Picture Vocabulary Test; Dunn, 1965) to ascertain that estimated intellectual functioning fell above IQ 85. Subjects then completed the six CAK subtests, followed by causality questions, which were interspersed with items from the role-taking task.

RESULTS

In order to enhance the statistical summary to follow, illustrative examples of children's responses are given to exemplify the qualitative categories. Stage I: responses scored for this stage reflected global and undifferentiated conceptions of illness and health. In response to the question, "What does medicine do?" a boy (age 5-9) responded, "Sometimes kills them." To the question, "How do children get sick?" one girl (age 5-8) suggested, "When you kiss old people and women," while another girl (age 4-10) responded, "When they need pills." The above three examples suggest that conceptions of illness causality at this stage are undifferentiated, magical, and superstitious (first two responses) and/or reflect circularity of reasoning in which cause and effect become confused (last response). Stage II: responses were scored according to the presence of concrete and specific conceptions of illness in this stage. A boy (age 6-1) responded to "How do children get sick?" by stating, "Peanuts goes in the wrong pipe, getting finger cut, getting electrocuted." A girl (age 6-3) given the same question, responded, "Go to the medicine cabinet and take medicine you're not supposed to, eat poison." These responses are typical of many Stage II responses in that they reflected conceptions dealing with the violation and/or observation of specific rules. Causality of illness and health was often associated with the enumeration of acts or events without the presence of an organizing or generalizing principle. Stage III: responses were assigned to this stage when there was evidence of an abstract and/or generalizable principle. A boy (age 9-4) suggested in response to the question "When sick, how do children get better again?" by saying, "Take medicine and do what the doctor tells you to do." Another boy (age 8-4) responded to the question "How do children get sick?" by saying, "Sometimes you catch it from other people from germs." These two responses illustrate a relative understanding of disease states and treatment and suggest awareness of causal factors for

Table I. Mean Scores on Questions Concerning Illness

Age group	Questions[a]					
	b	c	d	e	f	g
5	1.50	1.78	1.67	1.50	1.55	1.61
7	1.96	1.86	1.95	1.66	1.66	1.90
9	2.09	1.85	2.20	1.90	1.76	2.10

[a] The questions were as follows:
(b) How can children keep from getting sick?
(c) What does medicine do?
(d) How do children get sick?
(e) How do children yet stomachaches?
(f) How do children get bumps or spots?
(g) When children are sick, how do they get better again?

illness which extend beyond specific acts, events, and/or violation of rules. All of the responses were classified into one of the three categories specified previously. The inclusion of "don't know" responses (less than 10% of all responses) in Stage I seemed appropriate in light of the fact that such responses were more than 2 1/2 times as frequent in the youngest age group as in either of the other two groups. Interrater agreement was found to be 86% on a sample of 23 protocols.

Mean scores for each of the six illness-conception questions are given in Table I. Multivariate analysis of variance (Presentation Mode × Age × Questions) revealed that neither the effects for Presentation Mode nor the Presentation Mode × Age interaction reached the .05 level of significance. The data are reviewed, first, by focusing upon the developmental nature of illness and health concepts and, second, by examining the relationship between these concepts and the cognitive indices of conservation, role taking, and physical causality concepts.

A significant multivariate effect, however, was found for Age, $F = 2.22, p < .02$. Examination of univariate F tests indicated that four of the six illness causality questions reflected significant age effects. These questions concerned how children (b) keep from getting sick, $F(2, 54) = 9.33, p < .001$; (d) get sick, $F(2, 54) = 5.32, p < .008$; (e) get stomachaches, $F(2, 54) = 4.40, p < .02$; and (g) get better, $F(2, 54) = 8.43, p < .001$. These findings not only suggest developmental differences in children's illness causality conceptions but also that some questions are more developmentally sensitive than others. Inspection of the Table I shows minimal mean age differences for questions (c) "What does medicine do?" and (f) "How do children get bumps and spots?" whereas more distinct transitions are evident for the remaining questions. It appears that questions dealing with causes for illness and stomachaches as well as con-

Table II. Mean Scores for Cognitive and Overall Illness
Measures

Measure	Age group		
	5	7	9
Conservation	1.17	6.00	8.90
Egocentrism	7.78	7.43	3.00
Causality	3.50	3.62	3.57
Overall illness	1.60	1.83	1.98

Table III. Intercorrelation of Variables

	Chronological age	Conservation	Egocentrism	Physical causality	Total illness
Chronological age		$.63^c$	$-.47^c$		$.49^c$
Conservation			$-.37^b$		$.53^c$
Egocentrism					$-.56^c$
Physical causality					$.27^a$
Total illness					

$^a p < .05.$
$^b p < .005.$
$^c p < .001.$

ditions identified for recovery or the maintenance of health are most sensitive to developmental differences in the age range tested.

Support for a developmental progression was evident in that Stage I responses characterized 39% of all responses of 5-year-olds, whereas it dropped to 20% and 10% for the two older age groups. Stage II responses accounted for 61%, 74%, and 84% of all responses for the 5-, 7-, and 9-year age groups, respectively. Stage III responses, on the other hand, were nonexistent for the youngest population and accounted for small percentages (6 and 6) in the middle and oldest age groups. Children's conceptions of illness causality thus appear to have some uniformity at different developmental levels and to progress from global to abstract with age.

Table II presents the mean scores of the three age groups on conservation, role taking, illness (averaged over questions), and physical causality. Conservation and role-taking scores reflect developmental differences for age groups, whereas scores for physical causality concepts do not.

A correlation matrix was constructed to clarify the relationships among variables examined in this study. This is presented in Table III. Mean illness causality scores correlated significantly with measures of egocentrism, conservation, and chronological age. Furthermore, an overall trend of qualitative shifts in cognition, whether it involved physical aspects (i.e., conservation of space and number), social cognition (role taking), or conceptions of phenomena such as illness and health, is supported by the substantial intercorrelations among these measures as well as their correlation with the developmental index of chronological age. The commonality of cognitive growth across measures is further supported by first-order partial correlations in which the effect of chronological age is controlled. The partial correlations of mean illness causality scores with several variables were as follows: conservation, $r = .33$, $p < .006$; egocentrism, $r = -.44$, $p < .001$; and physical causality, $r = .27$, $p < .02$.

DISCUSSION

The results have shown that the conceptions of illness causality follow a developmental progression of stages similar to that reported for other domains (Elkind, 1962, 1967; Koocher, 1973; Piaget, 1929).

The first stage identified was global and undifferentiated in its structure and reflected responses which were magical, superstitious, and/or circular in their logic. The magical and circular aspects of reasoning have been pointed out by Piaget (1930) to be characteristic of young children in areas of causality and moral judgment. At the second stage, causality of illness was attributed to a variety of specific acts and/or events associated with illness and health. An association was very frequently made between becoming ill or getting well and the enumeration of breaking or keeping rules and regulations. This focus is in keeping with Piaget's (1932) and Kohlberg's (1963) proposed stages of moral judgment in which evaluations by the young child are strongly based on respect for authority and rules. The third stage of illness-conceptions provided evidence for generalized, relative, and/or abstract notions in that the phenomena of illness or health were generalized to basic concepts of infection, health maintenance, differentiated and relative bases for treatment.

The predominance of Stage I and Stage II responses may be due to the age range and the level of measurement selected for this study. It is clear that only a small portion of the 9-year-old group was demonstrating consistent Stage III responding. Based on the results of this exploratory study it may be useful to explore expansion of stages to be scored, particularly of responses scored as concrete differentiated. Documentation of Stage I and Stage II responses, however, is in keeping with the specific intent of this study, i.e., to probe the young child's understanding of illness and hospitalization.

The demonstration that illness causality conceptions were significantly related to conservation, decentration, and physical causality provides generalized support for the commonality of cognitive development across a range of phenomena. It suggests that conceptual development is characterized by children's increasing ability to free themselves of egocentric and intuitive reasoning in the domains of physical, social, and personal experiences.

A major contribution of Piaget (1970) and research based on his theory has been to sensitize us to the fact that children at every stage of development actively construct the world in order to understand it and thereby cope with it accordingly. The demonstration that children's conceptions of causality of illness and health show qualitative shifts in development is not an unexpected finding. Parents, nurses, and doctors often ask the child to be a "good patient." Perhaps it is of greater importance to explore how children perceive themselves as "patients" and to provide them with information about treatment which is consistent with their level of understanding. This may be particularly true for hospitalized children under 6 or 7 years old whose conceptions are prone to be egocentric, magical, and/or superstitious and who, therefore, lack not only a realistic understanding of illness but also of their role as patients in the treatment process. Further explorations of children's conceptions of illness and health are needed to form a basis for more effective patient–staff relationships to enhance the child's participation in treatment, an essential aspect of the recovery process.

REFERENCE NOTE

1. Chandler, M. J. *Role theory and developmental research.* Paper presented at the meeting of the American Psychological Association, Montreal, August 1973.

REFERENCES

Adams, M. L., & Berman, D. C. The hospital through a child's eyes. *Children,* 1965, *12,* 102-104.

Blacher-Dixon, J., & Simeonsson, R. J. Effect of shared experience on role-taking performance of retarded children. *American Journal of Mental Deficiency,* 1978, *83,* 21-28.

Campbell, J. D. Illness is a point of view: The development of children's concepts of illness. *Child Development,* 1975, *46,* 92-100.

Childers, P., & Wimmer, M. The concept of death in early childhood. *Child Development,* 1971, *42,* 1299-1301.

Dunn, L. *Peabody picture vocabulary test: Expanded manual.* Minneapolis: American Guidance Service, 1965.

Elkind, D. The child's conception of his religious denomination II: The Catholic child. *Journal of Genetic Psychology*, 1962, *101*, 185-193.

Elkind, D. The child's conception of prayer. *Journal for the Scientific Study of Religion*, 1967, *6*, 101-109.

Goldschmid, M. L., & Bentler, P. M. *Concept assessment kit—Conservation*. San Diego: Educational and Industrial Testing Service, 1968.

Goochman, D. S. Some correlates of children's health beliefs and potential health behavior. *Journal of Health and Social Behavior*, 1971, *12*, 148-154.

Kohlberg, L. The development of children's orientation towards a moral order: I. Sequence in the development of moral thought. *Vita Humana*, 1963, *6*, 11-33.

Koocher, G. P. Childhood, death, and cognitive development. *Developmental Psychology*, 1973, *9*, 369-375.

Mechanic, D. The influence of mothers on their children's health attitudes and behavior. *Pediatrics*, 1964, *33*, 444-453.

Piaget, J. *The child's conception of the world*. New York: Harcourt Brace, 1929.

Piaget, J. *The child's conception of physical causality*. London: Kegan Paul, 1930.

Piaget, J. *The moral judgment of the child*. London: Kegan Paul, 1932.

Piaget, J. Piaget's theory. In P. H. Mussen (Ed.), *Carmichael's manual of child psychology* (3rd ed., Vol. 1). New York: Wiley, 1970.

11

Mom or Dad Says I Shouldn't
Supervised and Unsupervised Children's Knowledge of Their Parents' Rules for Home Safety

Lizette Peterson, Lisa Mori, and Cathy Scissors
University of Missouri–Columbia

An increasingly large number of children spend some portion of the day without adult supervision (Belsky & Steinberg, 1978) as an expanding number of primary caretakers join the work force each year. These children are often referred to as "latchkey children" because of the latchkeys they often wear on a chain or carry to let themselves into their homes after school, several hours before their parents return home from work (Gar barino & Sherman, 1980). There is increasing evidence that such children, left at home without adult supervision, experience a greater risk of accidents (Tokuhata, Colflesh, Digon, & Mann, 1972) which are the number one killer of young children (Gratz, 1979). In addition, there are emotional and motivational problems inherent in being unsupervised (Elkind, 1981).

Several clinical researchers have suggested the importance of training children to follow rules of safe conduct when encountering emergencies (e.g., Jones, Kazdin, & Haney, 1981) or strangers (e.g., Poche, Brouwer, & Swearingen, 1981). With the recent increase in emphasis on preventing child disorders rather than attempting to simply remediate them (e.g., Peterson & Mori, 1985; Roberts, Elkins, & Royal, 1984), it seems increasingly important for clinicians to assess the need for behavioral programs to train children in rules of safe conduct. However, there has been very little research to determine the extent to which parents, in the absence of any spe-

The authors thank the participating children and parents as well as the school, teachers, and principal.
Originally published in *Journal of Pediatric Psychology, 11*(2)(1986):177–188.

cific training programs, attempt to provide their children with a set of rules for appropriate home safety behavior whether or not the child is left alone at home. Few, if any, investigations have attempted to ascertain the kinds of provisions parents may make to ensure their children's safety at home and the extent to which children are aware of and able to implement their parents' wishes. The primary objective of the present study was to gather some preliminary answers to these questions by assessing rules that parents suggested they had constructed to ensure their children's safety and by ascertaining the extent to which their children were aware of these home safety rules. A secondary purpose was to determine if the degree of supervision a child experienced influenced the child's awareness of home safety rules. This survey is viewed as an important first step in documenting the need for home safety skills training, as well as a vehicle for indicating the most important areas for future clinical intervention to prevent child accidents.

METHOD

Subjects, Experimenters, and Raters

All children in the fourth and fifth grades from a predominantly white, middle-class elementary school were asked to take home a permission-to-participate request to their parents. This request noted that the investigator was interested in asking parents and their children about some of their rules for safe behavior around the home and asked that the parent who identified himself or herself as the primary caretaker agree to (a) allow the child to participate in a 20- to 30-min interview over the lunchtime recess and (b) complete a written questionnaire which the child would bring home from school. Forty parents (over 85% of the total sample) agreed to participate and 32 parents ultimately returned the questionnaire. Twenty-six mothers, four fathers, and two mother–father pairs completed the questionnaire as the primary caretaker.

All 40 children of the parents agreeing to participate were interviewed, but the data from only the 32 children (10 girls and 22 boys, ages 8 years to 10 years, 7 months; $\bar{x}$ = 9 years, 5 months) whose parents completed the questionnaire are reported here. Fourth- and fifth-grade children were selected as a sample because 8 years of age is the youngest age at which a child in this state can legally be left home alone without adult supervision (e.g., Masters, 1978).

Experimenters were an undergraduate man and woman who were blind to any of the experimental hypotheses. Experimenters conducted oral interviews with the child subjects, writing out the children's answers to the questions longhand. Both experimenters recorded data on approximately 20% of the children for reliability purposes. They also distributed the written questionnaires to the children after each interview and collected the written answers of the parents when the forms were returned to the school.

The first and second authors served as raters. These individuals independently categorized and summarized the longhand written answers for both the child and parent data for 25% of the sample.

Procedure

Children individually participated in a 20- to 30-min interview and parents later completed a written questionnaire over the same material. Five general types of questions were posed. The interview questions began with a multiple-choice question concerning how frequently the children remained unsupervised at home (e.g., never, once a week, two–three times a week, more than four times a week). This question was later used to group children according to level of child supervision. The next question asked children to rate themselves on how well prepared they were to stay at home alone (1 = very well prepared, 5 = as prepared as the average child, and 10 = not at all prepared). Then, the children responded to open-ended questions which began with very general issues and gradually became more focused (e.g., a tightly focused question asked "Do your parents have specific rules about how you are to answer the phone, take messages, etc.? Can you tell me about them?"). The child was asked to enumerate any specific rules about preparing and eating certain foods, answering the telephone, answering the door, performing chores, and reacting to emergencies (a fire, a cut hand). The child was then presented with rules for safe behavior in the home and asked if the parent advocated the rule. The topics covered were the same as the open-ended questions: food (e.g., "I am allowed to have candy after school"), strangers (e.g., "I am allowed to tell someone who comes to the door that my parent(s) aren't home"), and emergencies (e.g., "If I cut my hand badly, I should wait until my parent gets home."). The children were prompted and encouraged to think about each answer and after the interviews were concluded, they were asked not to discuss the project with any of the other children. The questionnaire attempted to cover the wide range of problems suggested by individuals involved in latchkey intervention programs (e.g., Swan, Briggs, & Kelso, 1982) and past child safety training studies (e.g., Jones et al., 1981; Peterson, 1984a, 1984b; Poche et al., 1981; Rosenbaum, Creedon, & Drabman, 1981). Finally, external validation of the categories selected was sought and obtained from local experts such as a family practice physician, a policeman involved in crime prevention, a fire department official, and a pediatric nutritionist. Parents were also asked to rate each of the areas of concern described by the questionnaire in terms of importance (1 = extremely important and 10 = not at all important) and how much the parent worried about the topic (1 = worry constantly and 10 = never worry) and to suggest additional areas of concern.

Each child was given a sealed envelope to deliver to the parent at the end of the interview. The envelope contained an 11-page questionnaire comprising items identical to the 40 questions the children had just answered, except that the items were worded for the parent. Of the parents receiving the questionnaires, 80% returned the questionnaires completed, constituting the present sample. Most of the parents asked for and subsequently received the results of the study.

RESULTS

Reliability of Experimenters and Raters

The two experimenters repeatedly demonstrated high (95–100%) reliability in their longhand recording of the children's responses to the open-ended questions and four option responses (agreement was coded only if all words except articles such as "a" and "the" were recorded exactly the same). The raters demonstrated acceptable (87%) reliability in their categorizing of the longhand responses into the rule agreement categories. An agreement on rule categories was scored whenever the raters independently listed that parent and child had the same behavioral response or rule to a given question.

Descriptions of Survey Results

Parents and children rated how often the child remained home unsupervised by an adult into four categories: never, once a week, two–three times a week, or more than four times a week. Children and parents tended to agree on these categorizations ($r = .59, p < .05$); where disagreements occurred, the majority ($n = 5$) were within one category of one another, with the child indicating being left at home alone more often than the parent. Where such disagreement occurred, the parents' rating was used to categorize the child's responses. This resulted in six boys and four girls categorized as never unsupervised, four boys and four girls categorized as unsupervised two or three times a week, and six boys and one girl categorized as unsupervised four or more times a week.

For each of the four categories of survey answers, the means for parent–child agreement within each of the four levels of weekly child supervision were compared on a question by question basis. Because this process involved multiple comparisons, only those findings of $p < .02$ will be regarded as significant. With few exceptions,[1] there were no differences among the four levels of supervision on the degree of parent–child agreement for Ratings of Preparation, Open-Ended Listing of Parents' Rules, and Responses to Suggested Rules. Therefore, an overall group mean best represents these data and is reported here. There were some scattered differences in the four levels of supervision on parents' listing of Rule Areas of Concern, and so these data are shown with separate means for each of the supervision levels.

Ratings of Preparation to Stay Alone. Children and parents showed fairly close agreement in rating how well prepared the child was to stay at home alone, with both parents ($M = 3.45$) and children ($M = 4.09$) rating the child as better prepared than the average child to stay at home alone. Interestingly, parents tended to rate the children as better prepared than even the children rated themselves.

Open-Ended Listing of Parents' Rules. All parents listed from one to six specific rules for their children for the preparation of food, 29 of 32 parents had rules concerning what the child should do when answering the telephone, all parents listed from one to five rules in regard to procedures for answering the door, 23 parents had rules about doing chores, and all but 2 listed rules concerning how to respond to emergencies.

As shown in Table I, the mean number of parent rules correctly recalled by children for each of the six problem areas was less than 1, and a very small proportion of parents' rules were recalled.

Responses to Suggested Rules. In addition to examining children's free recall of parental rules in the open-ended listing, this category utilized a

---

[1]The few differences noted between groups under differing levels of supervision did not seem to form any clear or predictable patterns. For the six open-ended listing of parents' rules (Table I), the only mean difference at $p < .02$ was found on the "Chores" question and was between the never unsupervised ($M = 0.20$) and the 2–3 times a week unsupervised ($M = 1.14$) groups. On parent–child agreement on the 44 responses to suggested rules listed in Table II, the 2–3 times a week ($M = 29\%$) and 4 times a week ($M = 86\%$) groups differed on use of knives (Item 3), the never group ($M = 50\%$) and 1 time a week group ($M = 88\%$) differed on responsibility for younger siblings (Item 7), all four groups differed ($M = 13\%$, 1 time a week; $M = 28\%$, 4 times a week; $M = 20\%$, never; and $M = 865$, 2–3 times a week) on dealing with a neighbor at the door (Item 16), and the 1-time-a-week group ($M = 38\%$) differed from the 2–3 times a week group ($M = 100\%$) on contacting a parent in case of trouble (Item 19).

Table I. Open-Ended Questions

	Mean no. of rules listed by both parent and child	% of parental rules listed by children
1. What rules for being alone (in general)	0.59	18.0
2. Food rules	0.25	12.5
3. Rules for answering phone	0.59	38.9
4. Rules for who to admit when person comes to the door	0.68	39.0
5. Rules about chores	0.47	28.8
6. Rules about emergencies like fires and cuts	0.65	37.6

recognition strategy in which children were given a concrete rule and asked if their parent would agree, disagree, or didn't care about the rule. Children were also allowed to respond that they did not know. In fact, most children tended to respond that their parent agreed or disagreed. Thus, the level of chance agreement between parent and child ranged from 25% (if all four answer categories were used) to 50% (if answers were restricted to agree or disagree).

As can be seen in Table II, there was a large amount of disagreement between parents and children. On a few items (e.g., cannot punish younger siblings, cannot allow an adult stranger in the house, cannot play with cigarettes or fireworks), children were well aware of their parents' rules. However, for very serious issues such as what to do in case of fire, tornado, a serious cut, or a sharp cinder in the eye, disagreements were often above 90%. This suggests not only a lack of awareness of parental rules but also some serious misinformation on the part of the children.

Overall, the data in Table III show a profound lack of parent–child agreement on most items, especially given the high potential level of chance agreements and parents' almost universal acquiescence to the question "Does my child know what my decision is?" asked after each rule.

Rule Areas of Concern. As can be seen in Table III, there was more consensus than difference among parents in the four different supervision areas. All parents indicated responses to emergencies like fires, tornadoes, and accidental injury as being very important and as provoking at least moderate worry. Children's after-school snacks, disciplining younger siblings, responses to well-known people on the telephone, and the child making a mess were not rated as very important or worry provoking. Where group differences occurred, the most consistent difference was for parents who leave their children unsupervised at home more often to worry more

Table II. Responses to Suggested Rules — Percentage of Disagreement Between Parent and Child Answers Categorized as Yes, No, Undecided or Don't Know

Question[a]	% disagreement
1. Eat candy after school	41
2. Eat potato chips after school	38
3. Use knives to make snack	37
4. Use stove to make snack	25
5. Open cans to make snack	41
6. Use blender to make snack	22
7. Responsible for younger sibs	19
8. Physically punish younger sibs	3
9. Answer phone, take message	29
10. Answer phone and say home alone	29
11. Tell a stranger on the phone your address	16
12. Dial 911 in an emergency	44
13. Have same age friends over	41
14. Have much older friends over	31
15. Tell adult at door no one home	38
16. Allow adult neighbor to come in home	60
17. Allow stranger to come in home	04
18. Should contact neighbor if trouble	91
19. Should contact parent if trouble	32
20. Must do homework after school	50
21. Is allowed to play after school	22
22. Is allowed all TV wanted after school	41
23. If sees fire, should contact an adult	88
24. If sees fire, should call fire department	45
25. If sees fire, should contact parent	100
26. If power goes out, child can use candles	91
27. If power goes out, child can use flashlight	13
28. If tornado, seek shelter with neighbor	75
29. If tornado, seek shelter in our home	53
30. If tornado, contact parent	97
31. Bad cut, contact parent	91
32. Bad cut, wait for parents to get home	100
33. Bad cut, contact another adult	60
34. Cinder in eye, get it out by self	97
35. Cinder in eye, contact neighbor	66
36. Cinder in eye, contact parent	60
37. Cinder in eye, wait for parent to come home	100
38. Can play with fireworks	4
39. Can play with cigarettes	0
40. Allowed access to parents' things	13
41. Allowed access to sibs' belongings	29
42. Allowed to go to playmates' house after school	47
43. Allowed to play in neighborhood after school	41
44. Allowed to go anywhere after school	25

[a] All questions presume that there is no adult in the house and ask if the child is allowed to engage in the specific behaviors listed.

Table III. Parents' Mean Ratings (and Standard Deviations) of the Importance and the Degree to Which They Worry Over Select Problems[a]

Problem	Important (1 = Extremely important, 5 = kind of important, 10 = not at all important)				Worry (1 = I worry about it constantly, 5 = I occasionally worry about it, 10 = I never worry about it)			
	Degree of Child Supervision				Degree of Child Supervision			
	Never	1 × /wk	2-3/wk	4+/wk	Never	1 × /wk	2-3/wk	4+/wk
1. The food my child eats after school	4.4 (2.6)	4.2 (2.8)	5.7 (2.2)	4.6 (0.7)	7.1 (2.4)	8.0[a] (2.0)	6.5 (2.6)	4.9[b] (3.5)
2. The kitchen utensils/appliances my child uses	3.0 (2.9)	3.2 (2.3)	2.3 (1.0)	3.9 (2.1)	5.8 (3.2)	6.4 (1.7)	7.2 (1.7)	5.9 (2.5)
3. My child's behavior in case of a fire	1.1 (0.3)	1.0 (0)	1.0 (0)	1.0 (0)	3.4 (2.1)	5.4[a] (2.4)	4.7 (2.4)	2.6[b] (1.0)
4. My child's behavior in a bad storm/tornado	1.3 (0.6)	1.6 (1.3)	1.0[b] (0)	1.9[a] (0.8)	3.4 (2.3)	4.5 (2.5)	5.5 (2.6)	3.3 (1.0)
5. My child's behavior if he or she injures himself or herself	1.0 (0)	1.7 (1.4)	1.9 (1.5)	1.3 (0.4)	3.2[b] (2.1)	4.7 (1.9)	5.6[a] (1.1)	2.6[b] (0.5)
6. My child's looking after younger siblings	3.3[b] (2.9)	3.0[b] (1.4)	8.2 (3.6)	10.0[a] (0)	5.4[b] (2.0)	4.8[b] (2.1)	8.3 (3.0)	10.0[a] (0)
7. My child's disciplining younger siblings	6.5 (3.6)	4.2[a] (2.0)	9.0 (2.0)	10.0[b] (0)	7.6 (2.9)	7.3 (1.7)	9.3 (1.3)	10.0 (0)
8. My child's response to people I know on the phone	6.1 (3.7)	6.1 (3.0)	4.0 (2.1)	5.0 (2.3)	9.1[a] (1.2)	7.6 (2.7)	6.0[b] (2.6)	6.4[b] (2.6)
9. My child's response to people I don't know on the phone	2.9 (2.6)	3.6 (2.9)	3.0 (1.2)	3.0 (1.4)	7.4[a] (2.5)	6.1 (2.6)	5.7 (3.3)	3.8[b] (2.0)
10. My child's response to people I know who come to the door	5.7 (4.0)	5.6 (3.1)	3.0 (2.0)	3.0 (1.4)	7.4 (3.4)	7.5 (2.6)	6.7 (1.7)	5.7 (2.4)
11. My child's response to people I don't know who come to the door	2.0 (1.6)	1.6 (0.9)	2.1 (1.4)	2.7 (1.6)	5.6[a] (2.2)	5.1 (2.4)	4.5 (2.5)	3.2[b] (1.6)
12. My child completing his/her chores	4.1 (2.6)	5.5 (3.7)	5.9 (2.2)	5.4 (2.0)	6.9 (2.6)	6.0 (4.0)	4.0 (2.3)	6.1 (2.6)
13. My child getting into mischief	1.7[b] (1.3)	3.4[a] (1.6)	3.4[a] (1.2)	2.4 (0.7)	5.1 (2.2)	6.2 (2.0)	5.5 (2.0)	5.0 (2.8)
14. My child not completing homework	1.1[b] (0.3)	4.2[a] (1.8)	4.7[a] (2.7)	5.4[a] (2.4)	7.0[a] (2.6)	3.0[c] (2.2)	7.3[a] (1.8)	6.3[b] (2.4)
15. My child making a mess	5.9 (2.7)	5.3 (2.8)	5.4 (2.7)	5.7 (1.5)	5.4 (3.7)	6.4 (3.6)	4.3 (3.5)	6.3 (2.0)
16. Where my child is after school	1.8 (1.3)	3.3[a] (2.4)	3.3 (3.1)	1.3[b] (0.5)	4.8 (2.7)	5.8 (2.6)	3.8 (1.5)	3.7 (2.1)

[a,b,c] Means with differing superscripts differ by $p < .02$. Where no superscripts appear, means do not differ.

than parents who leave their children unsupervised at home less frequently. However, no clear anticipated differences in supervision levels were noted for most of the items on the importance or worry questions.

DISCUSSION

The absence of an awareness of appropriate at-home rules can have a variety of kinds of impact upon a child, ranging from boredom and poor nutrition to child molestation and fire-related death. The present survey presents four important conclusions. First, both parents and children believed the children to be well prepared to stay at home alone. Second, parents did not ignore the need for appropriate at-home rules; they uniformly reported a set of rules for a variety of situations in preparation of their child's being unsupervised at home. Third, the parents believed that their children were fully informed of the rules they had devised. Finally, and most important, the children were not aware of most of their parents' rules and did not appear well prepared to be left at home unsupervised. Not only were they unable to recall their parents' rules, they failed to recognize what behaviors were and were not acceptable, even when the behavioral rules were presented. This study provides the first empirical evidence of children's general need for home safety rule training recently suggested by clinicians (e.g., Jones et al., 1981; Peterson, 1984a, 1984b; Poche et al., 1981). Further, the data obtained indicate that parents are very likely to be unaware of their children's need for such training.

Because the number of young children left unsupervised for some portion of the day is growing rapidly (Belsky & Steinberg, 1978), it becomes increasingly important to assess children's ability to behave safely and sensibly in their parents' absence. Although the data from the present study are from a relatively small sample, they demonstrate consistently a disturbing gap between what parents and children think children know and what children actually know. A larger sample would scarcely yield more robust conclusions regarding the very low level of parent–child agreement. Surprisingly, children who were typically left unsupervised did not appear to be demonstrably more knowledgeable about how to deal with daily self-care problems than did children who were never left alone. For all four groups of subjects, the parents and the children gave the children high marks for how well prepared they believed the child to be. Yet the results indicated that children clearly lack awareness of parental rules concerning problems parents rate as important and worrisome.

It could be argued that some differences in parents' and children's answers might have been a product of the different manner in which the data were collected, but this is unlikely to have been the case. Children received an oral interview not only to control for differences in their abilities to read and write but more importantly to assure that children thought about each question and responded to it completely and carefully. For example, on the open-ended questions, children were inclined to list one rule and then to quit; interviewers were trained to probe further, to ask the child to try and remember other rules, and to elicit the child's "best," most accurate performance. If anything, the method of data collection was weighted in favor of the children recalling more rules than the adults, the opposite of what actually occurred.

Similarly, it could be argued that children actually knew the rules but were simply unable to verbally or behaviorally access them in the interview. Although it is impossible to rule out such an explanation, it seems unlikely that in a quiet room with no time pressure and with a responsive interviewer who allowed the child to "tell me or show me" that the child would perform less well than when in an actual, time-pressured emergency or when encountering an actual stranger. Studies that have examined children's verbal listing and actual behavioral adherence to home safety rules suggest that the actual behavior is less rule-bound than the verbal report (e.g., Peterson, 1984a). Thus, it is unlikely that the present method of assessing children's understanding of the home safety rules underestimated children's actual working knowledge.

It is possible that parents gave socially appropriate answers to the questionnaire but suggested alternate rules to their children. This would not explain why, for the most part, children failed to list any rules. Furthermore, it seems somewhat unlikely that parents would suggest less than "socially appropriate" rules to their children simply because less socially appropriate rules would be likely to be less safe.

It could also be argued that children were cared for by older siblings who were, in turn, aware of the rules. The majority of parents did not report such an arrangement, however, and this explanation neglects the fact that parents universally indicated that the children were aware of their rules.

What can account for the discrepancy in what parents believe the children know and what the children actually know? The most obvious answer seems to be the absence of any formal parental training of these behavioral rules, accompanied by a lack of perceived contingencies for appropriate and inappropriate behavior. That is, no one is there at home to object if the child behaves in an unsafe manner or to congratulate the child for behaving safely. Unless the child is actually injured, molested by a stranger, or causes property damage, the parent is unaware of the child's behavior. Further, recent research suggests that merely discussing home safety rules with children does not improve their home safety behavior; instead, behavioral rehearsal is needed (e.g., Peterson, 1984b). In addition, it is very typical for parents to afford lip service to actions on their part which could ensure their child's safety (e.g., child car seats or poison-proofing a home) but to do little behaviorally about it (Roberts et al., 1984). Thus, this discrepancy should not be surprising. The parents in the present survey received the results reported here several months prior to this manuscript's submission and with the results they received the principal investigator's telephone number. No parent contacted the investigator to discuss the accuracy of the results or to determine a method by which children's understanding of home rules could be improved.

Finally, it is legitimate to question the generality of the present findings. Although it is highly unlikely given the clear and robust findings of the present survey that adding additional subjects from this population would alter the findings, it is certainly possible that they are limited to a middle-class Midwestern population. Only similar studies with differing populations will be able to comment on this possibility. However, if one were to speculate about the degree to which such parent–child disagreement about rules exists in other populations, it might be anticipated that the present population would show lower, not higher, rates of parent–child disagreement than more urban or lower SES populations. Such speculations, however, await further research.

Depending upon the generality of the present results, they suggest a problem that is at once very serious and potentially underestimated by parents. It is clear that if children are unsupervised, as were the majority of the children in this survey at least part of the time, and unaware of appropriate behavior, they are at risk for a variety of kinds of injury and misfortune (e.g., Roberts et al., 1984). A few researchers have suggested that such problems can be prevented by training appropriate rules to apply when dealing with strangers (e.g., Poche et al., 1981), escaping from fires (e.g., Jones et al., 1981), and dealing with home situations in which personal injury might occur (e.g., Peterson, 1984a, 1984b). Such training programs show much promise in eliminating unsafe behavior in unsupervised children. However, before such programs can become accepted by parents and implemented on a widespread basis, the need for such programs must be demonstrated. Paradoxically, this survey, which is the first empirical attempt to document children's generally poor knowledge of home safety rules, also documents that parents are unaware of their children's need for safety rule training.

REFERENCES

Belsky, J., & Steinberg, L. D. (1978). The effects of day care: A critical review. *Child Development, 49,* 929-949.

Elkind, D. (1981). *The hurried child.* Reading, MA: Addison-Wesley.

Garbarino, J., & Sherman, D. (1980). High-risk neighborhoods and high-risk families: The human ecology of child maltreatment. *Child Development, 51,* 188-190.

Gratz, R. R. (1979). Accidental injury in childhood: A literature review on pediatric trauma. *Journal of Trauma, 19,* 551-555.

Jones, R. T., Kazdin, A. E., & Haney, J. I. (1981). Social validation and training of emergency fire safety skills for potential injury prevention and life saving. *Journal of Applied Behavior Analysis, 14,* 249-260.

Masters, M. (1978). *Revised statutes of the state of Missouri, 4,* 4707.

Peterson, L. (1984a). The "Safe at Home" game: Training comprehensive prevention skills in latchkey children. *Behavior Modification, 8,* 474-494.

Peterson, L. (1984b). Teaching home safety and survival skills in latchkey children: A comparison of two manuals and methods. *Journal of Applied Behavior Analysis, 17,* 279-294.

Peterson, L., & Mori, L. (1985). Prevention of child injury: An overview of targets, methods and tactics for psychologists. *Journal of Consulting and Clinical Psychology, 53,* 586-595.

Poche, C., Brouwer, R., & Swearingen, M. (1981). Teaching self-protection to young children. *Journal of Applied Behavior Analysis, 14,* 169-176.

Roberts, M. C., Elkins, P. D., & Royal, G. P. (1984). Psychological applications in the prevention of accidents and illnesses. In M. C. Roberts & L. Peterson (Eds.), *Prevention of problems in childhood: Psychological research and applications* (pp. 173-199). New York: Wiley-Interscience.

Rosenbaum, M. S., Creedon, D. L., & Drabman, R. S. (1981). Training preschool children to identify emergency situations and make emergency phone calls. *Behavior Therapy, 12,* 425-435.

Swan, H., Briggs, S. M., & Kelso, M. (1982). *"I'm in charge": A self-care course for parents and children.* Olathe, KS: Johnson County Mental Health Center.

Tokuhata, G. K., Colflesh, V., Digon, E., & Mann, L. (1972, May). *Childhood injuries caused by consumer products. Pennsylvania Department of Health, Division of Research and Biostatistics.* Harrisburg.

12

Cognitive Characteristics as Predictors of Children's Understanding of Safety and Prevention

Nina M. Coppens

College of Health Professions, University of Lowell

An understanding of children's characteristics that might contribute to their injury proneness should provide direction for recognizing children at risk and for taking preventive action. Compared to school-age children, preschoolers have a higher rate of accidents (Baker, O'Neill, & Karpf, 1984; International Children's Centre, 1979). In attempting to discover the reasons for this age-related difference in proneness to accidents, consideration of other differences between these two age groups may be helpful.

Differences in cognitive capabilities could be related to the relative degree of vulnerability to accidents found in children at different stages of development. Faber and Ward (1977) suggested that an association exists between the age-related differences they found in children's understanding of using products safely and children's ability to see cause and effect relationships. In the majority of accidents involving children predictable causal relationships between accident agents and injuries can be identified (e.g., fire causes burns) (International Children's Centre, 1979). Children's ability to engage in causal reasoning may be predictive of their accuracy in identifying these relationships. Children with an ability to make causal connections may use this information to differentiate situations as safe or unsafe. Avoidance of identified unsafe situations could reduce children's proneness for accidents. Furthermore, ability to

Based on doctoral dissertation research, Psychology Department, University of New Hampshire, May 1985. I gratefully acknowledge the guidance of my dissertation advisor Carolyn J. Mebert. This research was supported in part by a grant and a dissertation fellowship awarded to the author by the University of New Hampshire.
Originally published in *Journal of Pediatric Psychology, 11*(2)(1986):189–202.

assess the safeness of a situation may be affected by the cognitive style of the individual inasmuch as cognitive style reflects children's ability to systematically scan for critical features of the environment and to generate alternatives for preventing injury.

Causal Reasoning

Although Piaget (1960) observed that children did not have the ability to predict and to explain logically cause and effect sequences until they reached school age, he described transitional stages that existed during the preschool years. More recent research has indicated that preschoolers were able to make causal connections (Sharp, 1982; Siegler, 1975); however, limitations occurred in the children's reasoning abilities. Variability in the preschoolers' performance was present and distracting influences needed to be removed from the stimuli to enhance their causal reasoning ability.

Translating this into accident-related issues, it is expected that school-age children have a more accurate understanding of causal relations, safety, and prevention than their younger counterparts. Preschoolers may be able to make causal connections necessary to identify accident agents and their consequences when irrelevant information is kept to a minimum. Realistically it is impossible to remove all distracting, competing factors from the environment; therefore, limitations would be expected in preschoolers' reasoning. Shultz and Mendelson (1975) reported that preschoolers achieved greater success in identifying factors that caused an effect than identifying factors that prevented an effect from occurring. Thus, it is expected that children's scores on measures evaluating their ability to differentiate between safe and unsafe situations would be relatively high compared to their ability to specify measures for preventing unsafe situations.

In a previous investigation of preschoolers' understanding of safety and prevention, children scored significantly higher on the safety compared to the prevention task (Coppens, 1985). Results from this earlier work also indicated that even after controlling for the variability explained by age, level of causal reasoning was found to be a significant predictor of preschoolers' performance on the criterion measures of safety and prevention. However, most of the variability in the criterion measures was not accounted for by these predictors (i.e., 59% in safety and 76% in prevention scores). Children's cognitive style may have helped explain additional variability in these scores.

Cognitive Style

Based on a series of studies of children performing cognitive tasks, Kagan, Rosman, Day, Albert, and Phillips (1964) proposed the cognitive style continuum referred to as reflection–impulsivity. In comparison to reflective children, impulsive children responded more quickly and with more errors on the tasks. Subsequently Kagan and Kogan (1970) clarified this dimension as one concerned with the degree to which the child reflects on the validity of his/her solution hypothesis in problems that contain response uncertainty. The most common operational definition includes latency to first response and total errors on the Matching Familiar Figures Test (Kagan et al., 1964).

Research has revealed that reflectives systematically gather more information about the stimuli before offering an answer than do impulsives (Drake, 1970; Siegelman, 1969). Children's tendency to be reflective or impulsive has been shown to be predictive of their performance on other tasks that involve scanning and analysis of a visual field. On these tasks, reflectives perform consistently better than impulsives (Duryea & Glover, 1982; Messer, 1976). From a developmental perspective, research suggests that cognitive style in problem solving becomes more stable during the school years and children become increasingly more reflective (Messer, 1976). Hence, it is expected that school-age children are more likely to have a reflective cognitive style than preschoolers and that cognitive style will help explain differences in children's understanding of safety and prevention.

The present study, a follow-up of earlier research (Coppens, 1985), was designed to examine relations between preschool and school-age children's cognitive style, level of causal reasoning, differentiation of safe and unsafe situations, and specification of preventive measures. This extension of age range was included to increase the variability among scores and provide a better indication of developmental changes in children's performance. The inclusion of both age groups enables a comparison between preschoolers' and school-age children's responses that may help explain why preschoolers are relatively more accident prone. Because children's delay and their errors on the Matching Familiar Figures Test (MFFT) may be independent predictors of performance, they were examined as separate elements of children's cognitive style.

The following hypotheses were tested:

1. Children will be able to differentiate between safe and unsafe situations before they are able to specify preventive measures.

2. A positive correlation will exist between children's causal reasoning scores and their safety and prevention scores.

3. A positive correlation will exist between children's response time on the MFFT and their safety and prevention scores.

4. A negative correlation will exist between children's error score on the MFFT and their safety and prevention scores.

METHOD

Subject Selection

A written description of the study and the consent form were sent to all parents of children 3 years and older enrolled in a preschool day care center and children between the ages of 6 and 8 years enrolled in an after-school program in the same city. Parents of 29 out of 34 preschoolers and 52 out of 67 school-age children agreed that their child could participate in the study. Two additional preschool day care programs were sampled selectively for the ages needed to obtain a fairly equal representation of children at each age from 3 through 8 years. Oral consent was obtained from children prior to their being interviewed. None of the children refused to participate.

Subjects

The 112 children studied included 60 girls and 52 boys. The number of children at each age from 3 through 8 years was 19, 18, 18, 19, 20, and 18, respectively. The children ranged in age from 38 to 107 months, with a mean of 73 months ($SD = 21$).

Parental information was obtained for 66 children whose parents returned the demographic questionnaire (i.e., 59% of the sample). Three of the children lived with father only, 25 lived with mother only, and 38 lived with both parents. There were no significant differences in children's safety or prevention scores for children from one-parent compared to two-parent families. The median income of these families was $25,000.

Procedure

Children were interviewed individually at their school during two separate half-hour sessions.

Session 1. In Session 1, children's level of causal reasoning was determined by their temporal ordering of events in picture sequences and by their identification of factors relevant to gear movement. To determine cognitive style the children's version of the MFFT (Kagan et al., 1964) was administered.

Session 2. Understanding of safety and prevention was determined by responses to questions asked after viewing 4 × 6-inch color photographs of safe and unsafe situations. The potential injuries depicted in the unsafe situations represented those cited by the International Children's Centre (1979) as being the most frequent among children (e.g., poisoning, falls, and burns). Immediately following this session, the correct answers and reasoning concerning safety and prevention were discussed with each child. This same procedure was used in previous research (Coppens, 1985).

Measures and Scoring

The measures were piloted with 22 children from 3 through 8 years of age for clarity of instruction and interest level.

Temporal Ordering of Events Task. Children were presented 14 sets of picture sequence cards. The first two sets served as a practice trial to clarify directions and were not scored. In the practice trial the children were taken through the steps of placing the picture cards on the display board to tell a story. The directions for "first" and "next" were explained in terms of sequencing the story. The color photo sequences used, "Kids at Play" and "Everyday Skills," were produced by Lakeshore Company as curriculum materials. When questioned, none of the children indicated they had previously seen these pictures. An example of one set consists of a child going up and down a slide in a series of five progressive stages. In Part 1, four sets were shown one set at a time. For two of the four sets, the third and fourth picture cards of the sequence were placed on a display board; a card marked with an X on it was placed after the fourth picture. Children were asked to look at the three remaining cards and to place the card that shows what happens next on the X card. For the remaining two sets, the second and third picture cards were placed on the display board with the X card before the second picture. Children were asked to look at the three remaining cards and to place the card that shows what happens first on the X card. This procedure was continued in Parts 2 and 3 except now four sets were shown simultaneously. The total possible score was 12 points. The range of scores for these children was 1 to 12, with a mean of 7.7 ($SD = 3$).

Gear Movement Task. The gears and figures used in this task came from two "Gear Circus" sets available from Chaselle Inc., a supplier of curriculum materials. When questioned, none of the children indicated they had seen this toy before. Children were shown a colorful network of gears designed in the shape of a T. On one side there were two areas where gears did not mesh which prevented the gear movement from continuing to the end. On the other side all the gears did mesh and the movement could continue to the end. Animal and people figures were located on the penultimate gear of each branch. Their rotation or lack of rotation was the effect of interest. Part 1 tested children's ability to predict and explain this effect. After Part 1, the operation of the gears was demonstrated but not discussed with the children. Part 2 assessed children's ability to predict and explain the effect on the figures' rotation when the tester removed and added relevant and irrelevant parts to the gear display. A part was considered relevant if its removal or addition affected the rotation of the figures. An irrelevant part had no effect on their rotation. The total possible score was 25 points. The range in scores for these children was 0 to 25, with a mean of 10.1 ($SD = 8$).

Matching Familiar Figures Test (MFFT). This task was scored in the standard manner (Kagan et al., 1964). The range in total latency scores for these children was 23 to 381 seconds, with a mean of 99 seconds ($SD = 71$). And the range in total errors was 3 to 36, with a mean of 18.5 ($SD = 9$).

Differentiation of Safe and Unsafe Situations Task. A safe and unsafe situation was depicted within each of the 11 pairs of photographs (e.g., standing vs. sitting in a grocery cart, wearing a seat belt vs. leaning on the dashboard). After children made their initial decision on the safeness of the photographs, they were questioned to determine if they could describe the presence or absence of an accident agent and the potential injury. The scoring represented a possible 3 points per pair with a maximum total of 33 points (Coppens, 1985). The range in scores for these children was 4 to 33, with a mean of 28 ($SD = 6$).

Specification of Preventive Measures Task. Since children were told the five photographs shown in this task depicted unsafe situations, the prevention task always followed the differentiation of safe and unsafe situations task. After viewing each photograph, children were asked a series of five questions to probe for different types of preventive measures. A preventive measure was considered correct if it was an action that either prevented the unsafe situation or stopped the occurrence of injury. The scoring represented a possible 5 points per photograph with a maximum total of 25 points (Coppens, 1985). The range in scores for these children was 0 to 25, with a mean of 14 ($SD = 7$).

Reliability. The percentage agreement between this investigator's onsite scoring and an independent rater's scoring of 34 randomly selected audio tapes were 98% for the safety task and 97% for the prevention task. Because of the nonverbal indicators present in the other measures, reliability of their scoring could not be determined from the tapes (i.e., children's placement of cards in the temporal task and the tester's removal and addition of parts in random order for the gears task). The alpha reliability coefficients for the temporal, gears, safety, and prevention tasks were .84, .95, .93, .94, respectively.

RESULTS

Preliminary analyses indicated no sex differences in children's performance on the predictor and criterion measures. Therefore, scores for boys and girls were combined in all subsequent analyses.

In order to examine the developmental nature of children's performance on the measures, the means and standard deviations for each age are presented in Table I. A progression existed in that there was improvement in performance from 3 through 8 years of age. The reduced variability in the older children's safety scores probably reflects a ceiling effect for this measure. More than half of the children in the 6- to 8-year-old group had

Table I. Means (Standard Deviations) for Predictor and Criterion Measures by Age

Measures	Age in years					
	3	4	5	6	7	8
Causal reasoning						
Gears	2.8	2.2	7.4	13.2	14.9	19.6
	(3.3)	(2.4)	(5.4)	(7.4)	(7.3)	(4.5)
Temporal	3.9	4.6	7.3	9.8	10.2	10.5
	(1.8)	(2.3)	(2.9)	(2.1)	(1.4)	(1.6)
Cognitive style						
Latency	60.6	55.2	76.9	122.3	141.8	133.4
	(74.8)	(22.0)	(46.4)	(65.3)	(86.8)	(54.7)
Errors	27.2	26.8	22.1	14.9	10.6	9.9
	(5.5)	(5.4)	(8.7)	(6.2)	(3.1)	(4.1)
Criterion						
Safety	20.1	23.9	28.8	30.7	31.9	32.6
	(8.3)	(5.1)	(3.6)	(2.7)	(2.0)	(0.8)
Prevention	6.4	7.9	12.9	16.4	19.4	20.4
	(6.6)	(5.3)	(5.2)	(5.0)	(3.7)	(2.8)

a perfect safety score. On the other hand only one child, who was from the older age group, had a perfect prevention score. None of the children who scored in the lower 50% on the safety task scored in the upper 50% on the prevention task. In addition, the mean percentage score on the safety task was 85% compared to 56% on the prevention task. These data suggest that children's differentiation of safe and unsafe situations occurs prior to their specification of preventive measures.

The three hypotheses that referred to children's level of causal reasoning and cognitive style were tested with correlations. Prior to conducting these correlations, each measure's scores were checked for normality of distribution. The safety and MFFT latency scores were significantly skewed (i.e., −1.7 and 1.9, respectively) whereas all the other measures were skewed less than 0.5. To reduce their skewness, logarithmic transformations were performed on the safety and latency scores. The correlation coefficients for the entire group and separate analyses for the 3- to 5-year-old and 6- to 8-year-old groups are presented in Table II.

Causal Reasoning

The coefficients for the total and separate groups provided support for the hypothesis that a positive correlation exists between children's causal reasoning scores and their safety and prevention scores. Although the correlations for the older group were significant, they were relatively lower in magnitude than those of the younger group.

Next, stepwise multiple regression analyses were conducted to examine the unique variance of the causal reasoning measures in predicting safety and prevention scores. Because children's age was significantly correlated with safety and prevention scores it was entered first in all regression analyses to determine how much variance the predictors could explain in addition to this general index of development (see Table III). For all of the regression analyses causal reasoning contributed a significant amount of variance in explaining safety and prevention scores.

Cognitive Style

The correlations for the total group provided support for the hypothesis that a positive relationship exists between children's response time on the MFFT (latency score) and their safety and prevention scores (see Table II). However, when examined separately for the younger and older age groups, latency was no longer significantly related to safety score. In con-

Table II. Correlations of Predictor and Criterion Measures for Total Group, 3- to 5-Year-Olds, and 6- to 8-Year Olds

Measures	1	2	3	4	5	6
Total group (N = 112)						
1. Age (months)						
Causal reasoning						
2. Gears	.75^c					
3. Temporal	.77^c	.79^c				
Cognitive style						
4. Latency	.59^c	.59^c	.63^c			
5. Errors	−.78^c	−.71^c	−.74^c	−.73^c		
Criterion						
6. Safety	.77^c	.77^c	.75^c	.55^c	−.69^c	
7. Prevention	.75^c	.76^c	.79^c	.56^c	−.67^c	.82^c
3-, 4-, and 5-year-olds (n = 55)						
1. Age (months)						
Causal reasoning						
2. Gears	.54^c					
3. Temporal	.61^c	.68^c				
Cognitive style						
4. Latency	.26^a	.33^b	.35^b			
5. Errors	−.35^b	−.51^c	−.48^c	−.54^c		
Criterion						
6. Safety	.56^c	.65^c	.60^c	.21	−.44^c	
7. Prevention	.52^c	.69^c	.63^c	.23^a	−.30^a	.74^c
6-, 7-, and 8-year-olds (n = 57)						
1. Age (months)						
Causal reasoning						
2. Gears	.29^a					
3. Temporal	.09	.55^c				
Cognitive style						
4. Latency	−.01	.25^a	.30^a			
5. Errors	−.40^b	−.31^b	−.29^a	−.46^c		
Criterion						
6. Safety	.30	.49^c	.30^a	.20	−.23^a	
7. Prevention	.35^a	.51^c	.46^c	.29^a	−.36^b	.56^c

$^a p$ < .05.
$^b p$ < .01.
$^c p$ < .001.

Table III. Multiple Regressions with Children's Level of Causal Reasoning and Cognitive Style Regressed After Age on Safety and Prevention Scores

Criterion	Step Predictor	Beta	F^a	r	R	R^2
Total group (N = 112)						
Safety	1 Age	.77	155.3^c	.77	.77	.59
	2 Gears	.44	27.9^c	.77	.82	.67
	3 Temporal	.22	4.9^b	.75	.83	.68
	2 Errors	−.25	6.8^b	−.69	.78	.61
	3 Latency	.06	0.5	.55	.78	.61
Prevention	1 Age	.75	140.5^c	.75	.75	.56
	2 Temporal	.52	15.2^c	.79	.82	.67
	3 Gears	.29	9.7^c	.76	.83	.70
	2 Latency	.18	5.7^b	.56	.76	.58
	1 Errors	−.12	1.1	−.67	.77	.59
3-, 4-, and 5-year-olds (n = 55)						
Safety	1 Age	.56	24.8^c	.56	.56	.32
	2 Gears	.48	16.4^c	.65	.69	.48
	3 Temporal	.19	1.6	.60	.71	.50
	2 Errors	−.27	5.4^b	−.44	.62	.38
	3 Latency	.08	0.4	.21	.62	.39
Prevention	1 Age	.52	19.3^c	.52	.52	.27
	2 Gears	.57	24.1^c	.69	.71	.50
	3 Temporal	.25	3.1	.63	.73	.53
	2 Errors	−.14	1.2	−.30	.53	.28
	3 Latency	.05	0.1	.23	.53	.29
6-, 7-, and 8-year-olds (n = 57)						
Safety	1 Age	.30	5.5^b	.30	.30	.09
	2 Gears	.44	13.2	.49	.52	.27
	3 Temporal	.05	0.1	.30	.52	.27
	2 Latency	.20	2.5	.20	.36	.13
	3 Errors	.03	0.0	−.23	.36	.13
Prevention	1 Age	.35	7.5	.35	.35	.12
	2 Gears	.45	14.4	.51	.55	.31
	3 Temporal	.28	4.4^b	.46	.60	.36
	2 Latency	.29	5.8^b	.29	.45	.21
	3 Errors	−.14	0.8	−.36	.47	.22

[a] Test for increment in proportion of variance accounted for.
[b] $p < .05$.
[c] $p < .01$.

trast, the hypothesis that a negative correlation exists between children's MFFT error score and their safety and prevention scores was supported for both the total group and separate age groups (see Table II).

After entering age, stepwise multiple regression analyses were conducted to determine the relative importance of errors and latency as predictors of safety and prevention scores. Because the interaction terms were not significant as predictors, they were not included in Table III. When the total group was considered, errors was the preferred predictor for safety score and latency preferred for explaining prevention scores. The zero-order correlations indicated MFFT errors should have been the preferred predictor for both criterion measures; however, it was also more highly correlated with age than latency. Regression analyses conducted separately for 3- to 5-year-olds and 6- to 8-year-olds, indicated error score was the preferred predictor for the younger group and latency for the older group. For this older group, error score was significantly correlated with age whereas latency was not (see Table II).

Significant Causal Reasoning and Cognitive Style Predictors

In order to determine the unique variance contributed by the significant causal reasoning and cognitive style predictors, multiple regression analyses were conducted entering them in stepwise fashion after age. For all of the regression analyses the causal reasoning measures entered before cognitive style and therefore remained as significant predictors of safety and prevention scores. Because none of the measures of cognitive style remained significant as predictors, this suggested the variance they explained was shared with causal reasoning. When cognitive style was forced to enter after age and before causal reasoning, the measures of causal reasoning still accounted for a significant increment in explained variance. Thus, measures of causal reasoning appear to be the preferred predictor of safety and prevention scores.

DISCUSSION

The results of this study were consistent with previous research (Coppens, 1985) and indicate that there are age-related differences in children's understanding of safety and prevention which parallel cognitive development. The present findings, based on preschool and school-age children from a range of socioeconomic levels, support the view that both children's level of causal reasoning and their cognitive style are related to their understanding of safety and prevention. Examination of children's safety and prevention scores indicated that an understanding of safety occurs before children are able to specify measures for preventing accidents.

The cognitive style results are consistent with other studies from which researchers have concluded that MFFT errors is a preferred predictor over MFFT latency (Gjerde, Block, & Block, 1985; Victor, Halverson, & Montague, 1985). The reflection-impulsivity dimension is concerned with children's solution hypotheses in problems that contain response uncertainty (Kagan & Kogan, 1970). Because so many of the older children had a perfect score on the safety measure, the uncertainty issue of this task for the older group could be questioned. This may help explain why level of causal reasoning was a preferred predictor over cognitive style. Videotapes would have provided a more challenging task by depicting moving environments.

The magnitude of the correlations between components of cognitive style, level of causal reasoning, and age were higher for 3- to 5-year-olds compared to 6- to 8-year-olds. The interrelations between these characteristics indicate the developmental flux within the younger age group. In comparison with the older children, differences in these characteristics explained more of the variance in preschoolers' safety and prevention scores. This finding provides support for the possibility that proneness to accidents may be related to stage of psychological development. The limitations inherent in younger children's causal reasoning and in their cognitive style place restrictions on their abilities to process information provided in the environment. Children's misunderstandings concerning the concepts of safety and prevention may increase the probability of their being in unsafe situations. Also, once in these situations, the children may have difficulty recognizing measures for preventing injury.

The present results suggest that the focus of safety education programs be on helping children identify preventive measures through encouraging the development of an understanding of cause-effect relationships existing between accident agents and potential injury. If safety education programs assume children can initially make and then reverse cause-effect connections, these programs might be either ineffective or confusing for those children who are limited in these abilities. Videotaping children in multiple environments might be particularly effective for guided experiences in preventive thinking. This approach would make the abstract concepts of safety and prevention more concrete. Environments (e.g., street, playground, home) could be scanned with close-ups on critical features that define the situations as safe or unsafe. Special effects could portray children in unsafe situations, reverse the unsafe activity, and show safe actions that would prevent injury.

Pediatric well-child visits are an ideal time to screen for children's understanding of causal relationships, safety, and prevention and for presentation of an injury prevention program directed toward children's cognitive abilities. Pediatric psychologists could also assist children (who receive health care following injury) to transform the realities of the accident situation into a learning experience by identifying elements of the environment critical in calculating risk and how injury could have been prevented.

Despite strong evidence both from this study and the previous research (Coppens, 1985) that level of causal reasoning is related to children's understanding of safety and prevention, limitations on the present findings should be emphasized. Care must be taken in generalizing the results of the current study to other age groups and unsafe situations in which injury is neither foreseeable nor preventable. It must also be stressed that the correlational nature of the study precludes making causal links between the variables investigated. A longitudinal examination of children's cognitive characteristics, understanding of safety and prevention, and frequency of accidents would clarify the relationship among these variables.

Incorporating additional predictor and criterion measures in future studies might help explain statistical differences in rate of accidents not examined in the current study. For example, although a sex difference was not present in children's understanding of safety and prevention, statistically boys have a higher rate of accidents than girls (International Children's Centre, 1979). Observations made by Ginsburg and Miller (1982) indicated that more 3- to 11-year-old boys than girls engaged in risk-taking behavior. The extent to which children expose themselves to unsafe situations may be related to their frequency of accidents. Future studies that examine children's proneness to injury should consider not only psychological characteristics which vary as a function of development but also the extent to which children expose themselves to risk. Knowledge gained from this research would guide pediatric psychologists and other health professionals in identifying children at risk for accidents and in the development of effective intervention programs.

REFERENCES

Baker, S., O'Neill, B., & Karpf, R. (1984). *The injury fact book.* Lexington, MA: D.C. Heath.

Coppens, N. (1985). Cognitive development and locus of control as predictors of preschoolers' understanding of safety and prevention. *Journal of Applied Developmental Psychology, 6,* 43-55.

Drake, D. (1970). Perceptual correlates of impulsive and reflective behavior. *Developmental Psychology, 2,* 202-214.

Duryea, E., & Glover, J. (1982). A review of the research on reflection and impulsivity in children. *Genetic Psychology Monographs, 106*, 217-237.

Faber, R., & Ward, S. (1977). Children's understanding of using products safely. *Journal of Marketing, 41*, 39-46.

Ginsburg, H., & Miller, S. (1982). Sex differences in children's risk-taking behavior. *Child Development, 53*, 426-428.

Gjerde, P., Block, J., & Block, J. H. (1985). Longitudinal consistency of matching familiar figures test performance from early childhood to preadolescence. *Developmental Psychology, 21*, 262-271.

International Children's Centre (1979). *Prevention of child accidents at home.* Paris. (ERIC Document Reproduction Service No. ED 187 479)

Kagan, J., & Kogan, N. (1970). Individual variation in cognitive processes. In P. H., Mussen (Ed.), *Carmichael's manual of child psychology* (Vol. 1, pp. 1273-1365). New York: Wiley.

Kagan, J., Rosman, B., Day, D., Albert, J., & Phillips, W. (1964). Information processing in the child: significance of analytic and reflective attitudes. *Psychological Monographs: General and Applied, 78*(1, Whole No. 578).

Messer, S. (1976). Reflection-impulsivity: a review. *Psychological Bulletin, 83*, 1026-1052.

Piaget, J. (1960). *The child's conception of physical causality.* Paterson, NJ: Littlefield Adams.

Sharp, K. (1982). Preschoolers' understanding of temporal and causal relations. *Merrill-Palmer Quarterly, 28*, 427-436.

Shultz, T., & Mendelson, R. (1975). The use of covariation as a principle of causal analysis. *Child Development, 46*, 394-399.

Siegelman, E. (1969). Reflective and impulsive observing behavior. *Child Development, 40*, 1213-1222.

Siegler R. (1975). Defining the locus of developmental differences in children's causal reasoning. *Journal of Experimental Child Psychology, 20*, 512-525.

Victor, J., Halverson, C., & Montague, R. (1985). Relations between reflection-impulsivity and behavioral impulsivity in preschool children. *Developmental Psychology, 21*, 141-148.

IV

Pain and Distress in Children

Donald K. Routh

University of Miami

Like all of the articles reproduced in this book, the five in the following section were selected because they were considered to be some of the most influential ones published so far in the *Journal of Pediatric Psychology*. That means both that they addressed important themes and that the research they reported had an impact on others. The present chapter attempts to indicate how these papers relate to the previous and subsequent history of research and professional developments in the area of pain and distress. The chapter also considers briefly some of their implications for the future focus of research and practice in pediatric psychology.

BACKGROUND

Let us begin with a definition. What is pain? According to the International Association for the Study of Pain's Subcommittee on Taxonomy (1979), *pain* is best defined as "an unpleasant sensory and emotional experience associated with actual or potential tissue damage, or described in terms of such damage" (p. 249). Thus, pain is essentially seen as a subjective experience, although it has well-known behavioral and physiological components. The above definition of pain applies to children just as it does to adults, although it has proved to be more difficult to appraise the subjective as well as the neurophysiological components of a child's pain. Probably for this reason, research in pediatric psychology has tended to focus on behaviors associated with pain rather than on its subjective or physiological aspects.

Pain inherently involves an affective experience, which can include positive as well as negative components. Compare, for example, the emotions that might be experienced by a woman during the pain of childbirth with those of one suffering equally intense pain resulting from cancer.

Notice also that in some cases pain may be associated with potential rather than actual tissue damage or that it may be only *described* in terms of such damage. In other words, by definition, pain can occur in the absence of any known tissue damage. This is important to keep in mind when thinking about chronic pain syndromes such as phantom limb pain or the phenomena such as headache and recurrent abdominal pain in children. The experience of pain seems to be just as "real" to the individuals involved as when obvious tissue damage is involved.

Distress is a broader term including pain, fear, and other such unpleasant experiences. Part of what all these states have in common is stress. According to Lazarus and Folkman (1984), perhaps the most influential modern authorities on the topic, *stress* can be defined as "a particular relationship between the person and the environment that is appraised by the person as taxing or exceeding his or her resources and endangering his or her well-being" (p. 19). Stress also has well-established physiological concomitants (e.g., Selye, 1936, 1956), notably involving the hypothalamus, the adrenal glands, and arousal of the sympathetic nervous system. Pain and stress are linked in that intense pain or pain associated with high levels of negative affect inevitably involve stress. As was the case for pain, the definition of stress applies to children as well as adults, although it is more difficult to acquire information on children's appraisal of their environments and their psychological coping strategies, that is, the cognitive components of stress. One common example of a stressful situation is public speaking. Brown, O'Keeffe, Sanders, and Baker (1986) studied children's responses to giving a class report and also their experience of going to the dentist. The proportion of subjects engaging in positive coping responses, especially self-talk, in these situations increased with age, as did the number of different coping strategies used. Some children, especially the more anxious ones, tended to "catastrophize" instead. Another example of distress is provided by Peterson and Shigetomi's (1982) finding that for children undergoing a tonsillectomy, the most frequent hospital stressor mentioned by parents was overnight separation of mother and child. Johnson (1986) has written in some detail on the use of life events scales as measures of stress in children and adolescents and discusses a number of possible moderator variables such as social support, locus of control, sensation seeking, and hardiness.

In tracing the history of the study of pain and distress, it might be well to begin by considering the evolutionary history of the phenomena themselves. Pain is presumed to have some biologically adaptive value in that it leads the organism to escape or avoid harmful stimuli. Consider the case of children with congenital insensitivity to pain and how they tend to sustain serious or even life-threatening injuries because of the absence of this protective mechanism (e.g., Dyck et al., 1983). Insofar as pain is adaptive for children, it would be a serious mistake to try to do away with all of it by treatment measures we might devise. Similarly, the stress response exists in a variety of species and also has obvious adaptive value insofar as it prepares the organism physiologically for a "fight or flight" response or other types of coping strategies requiring the expenditure of large amounts of energy (e.g., Selye, 1956). Ross and Ross (1985), in developing curriculum materials about pain for third- and fourth-grade children, found that most children were unaware of the early warning value of pain and also did not realize how it could be used in a maladaptive way. Their instructional program produced a significant increase in such knowledge in these children and also gave them suggestions about handling needle procedures and general coping strategies.

The study of pain is an interdisciplinary field, with important biological underpinnings. Neurophysiologists and psychologists have cooperated in the discovery and description of some of the neurosensory mechanisms underlying pain perception. For example, it is known that there are at least two different neurological components in the peripheral reception of pain, a fast-conducting and a slow-conducting one, subserved by different types of nerve fibers. Analgesic drugs such as aspirin have their effects at this peripheral level at least in part by inhibiting an enzyme called cyclooxygenase (Fields, 1987). There also appears to be a "gate" mechanism within the spinal cord capable of sensitizing a person to pain or inhibiting the reception of pain impulses (Melzack & Wall, 1982). Within the central nervous system there is also a network mediated by endogenous opioid peptides that can selectively inhibit pain. This opioid-mediated analgesic system can be activated by pain, stress, or suggestion and also, of course, by opiate drugs such as morphine (Fields, 1987).

One of the important technical changes within nineteenth-century medicine, from 1846 onward, was the development of effective and relatively safe chemical anesthetics and analgesics which permitted types of surgery that had previously been undreamed of (Pernick, 1985). Anesthesiology continues to make rapid technical progress in using chemical means to control pain. One related topic that is emerging in pediatric psychology concerns factors that affect the postoperative use of analgesic drugs by medical and nursing personnel, for example, the seriousness of a surgical procedure in terms of anticipated sequelae (Bush, Holmbeck, & Cockrell, 1989).

The further elucidation of peripheral and central neurophysiological mechanisms underlying pain and stress is important but for the most part requires invasive research strategies. Therefore, most such research has proceeded with nonhuman animal species rather than with humans. Research seeking linkages between these neurophysiological phenomena and the subjective sensory, affective, or cognitive components of pain, stress, and coping has taken place mostly with adults, who can ethically and legally consent to participate, rather than with children. An example along these lines was set by Boring's (1916) heroic experiment in which he deliberately cut a nerve in his own arm in order to study how cutaneous sensation recovered as the nerve regenerated.

ARTICLES IN THE JOURNAL OF PEDIATRIC PSYCHOLOGY

From the beginnings of their field, pediatric psychologists have been interested in helping children with pain and distress. For example, Wright, Schaefer, and Solomons (1979), in their *Encyclopedia of Pediatric Psychology,* included an eight-page section on pain. This interest probably derived from observations in clinical settings and the realization that psychologists had much to offer to the study of and interventions into children's pain and distress. The *Journal of Pediatric Psychology* from its origins as a newsletter until the present has published a variety of articles on this topic. In the very first volume of the *Journal,* Ack (1976) discussed the importance of correcting children's fantasies and misconceptions about medical experiences and described a program in which mental health staff members were called in if routine preparation procedures for painful medical experiences did not seem adequate. Siegel (1976) reviewed the literature on preparation of children for hospitalization, including giving information, encouraging emotional expression, and building supportive relationships. One of the topics covered in Johnson's (1979) review of mental health interventions with medically ill children was preparation of children for painful medical experiences. Many other articles along these lines will be described as a background for the articles reprinted in this section.

One of the best known studies on children's pain and distress in the general literature appeared shortly before the *Journal of Pediatric Psychology* began, that is, the now classic article by Melamed and Siegel (1975) on preparing children for hospitalization. These authors found that watching a modeling film, "Ethan Has an Operation" (of a child's hernia repair surgery), enabled children 4–12 years old to cope significantly more effectively with hospitalization than did watching a control film entitled "Living Things Are Everywhere." Dependent measures included palmar sweating, hospital-related fears, and behavioral distress as rated by observers blind to the treatment assignment of the children. Melamed was honored for her work by the Research Contribution Award of the Society of Pediatric Psychology in 1991. The first of the articles reprinted in this section of the book, by Melamed, Meyer, Gee, and Soule (1976), "The Influence of Time and Type of Preparation on Children's Adjustment to Hospitalization," was a sequel to the Melamed and Siegel (1975) study mentioned above and in fact used the same film, "Ethan Has an Operation." In the Melamed et al. (1976) study, younger children who viewed the film a week before their own surgery scored higher than children who viewed the film upon admission, at least for the palmar sweating measure. For the older children the reverse was true; that is, the earlier viewing of the film was more effective.

Peterson and Mori (1988), who provide a thorough review of the topic of preparation of children for hospitalization, acknowledge that the Melamed et al. (1976) study is the most widely cited one on the issue of timing of such preventive treatment. They point out, however, that the results of Melamed et al. (1976) need to be taken as tentative until they are confirmed by further research. In fact, this represents Melamed's own view of this study. The study *raised the question* of the importance of the timing of preparation procedures, especially in relation to the age of the child. This question is still under active study, and much more research is needed before it is settled.

In terms of professional developments, Peterson and Ridley-Johnson (1980) surveyed nonchronic care pediatric hospitals in the U.S. and found that 70% of them used some kind of procedures for preparing children for hospitalization. An interdisciplinary organization, the Association for the Care of Children's Health, is involved in trying to maintain standards for the delivery of care in this area. It seems to be an important role of pediatric psychologists to try to coordinate such activities with what the research literature says are the most effective types of preparation. Unfortunately, Azarnoff (1982) found that many of the preventive preparation programs that had been begun in the 1970s were later discontinued. Peterson, Ridley-Johnson, Tracy, and Mullins (1984) therefore felt it to be important to concentrate on *cost-effective* presurgical preparation. This study found puppet modeling to be a particularly efficacious (and relatively inexpensive) component of preparation. A recent trend in medical care is the move toward short-stay and outpatient surgical procedures as a cost-cutting measure. Presurgical preparation needs to be adapted to this change (Atkins, 1987).

One particularly painful experience that some children have to undergo is treatment for burns, which can include daily sessions in the tub and the "debridement" of the child's wounds. Walker and Healy (1980), for example, discussed how the 8-year-old girl they treated would "procrastinate, whine, cry, scream uncontrollably, and kick the nurses during these procedures" (p. 397). Their treatment procedures, by increasing the child's tolerance, successfully reduced the time taken by such sessions from two hours to 30 minutes. Tarnowski, McGrath, Calhoun, and Drabman (1987) in an ingenious single-subject reversal study, found that their patient, a 12-year-old boy, showed significantly less behavioral distress when he was allowed to debride part of his own burn rather than having the physical therapist do it, and he preferred this procedure as well. In a similar single-case report, Dash (1981) described the rapid hypno-behavioral treatment of a needle phobia in a 5-year-old cardiac patient, using in vivo participant modeling.

Nocella and Kaplan (1982) trained children to cope with dental treatment, using a combination of relaxation and self-talk. Children in this study were randomly assigned to receive either this treatment, an attention control group procedure, or no treatment. Treatment was associated with significantly fewer body movements and verbalizations during dental treatment compared to the control groups. One subsequent study published in the *Journal of Pediatric Psychology,* however, did not find psychological preparation (filmed modeling) to be effective in helping children cope with dental treatment (Zachary, Friedlander, Huang, Silberstein, & Leggott, 1985). These investigators speculated that perhaps their subjects had low levels of fear to begin with (cf. Elkins & Roberts, 1985).

One of the most excruciating types of pain experienced by children receiving medical procedures is that associated with bone marrow aspirations and lumbar punctures so often required by children with leukemia. Variations of hypnotic procedures are often used to help these children cope with pain, with mixed results (e.g., Katz, Kellerman, & Ellenberg, 1987). A recent study focusing on bone marrow aspirations revealed some cultural differences in children's reactions: U.S. children showed higher levels of anticipatory distress than children from the Netherlands, though their distress during the procedure itself did not differ from that of the Dutch children (van Aken, van Lieshout, Katz, & Heezen, 1989). The explanation of these differences is not yet apparent.

Many children who undergo painful medical procedures do so in the emergency room or otherwise under circumstances making specific psychological preparation impractical. For these situations, some kind of preventive approach aimed at the general population of children seems to be the only answer. Roberts, Wurtele, Boone, Ginther, and Elkins (1981) pioneered such an approach. Their subjects were ordinary school children attending the second to fifth grades. The experimental condition consisted of a slide and audiotape package featuring coping peer models, while the control condition was a travelogue. A significant reduction in children's self-reported medical fears was found to result from this treatment, with further fear reduction seen at follow-up two weeks later. The children's general trait anxiety was not affected. In a sequel to this study, Elkins and Roberts (1985) compared three different audiovisual procedures designed to prepare children for hospitalization and a control film. In this case the preparations were only successful in decreasing the medical fears of those who had relatively high levels of fear to start with. Children who already had low levels of fear did not benefit significantly. Peterson and Ridley-Johnson (1984) found, to their surprise, that an academic lecture was actually more effective than a filmed model in reducing school children's hospital fears. Psychology students and medical students, however, had judged that such an academic presentation might even have negative effects as a method of preparation (Peterson, Everett, Farmer, Mori, & Chaney, 1988).

Research on the preparation of children for painful medical procedures is beginning to move in a more theoretical direction lately. The work of Karen Smith, who won the 1988 Student Award of the Society of Pediatric Psychology, provided an example of this trend. She and her colleagues (Smith, Ackerson, & Blotcky, 1989) hypothesized that preparation would be more effective if it matched the child's coping style. However, their results came out significantly in the opposite direction than that predicted; that is, children with a "repressive" style reported more pain with a distraction intervention, than with sensory information, while those with a "sensitizer" style reported more pain with a sensory information intervention.

The second research article reproduced in the following section is by Shaw and Routh (1982) and is entitled, "Effect of Mother Presence on Children's Reaction to Aversive Procedures." Shaw and Routh began with the clinical observation that some pediatricians in an emergency room setting preferred to have parents present when carrying out a painful procedure on the child, and others preferred to have the parents absent under these circumstances. Shaw and Routh carried out two experimental studies, one with 18-month-old children and one with 5-year-olds, randomly assigning them to receive routine injections with mother either present or absent. In each study it was found that the children expressed significantly more behavioral distress with the mother present than with the mother absent.

Like the Melamed et al. study, the one by Shaw and Routh did not produce a final answer but proved to be one milestone on the road to such answers. The overall literature is equivocal as to whether parents' presence produces greater or lesser distress than their absence. Nevertheless, Shaw and Routh's basic findings of greater behavioral distress with parent presence were replicated by Gross, Stern, Levin, Dale, and Wojnilower (1983) the next year, albeit with venipuncture rather than injections. More recently, Gonzalez et al. (1989) carried out a similar study of children receiving injections involving physiological and self-report as well as behavioral measures. At least for the older children in this study, parent presence was again associated with more behavioral distress than parent absence. However, when asked for their preference in regard to future injections, 86% of these children said that they would rather have their parents present. These divergent findings can be explained on the hypothesis that children cry more when parents are there because only then can the parents provide effective comforting. One is reminded of the story of the child who skinned his knee, got up, ran all the way home, and only then, when his mother opened the door, began to cry. (What was the point of crying when no parent was present to help?)

Present research has probably moved beyond the question of the effects of mere parent presence or absence to the issue of exactly what parents and other adults do when they are in the room with their child during an aversive medical procedure, and how that relates to their previous history with the child. For example, Blount et al. (1989) coded interactions between children and various adults during bone marrow aspirations and lumbar punctures and found that certain adult behaviors such as humor or nonprocedural talk were associated with low child distress. Other adult behaviors such as reassuring comments were actually associated with high child distress.

Other recent research has suggested that the presence of the parent may be associated with greater communication of other kinds of affect than pain, namely smiling. In two separate studies with infants approximately 18 months old, Jones and Raag (1989) allowed their subjects to see attractive toys. The frequency of smiling by the infants in reaction to these toys was significantly greater if the mother was attentive than if she was reading a magazine. If the mother was inattentive, however, the infant would accept a friendly stranger as the target of such smiling.

The next article reproduced in the following section is by Lollar, Smits, and Patterson (1982) and is entitled, "Assessment of Pediatric Pain: An Empirical Perspective." This study assessed children's *concepts* of pain rather than their actual pain experiences. Lollar et al. (1982) developed the Pediatric Pain Inventory, an instrument with 24 pictures representing potentially pain-evoking situations in four settings: medical, recreational, activities of daily living, and psychosocial. A sample of 240 children and adolescents, ages 4–19 years, responded to the Inventory, rating both the intensity and the duration of pain that would be associated with these situations. Psychometric data were presented on the internal consistency of these measures in the different situations. Significant differences in means were found to be associated with the different situations, with the psychoso-

cial one being notably less intense and also involving pain of shorter duration. A factor analysis was also reported. Lollar et al. (1982) presented
their results with the Pediatric Pain Inventory as preliminary findings, and
hoped that the Inventory might turn out to have some validity for clinical
purposes. A personal communication from Donald Lollar at the time this
chapter was written indicated that indeed some other investigators had used
the Inventory. For example, one unpublished study found a series of significant positive correlations between the Inventory and pain ratings by
nurses of children in a hospital intensive care unit.

To the present author, the most interesting extension of the general
method of Lollar et al. (1982) was a recent paper by Belter, McIntosh,
Finch, and Saylor (1988). They devised their own set of 17 pictures, called
the Charleston Pediatric Pain Pictures, intended to represent either no pain
or low, moderate, or high levels of pain. A sample of 50 preschool children
aged 3 to 6 years then reacted to the pictures with three different self-report pain measures, namely, a faces scale, a pain thermometer, and the
Oucher scale, which has both a numerical scale and one anchored by pho-
tographed facial expressions. This approach was used to demonstrate acceptable levels of test–retest reliability for clusters of picture-items
representing different levels of pain. The three self-report measures of pain
appeared to be comparable in their test–retest reliability. Probably the most
important conclusion of the study was that even these young children were
able to differentiate these basic levels of pain intensity. Thus, there is the
hope that in the future some kind of practical self-report measures of pain
might be devised for children as young as 3 years of age.

The fourth article reproduced in the following section is the paper by
Routh and Ernst (1984) entitled "Somatization Disorder in Relatives of
Children and Adolescents with Functional Abdominal Pain." The problem
of recurrent abdominal pain with no evident medical explanation studied
by this research is very common. It is estimated that 1 out of 10 children
suffer from such unexplained pain at one time or another (Apley, 1975).

Ernst, Routh, and Harper (1984) had approached the issue of recurrent abdominal pain primarily from a genetic standpoint (e.g., Arkonac &
Guze, 1963). Thus, they inquired whether recurrent abdominal pain might
not be a precursor of adult somatization disorder and a part of a psychopathological syndrome involving alcoholism, psychopathy, and somatization
disorder seen in certain families. Indeed, in a chart review study, they found
that children with chronic functional abdominal pain were likely to have
more unfounded physical complaints than children with chronic pain with
a clear organic basis.

Routh and Ernst (1984) extended this study by administering family
interviews to the mothers of 20 children with functional abdominal pain

and 20 children with abdominal pain with an obvious organic basis. The mothers were asked about the psychopathology of all of the child's first- and second-degree relatives. The main finding was that 10 of the 20 children with functional abdominal pain had one or more relatives (most often the mother herself or a grandmother) with somatization disorder, as compared to only 1 out of 20 children with organic pain.

Although a genetic hypothesis provides one way to interpret the above study, one can also take a social learning position (Bandura, 1977) and see the same data as evidence of a modeling effect. This was the approach taken by Osborne, Hatcher, and Richtsmeier (1989) in a *Journal of Pediatric Psychology* sequel to Routh and Ernst's (1984) research. Osborne et al. interviewed 20 children with medically unexplained pain and 20 children with pain due to sickle cell anemia. The children with medically unexplained pain identified significantly more pain models and also more positive consequences of their pain behavior. In this study, many of the identified models were not blood relatives of the children but instead were stepparents, step grandparents, or even classmates. In both the Routh and Ernst (1984) and Osborne et al. (1989) studies, the relatives with pain were more likely to be female than male, which seems consistent with the particular genetic hypothesis espoused by Routh and Ernst. In any event, the genetic and social learning approaches are not incompatible with each other; in fact, both could be correct.

Other researchers, while agreeing with the finding that the mothers of children with recurrent abdominal pain might be role models for the pain, have given greater emphasis to the importance of anxiety and depression, both in the children and in their parents (Walker & Greene, 1989). These investigators also found a high level of anxiety, depression, and somatic complaints among children in their control group with organic abdominal pain. One possibility is that children with recurrent abdominal pain are interpreting their anxiety and depressive symptoms in somatic terms. It is certainly true that some severe emotional pain "hurts" just as much as physical pain, and there is room for confusing the two.

Like recurrent abdominal pain, children's headaches are defined almost entirely in terms of the child's subjective symptoms. Labbé and Williamson (1983) provide an example of a relevant treatment study published in the *Journal of Pediatric Psychology*. Their subjects were three children with migraine headaches who were all given thermal biofeedback training (to produce hand warming). In a multiple baseline design across subjects, all three children increased their skin temperature. Their headaches decreased in frequency immediately after treatment and continued to be infrequent at follow-up two months later. This is a promising study with a small sample that is in need of replication and elaboration to confirm the specific value of the treatment. Larsson, Melin, Lamminen, and Ullstedt (1987) carried out a larger-scale study with 36 high school students in Sweden with chronic headache symptoms. These youngsters were randomly assigned either to a treatment group (self-help relaxation involving audiotapes) or to one of two control groups. The treatment group was superior on all measures, and the effects were even more pronounced at follow-up five months later.

Pediatric psychologists also deal with chronic pain in children of more clearcut organic origin. Walco and Dampier (1987), for example, discuss the problem of "treating chronically ill adolescents who cope poorly with pain and are therefore overly dependent on the medical system" (p. 215). They described a group of 12 "overutilizers" with sickle cell disease who accounted for over one-half of the days of hospitalization in a sample of 260 patients with sickle cell disease. These authors advised the use of a standard protocol to reduce the dependency of such patients upon the hospital and upon analgesics. In managing chronic pain in children, nursing staff evidently much prefer positive reinforcement or self-management interventions to ignoring or pharmacologic interventions (Tarnowski, Gavaghan, & Wisniewski, 1989).

The final study reproduced in the following section is that by Elliott, Jay, and Woody (1987), entitled, "An Observational Scale for Measuring Children's Distress During Medical Procedures." Katz, Kellerman, and Siegel (1980) originally developed a measure known as the Procedure Behavior Rating Scale (PBRS) based on the observation of 13 different pain and stress behaviors of pediatric cancer patients undergoing bone marrow aspirations and lumbar punctures. Jay and Elliott (1984) then developed the Observational Scale of Behavioral Distress (OSBD) as an 11-item revision of the PBRS. The study by Elliott et al. (1987) reprinted here reported a more refined 8-item version of the OSBD based on a larger sample of children ($N = 55$) and a new item analysis. All items of the revised scale met certain criteria of frequency and intercorrelation with other items. Also, the revised (8-item) OSBD was more highly correlated with nurses' ratings of behavioral distress than was the longer version.

As a rationally and empirically based, weighted combination of children's distress behaviors, the OSBD has subsequently proved to be a very convenient measure for other clinicians and researchers to use. The term *behavioral distress* is well chosen, in that the measure appears to tap expressions of fear or separation protest and not just pain (e.g., Gonzalez et al., 1989). The OSBD is especially useful for assessing distress in young children, who often are not able to produce reliable self-report data on their subjective pain experiences. For example, Elliott et al. (1987) found that OSBD scores correlated .51 with self-reported pain in children older than 7 years of age but were not significantly correlated with self-reports of pain in children younger than that. Jay (1988), who summarizes research on children's reactions to invasive medical procedures, notes that OSBD scores are significantly negatively correlated with age, with younger children expressing more distress in response to a particular procedure than older ones. This does not necessarily mean that older children *experience* less pain than younger ones, but only that they are less likely to express their distress openly. Thus, younger children appear to be more dependent on their parents and other people to help them cope with painful situations, while older children and adults rely more on their own resources in trying to cope with pain.

In addition to behavioral distress, it is important that clinicians and researchers attend to the subjective dimension of pain. The standard way of assessing this in adults is with a visual analog scale. Thompson, Varni, and Hanson (1987) demonstrated that this kind of measure, namely, a 10-cm horizontal line with "no pain" and "severe pain" as anchoring phrases at either end, was a reliable way of assessing pain repeatedly in a sample of 23 families with a child with juvenile arthritis. They also successfully used an instrument called the Varni/Thompson Pediatric Pain Questionnaire with this population.

FUTURE IMPLICATIONS

In summary, the *Journal of Pediatric Psychology* has clearly published some important papers on measuring subjective pain, on observing children's behavioral distress, on the effects of parent presence, on preparing children for hospitalization, and on social factors important in unexplained pain in children. Much further work is needed along all of these lines. From a practical standpoint, the most pressing issues seem to be those related to preparing children and their families to cope with various aversive medical experiences and devising effective clinical protocols for the treatment of unexplained pain in children. Research on some of these practical issues, such as helping children cope with burns, dental treatment, and recurrent abdominal pain is summarized elsewhere (Miller, Elliott, Funk, & Pruitt, 1988; Routh, Ernst, & Harper, 1988; Siegel, 1988).

Although, as noted above, all of the reprinted papers have made some measurable impact on subsequent research in the field and no doubt on clinical work, they are collectively noteworthy for their neglect of the physiological aspects of pain. Thus, none of the articles dealt with the pain associated with particular disease entities (e.g., sickle cell disease), with the psychophysiological or biochemical aspects of the pain experience, or with the behavioral aspects of chemical analgesia. Perhaps in the future the *Journal* will include some notable articles on the psychobiology of pain in children.

REFERENCES

Ack, M. (1976). New perspectives in comprehensive health care for children. *Journal of Pediatric Psychology, 1,* 9–11.

Apley, J. (1975). *The child with abdominal pain* (2nd ed.). Oxford: Blackwell Scientific Publications.

Arkonac, O., & Guze, S. B. (1963). A family study of hysteria. *New England Journal of Medicine, 268,* 239–242.

Atkins, D. M. (1987). Evaluation of pediatric preparation program for short-stay surgical patients. *Journal of Pediatric Psychology, 12,* 285–290.

Azarnoff, P. (1982). Hospital tours for school children ended. *Pediatric Mental Health, 1(4),* 2.

Bandura, A. (1977). *Social learning theory.* Englewood Cliffs, NJ: Prentice-Hall.

Belter, R. W., McIntosh, J. A., Finch, A. J., Jr., & Saylor, C. F. (1988). Preschoolers' ability to differentiate levels of pain: Relative efficacy of three self-report measures. *Journal of Clinical Child Psychology, 17,* 329–335.

Blount, R. L., Corbin, S. M., Sturges, J. W., Wolfe, V. V., Prater, J. M., & James, L. D. (1989). The relationship between adults' behavior and child coping and distress during BMA/LP procedures: A sequential analysis. *Behavior Therapy, 20,* 585–601.

Boring, E. G. (1916). Cutaneous sensation after nerve-division. *Quarterly Journal of Experimental Physiology, 10,* 1–95.

Brown, J. M., O'Keeffe, J., Sanders, S. H., & Baker, B. (1986). Developmental changes in children's cognition of stressful and painful situations. *Journal of Pediatric Psychology, 11,* 343–357.

Bush, J. P., Holmbeck, G. N., & Cockrell, J. L. (1989). Patterns of PRN analgesic drug administration in children following elective surgery. *Journal of Pediatric Psychology, 14,* 433–448.

Dash, J. (1981). Rapid hypno-behavioral treatment of a needle phobia in a five-year-old cardiac patient. *Journal of Pediatric Psychology, 6,* 37–42.

Dyck, P. J., Mellinger, J. F., Reagan, T. J., Horowitz, S. J., McDonald, J. W., Litchy, W. J., Daube, J. R., Fealey, R. D., Go, V. L., Kao, P. C., Brimijoin, W. S., & Lambert, E. H. (1983). Not 'indifference to pain' but varieties of hereditary sensory and autonomic neuropathy. *Brain, 106,* 373–390.

Elkins, P. D., & Roberts, M. C. (1985). Reducing medical fears in a general population of children: A comparison of three audiovisual modeling procedures. *Journal of Pediatric Psychology, 10,* 65–75.

Elliott, C. H., Jay, S. M., & Woody, P. (1987). An observational scale for measuring children's distress during medical procedures. *Journal of Pediatric Psychology, 12,* 543–551.

Ernst, A. R., Routh, D. K., & Harper, D. C. (1984). Abdominal pain in children and symptoms of somatization disorder. *Journal of Pediatric Psychology, 9,* 77–86.

Fields, H. L. (1987). *Pain.* New York: McGraw-Hill.

Gonzalez, J. C., Routh, D. K., Saab, P. G., Armstrong, F. D., Shifman, L., Guerra, E., & Fawcett, N. (1989). Effects of parent presence on children's reactions to injections: Behavioral, physiological, and subjective aspects. *Journal of Pediatric Psychology, 14,* 449–462.

Gross, A. M., Stern, R. M., Levin, R. B., Dale, J., & Wojnilower, D. A. (1983). The effect of mother–child separation on the behavior of children experiencing a diagnostic medical procedure. *Journal of Consulting and Clinical Psychology, 51,* 783–785.

International Association for the Study of Pain, Subcommittee on Taxonomy. (1979). Pain terms: A list with definitions and notes on usage. *Pain, 6,* 249.

Jay, S. M. (1988). Invasive medical procedures. In D. K. Routh (Ed.), *Handbook of pediatric psychology* (pp. 401–425). New York: Guilford Press.

Jay, S. M., & Elliott, C. H. (1984). Behavioral observation scales for measuring children's distress: The effects of increased methodological rigor. *Journal of Consulting and Clinical Psychology, 52,* 1106–1107.

Johnson, J. H. (1986). *Life events as stressors in childhood and adolescence.* Beverly Hills: Sage.

Johnson, M. R. (1979). Mental health interventions with medically ill children: A review of the literature 1970–1977. *Journal of Pediatric Psychology, 4,* 147–164.

Jones, S. S., & Raag, T. (1989). Smile production in older infants: The importance of a social recipient for the facial signal. *Child Development, 60,* 811–818.

Katz, E. R., Kellerman, J., & Ellenberg, L. (1987). Hypnosis in the reduction of acute pain and distress in children. *Journal of Pediatric Psychology, 12,* 379–394.

Katz, E. R., Kellerman, J., & Siegel, S. E. (1980). Behavioral distress in children undergoing medical procedures: Developmental considerations. *Journal of Consulting and Clinical Psychology, 48,* 356–365.

Labbé, E. E., & Williamson, D. A. (1983). Temperature biofeedback in the treatment of children with migraine headaches. *Journal of Pediatric Psychology, 8,* 317–326.

Larsson, B., Melin, L., Lamminen, M., & Ullstedt, F. (1987). A school-based treatment of chronic headache in adolescents. *Journal of Pediatric Psychology, 12,* 553–566.

Lazarus, R. S., & Folkman, S. (1984). *Stress, appraisal, and coping.* New York: Springer.

Lollar, D. J., Smits, S. J., & Patterson, D. L. (1982). Assessment of pediatric pain: An empirical perspective. *Journal of Pediatric Psychology, 7,* 267–277.

Melamed, B. G., Meyer, R., Gee, C., & Soule, L. (1976). The influence of time and type of preparation on children's adjustment to hospitalization. *Journal of Pediatric Psychology, 1,* 31–37.

Melamed, B. G., & Siegel, L. J. (1975). Reduction of anxiety in children facing hospitalization and surgery by filmed modeling. *Journal of Consulting and Clinical Psychology, 43,* 511–521.

Melzack, R., & Wall, P. D. (1982). *The challenge of pain.* New York: Basic Books.

Miller, M. D., Elliott, C. H., Funk, M., & Pruitt, S. D. (1988). Implications of children's burn injuries. In D. K. Routh (Ed.), *Handbook of pediatric psychology* (pp. 426–447). New York: Guilford Press.

Nocella, J., & Kaplan, R. M. (1982). Training children to cope with dental treatment. *Journal of Pediatric Psychology, 7,* 175–178.

Osborne, R. B., Hatcher, J. W., & Richtsmeier, A. J. (1989). The role of social modeling in unexplained pediatric pain. *Journal of Pediatric Psychology, 14,* 43–61.

Pernick, M. S. (1985). *A calculus of suffering: Pain, professionalism, and anesthesia in nineteenth-century America.* New York: Columbia University Press.

Peterson, L., Everett, K., Farmer, J., Mori, L., & Chaney, J. (1988). Perceived effectiveness of children's preparation for a stressful medical event. *Journal of Pediatric Psychology, 13,* 23–32.

Peterson, L. J., & Mori, L. (1988). Preparation for hospitalization. In D. K. Routh (Ed.), *Handbook of pediatric psychology* (pp. 460–491). New York: Guilford Press.

Peterson, L. J., & Ridley-Johnson, R. (1980). Pediatric hospital response to survey on prehospital preparation for children. *Journal of Pediatric Psychology, 5,* 1–7.

Peterson, L., & Ridley-Johnson, R. (1984). Preparation of well children in the classroom: An unexpected contrast between academic lecture and filmed modeling methods. *Journal of Pediatric Psychology, 9,* 349–361.

Peterson, L., Ridley-Johnson, R., Tracy, K., & Mullins, L. L. (1984). Developing cost-effective presurgical preparation: A comparative analysis. *Journal of Pediatric Psychology, 9,* 439–455.

Peterson, L., & Shigetomi, C. (1982). One-year follow-up of elective surgery child patients receiving preoperative preparation. *Journal of Pediatric Psychology, 7,* 43–48.

Roberts, M. C., Wurtele, S. K., Boone, K. R., Ginther, L. J., & Elkins, P. D. (1981). Reduction of medical fears by use of modeling: A preventive application in a general population. *Journal of Pediatric Psychology, 6,* 293–300.

Ross, D. M., & Ross, S. A. (1985). Pain instruction with third- and fourth-grade children: A pilot study. *Journal of Pediatric Psychology, 10,* 55–63.

Routh, D. K., & Ernst, A. R. (1984). Somatization disorder in relatives of children and adolescents with functional abdominal pain. *Journal of Pediatric Psychology, 9,* 427–437.

Routh, D. K., Ernst, A. R., & Harper, D. C. (1988). Recurrent abdominal pain in children and somatization disorder. In D. K. Routh (Ed.), *Handbook of pediatric psychology* (pp. 492–504). New York: Guilford Press.

Selye, H. (1936). A syndrome produced by diverse nocuous agents. *Nature, 138,* 32.

Selye, H. (1956). *The stress of life.* New York: McGraw-Hill.

Shaw, E. G., & Routh, D. K. (1982). Effect of mother presence on children's reaction to aversive procedures. *Journal of Pediatric Psychology, 7,* 33–42.

Siegel, L. J. (1976). Preparation of children for hospitalization: A selected review of the research literature. *Journal of Pediatric Psychology, 1,* 26–30.

Siegel, L. (1988). Dental treatment. In D. K. Routh (Ed.), *Handbook of pediatric psychology* (pp. 448–459). New York: Guilford Press.

Smith, K. E., Ackerson, J. D., & Blotcky, A. D. (1989). Reducing distress during invasive medical procedures: Relating behavioral interventions to preferred coping style in pediatric cancer patients. *Journal of Pediatric Psychology, 14,* 405–420.

Tarnowski, K. J., Gavaghan, M. P., & Wisniewski, J. J. (1989). Acceptability of intervention for pediatric pain management. *Journal of Pediatric Psychology, 14,* 463–472.

Tarnowski, K. J., McGrath, M. L., Calhoun, M. B., & Drabman, R. S. (1987). Pediatric burn injury: Self- versus therapist-mediated debridement. *Journal of Pediatric Psychology, 12,* 567–579.

Thompson, K. L., Varni, J. W., & Hanson, V. (1987). Comprehensive assessment of pain in juvenile rheumatoid arthritis: An empirical model. *Journal of Pediatric Psychology, 12,* 241–255.

van Aken, M. A. G., van Lieshout, C. F. M., Katz, E. R., & Heezen, T. J. M. (1989). Development of behavioral distress in reaction to acute pain in two cultures. *Journal of Pediatric Psychology, 14,* 421–432.

Walco, G. A., & Dampier, C. D. (1987). Chronic pain in adolescent patients. *Journal of Pediatric Psychology, 12,* 215–225.

Walker, L. J. S., & Healy, M. (1980). Psychological treatment of a burned child. *Journal of Pediatric Psychology, 5,* 395–404.

Walker, L. S., & Greene, J. W. (1989). Children with recurrent abdominal pain and their parents: More somatic complaints, anxiety, and depression than other patient families? *Journal of Pediatric Psychology, 14,* 231–243.

Wright, L., Schaefer, A. B., & Solomons, G. (1979). *Encyclopedia of pediatric psychology.* Baltimore: University Park Press.

Zachary, R. A., Friedlander, S., Huang, L. N., Silberstein, S., & Leggott, P. (1985). Effects of stress-relevant/irrelevant filmed modeling on children's response to dental treatment. *Journal of Pediatric Psychology, 10,* 383–401.

13

The Influence of Time and Type of Preparation on Children's Adjustment to Hospitalization

Barbara G. Melamed, Raymond Meyer, Carol Gee, and Lisa Soule

Case Western Reserve University

Previous research has demonstrated the effectiveness of filmed peer models undergoing preoperative preparation on the presurgical anxiety reduction of children about to undergo their first hospital experience (Melamed & Siegel, 1975; Vernon & Bailey, 1974). Current interest focused on defining the critical variables determining appropriate timing and type of preparation. The age of the child has been isolated as a theoretically meaningful variable. Most authors believe that older children may benefit from a longer interval between preparation and the occurrence of the procedure. Heller (1967) also suggested that older children need a more lengthy and detailed preparation. Mellish (1969) felt that younger children need only a few days of preparation since longer intervals may only increase their anticipatory anxiety. However, the ideal time has never been subjected to systematic research efforts. Robertson (1958) feels that preparation should begin no

This research project was conducted at Rainbow Babies' and Children's Hospital, Cleveland. The cooperation of Dr. Izant, Jr., Dr. Crumrine, Dr. Filston, Dr. Persky, Dr. Maloney, and Dr. Kursh made this project possible. Appreciation is especially expressed to Dr. Dennis Drotar and Dr. Ann Godfrey, Miss Zemaityte, and Mrs. Wolkov for facilitating the hospital's support. The nurses, childlife workers, and children of the pediatric surgery division enabled the investigation to be carried out. John Zdencanovic and Russ Freed assisted in data collection. The efforts of Dr. Detterman in computer analysis are recognized. Ethan Stein and his family, along with the staff of the Health Sciences Communications Center, made the film possible. The initial funding for the project was provided by the Cleveland Foundation, and the National Institute of Dental Research grant number 04243 has provided financial support.

Originally published in *Journal of Pediatric Psychology, 1*(4)(1976):31–37.

sooner than one week prior to admission, whereas Dimock (1960) recommended that preparation for all children should begin one to three weeks prior to admission. In an attempt to derive more concrete evidence to support the need for early preparation, half the children in this study viewed a preparatory film one week prior to their hospital admission, whereas the other children viewed it immediately preceding their admission to the pediatric ward the day before surgery.

A second point of interest was whether the film by itself without additional preoperative preparation would replicate the findings of the earlier study in which filmed preparation was combined with in-hospital preoperative teaching.

A third point of interest was whether the film effects would be more potent in children with more similar characteristics in common with the peer model.

METHOD

Subjects

The subjects were 48 children between the ages of 4 and 12 years who were admitted for elective surgery at Rainbow Babies' and Children's Hospital, Cleveland, Ohio. None had ever before been hospitalized. Subjects were selected from the Division of Pediatric Surgery, and had been admitted for tonsillectomies, hernia, or genital-urinary tract surgery. Length of hospital stay ranged from 2-4 days.

Subjects were assigned to one of two groups. One group saw the film the day of admission to the hospital, the other saw the film 6-9 days prior to admission. In each of these groups, one-half of the subjects were assigned to a condition in which they received minimal preoperative preparation and instruction from the hospital staff. The other half received standard preoperative preparation. Group assignment was conducted so as to counterbalance the groups for age, sex, race, and type of surgery (see Table I).

Measures of Anxiety

Seven measures of the child's emotional behavior were employed, in order to assess the various response classes indicative of anxiety. Two of these indices were designed to measure "trait" or chronic anxiety levels:

Table I. Sample Characteristics of Groups

Variable	IA	IB	IIA	IIB
Age in months				
Mean	96.00	89.83	78.42	87.50
SD	31.94	22.32	19.00	24.47
Sex				
Female	6	5	6	8
Male	6	7	6	4
Race				
Black	6	5	5	5
White	6	7	7	7
Service (Type of Operation)				
Hernia	5	7	4	7
Tonsillectomy	4	2	3	2
Urinary genital tract	3	3	5	3
No. mothers staying overnight	3	6	7	8
Type of Patient				
Private	5	7	8	10
Staff	7	5	4	2

the Anxiety Scale of the Personality Inventory for Children, and the Children's Manifest Anxiety Scale (CMAS). The Palmar Sweat Index (PSI), the Hospital Fears Rating Scale, and the Observer Rating Scale of Anxiety were used to measure "state" or situational anxiety. In addition, the Behavior Problem Checklist was used to assess the child's emotional and behavioral adjustment, and the Parent's Questionnaire was used to measure maternal anxiety related to the child's hospitalization.

The Anxiety Scale of the Personality Inventory for Children consists of 30 items which were derived from the Personality Inventory for Children (Wirt & Broen, 1958). These statements, which the mother rated as true or false about her child, are intended to measure chronic, stable anxiety.

The CMAS has 52 items which measure self-reported anxiety. The child responds yes or no to each statement read by the experimenter, as it applies to himself or herself. Total score is determined by the number of yeses on 42 of the items. The other 10 items are used to indicate a tendency to falsify answers.

The PSI (Thomson & Sutarman, 1953; Johnson & Dabbs, 1967) is a method of taking plastic impressions of the active sweat glands of the fingers. Since the sweat glands are primarily affected by emotion rather than temperature, the number of active sweat glands can be used as a measure of transitory physiological arousal. The PSI was recorded from the child's right index finger.

The Hospital Fears Scale has a total of 25 items, and is a self-report measure. Eight items are from the Medical Fears Subscale, factor analyzed from the Fear Survey Schedule for Children (Scherer & Nakamura, 1968). Another 8 items with face validity for assessing hospital fears were also included, as were 9 non-related filler items. Each subject rated his fear to the item read by the experimenter on a "fear thermometer" ranging from 1 (not afraid at all) to 5 (very afraid). The numerical total on the 16 medical fear scores determined the total score.

The Observer Rating Scale was the final measure of state anxiety. It is composed of 29 categories of verbal and skeletal-motor behaviors believed to be manifestations of anxiety. Examples of these are crying, talking about going home, stereotyped, repetitive behavior, etc. An observer marked at 3 minute intervals whether each behavior occurred during a 9-minute observation period. This measure was scored by totalling the number of anxiety-related behaviors in the 9-minute period. Inter-rater reliabilities gathered before and during data collection exceeded 94%. They were calculated by dividing the number of agreements by the total number of categories during the 9-minute period.

The Behavior Problem Checklist contained 55 behavior problems frequently observed in children (Peterson, 1961; Peterson et al., 1961), and was used to assess the effects of hospitalization on the child's emotional and behavioral adjustment. Both conduct and personality items were rated by the child's mother as 0 (no problem), 1 (mild problem), or 2 (severe problem).

The Parent's Questionnaire was used to obtain a global measure of maternal anxiety related to the child's hospitalization. The mother rated, on a 1-5 scale, ten statements about her own anxiety about being a hospital patient, her child's past reactions to medical procedures, and her expectations as to how her child would react to the hospitalization.

Procedure

Subjects in Group I reported to Rainbow Babies' and Children's Hospital one hour prior to their scheduled admission time. They were escorted to the research laboratory in another building. Subjects in Group II reported to the research building, in order to avoid the possible desensitizing effect of seeing the hospital lobby, 6-9 days prior to their scheduled admission date. They were then escorted downstairs to the lab.

In both groups, the parents and child were separated once they entered the lab, and were taken to adjoining rooms. The parents were questioned about the child's age and grade, whether he was on any medication, whether any siblings had been hospitalized, and whether the mother was planning to stay overnight in the hospital with the child. The research procedure was explained to the parents, and they signed a consent form in accordance with the approval granted by the University Hospital Human Subjects Review Committee. At this time, also, the mother filled out the Parent's Questionnaire, the Behavior Problem Checklist, and the Anxiety Scale of the Personality Inventory for Children.

The child was taken to another room by an experimenter in a white coat who introduced himself as "Dr." to the child. Mothers of reluctant youngsters were allowed to stay with the child until he was comfortable. The "Dr." seated the child, and placed electrodes on the child's chest and left arm, explaining that these would enable him to listen to the child's heart during the film. These electrodes recorded heart rate and Galvanic Skin Response (GSR), as well as providing a sample of behavior in a situation which resembled actual hospital procedures to be encountered by the child. The "Dr." left the room after this, and another experimenter began rating the child on the Observer Rating Scale. At this point, a third experimenter entered, and administered the CMAS, the Hospital Fears Rating Scale, and the PSI, in that order.

Following this, the observer left the room, and the experimenter remained with the child in the darkened room for a three-minute rest period, in which baseline physiological data were collected on the polygraph. At the end of three minutes, the subject was shown a videotape of *Ethan Has an Operation.*

This videotape is a 16-minute-long film depicting a 7-year-old white male entering the hospital, for his first time, for a hernia operation. There are 15 scenes which portray various events which confront a hospitalized child, from admission to discharge. In some scenes, hospital personnel explain the medical procedures going on, such as the blood test, and some scenes are narrated by Ethan, who describes his feelings and fears about the situation. Both his narration and behavior typify a coping model—i.e., he acknowledges his initial anxiety but is able to overcome this and deal with the situation in a nonanxious manner. The coping model has been shown to result in greater reduction of anxiety in the observer than mastery models, who show no fear (Meichenbaum, 1971).

Immediately following the film, the observer returned to the room, and proceeded to observe S for another 9-minute period. The experimenter took the child's PSI, and then readministered the Hospital Fears Scale. The child and his parents were then reunited and escorted from the lab. Children in Group II went home with their parents, while children in Group I were taken to the admitting desk of the hospital, and admission procedures were begun.

Children in Group II were seen again immediately before admission. The procedure was identical to the Prefilm session except that the film was not seen, and the Observer Rating Scale, the PSI, and the Hospital Fears Scale were administered only once. Following this, the child was admitted to the hospital. Once hospitalized, no differentiation was made between children on the basis of the time the film had been seen.

At the time each child was admitted, a marker was placed next to his name on the nurses' population board, indicating to which preparation group the child had been assigned. Children in Group B received standard preparation that afternoon and evening. This included the use of picture books, display of anesthesia and surgeons' masks, and often an explanatory visit by the surgeon and/or anesthesiologist. Children in Group A did not receive preparation with general materials such as the book or the masks. In both cases, information specific to the child's case was given. A preoperative Teaching Communications Sheet was filled out by the nursing staff on each child to record exactly what preparation had been given.

After supper and appropriate preparation were concluded, two experimenters again assessed the child in his room. At this time, one experimenter observed the child, while the second experimenter administered the PSI and the Hospital Fears Scale. A game about surgery, "Operation," was played with all children during the last few minutes of the observation.

All children returned to the hospital for a check-up by the doctor an average of 3-5 weeks after surgery. At this time, the child was seen immediately before his appointment with the doctor by two experimenters. Again, the child was observed for 9 minutes, and the PSI, the CMAS, and the Hospital Fears Scale were administered. During this time, the mother was in another room, filling out the Anxiety Scale from the Personality Inventory for Children, and the Behavior Problem Checklist. She was instructed to rate the child's behavior since leaving the hospital.

Assessment during the preoperative medical procedures and the morning of surgery would have been ideal, but was not possible due to the wide variation in time that these events occurred. However, the nursing staff in the operating room did complete a form indicating the child's anxiety and cooperativeness upon arrival in the operating room. In addition, a Global Postoperative Recovery Scale was completed by the floor nurses, in order to assess the effect of immediate recovery from surgery.

Design

A repeated measures analysis of variance was used to evaluate the main effects of time of preparation, type of preparation, time of assessment and interactions between these variables. Trait measures of anxiety, including the Childrens' Manifest Anxiety Scale, the Anxiety Scale of the Personality Inventory for Children, and the Behavior Problem Checklist, were analyzed at prefilm and postoperative assessments. The measures of situational anxiety, including the Palmar Sweat Index, the Hospital Fears Rating Scale, and the Observer Rating Scale of Anxiety, were assessed at: 1. *prefilm* while the child was being hooked-up to the polygraph; 2. *post-film* immediately after the viewing of the film; 3. *pre-operatively* the night prior to surgery after preoperative preparation had been completed for those subjects assigned to standard inhospital preparation; and 4. *postoperatively* immediately before the surgeon's follow-up examination which took place 3-5 weeks following discharge. It should be noted that children who saw the film one week in advance had an extra measurement at preadmission time and the results of any significant tests between prefilm assessment and preadmission time were reported.

The attempt at counterbalancing did not yield equal cell frequencies of younger and older males and females in order to include age, sex, and race within the repeated measures analyses. Therefore, multiple t-tests were performed in those comparisons pertinent to the hypotheses. Two-tailed critical values which obtained an alpha level of at least $p < .05$ were used in reporting these effects.

RESULTS

Trait Anxiety Measures

The Children's Manifest Anxiety Scale revealed a significant reduction in overall anxiety from prefilm to postoperative assessment $F (1, 44) = 13.03, p < .001$. The group viewing the film one week in advance reported considerably less anxiety when arriving for hospital admission than they did prior to seeing the film six to nine days in advance of their hospital admission $t(23) = 2.63, p < .05$. The group coming for admission and not yet seeing the film showed significantly more anxiety at that time than the group that had seen the film one week before (Group × Time) $F (1, 44) = 4.42, p < .05$.

Subsequent t-tests revealed that black children reported greater manifest anxiety than white children at both prefilm and postoperative assessments $t(46) = 2.62, p < .05$ both. These racial differences were already significant a week in advance at the prefilm assessment $t(22) = 2.50$,

$p < .05$. This also achieved significance at preadmission $t(22) = 2.25$, $p < .05$ and at the postoperative assessment $t(22) = 3.40, p < .05$.

The Anxiety Scale of the Personality Inventory for Children revealed a significant Group × Type of Preparation effect. The group who viewed the film one week in advance reported the lowest anxiety when they also received standard preparation during their hospital stay. The group who viewed the film at the time of admission exhibited the highest overall ratings of anxiety when this was combined with standard preparation in the hospital. There were prefilm differences with mothers reporting lower anxiety in boys than in girls $t(46) = 3.27, p < .005$. This finding remained at the postoperative assessment $t(46) = 2.34, p < .05$ and may simply reflect a bias in social desirability as influencing mothers' reports.

The Behavior Problems Checklist yielded a significant overall reduction in the severity of behavior problems reported by parents from prehospital to posthospital assessment F (1, 44) = 4.12, $p < .05$. The age and sex differences revealed that the significant reduction in posthospital behavior problems was greater for older children viewing the film one week in advance as compared with older children who viewed the film on the day of admission $t(23) = 3.05, p < .01$. In addition, boys viewing the film at the time of admission regardless of age, showed fewer behavior problems than girls at the posthospital assessment $t(22) = 3.08, p < .01$. For boys there was no significant difference in severity of behavior problems regardless of whether after viewing the film they received minimal or standard preoperative preparation. However, within the immediate film group receiving standard preoperative preparation, boys did show significantly fewer posthospital behavior problems than girls $t(10) = 2.45, p < .05$. Further, when racial differences were examined, of those who had seen the film one week prior to hospitalization, white children showed fewer behavior problems than blacks at the time of actual admission $t(22) = 2.26, p < .05$.

The Parents Questionnaire did not reveal any initial differences between groups.

Situational Anxiety Measures

Palmar Sweat Index. There were no significant main effects on this measure of physiological arousal. When the data were analyzed for preoperative and postoperative assessments alone, there was a significant interaction between the time of preparation and the type of preparation. The children who viewed the film on the day of admission showed lower palmar sweat arousal when they also received standard preparation in the hospital, whereas the children viewing the film one week in advance showed least anxiety when minimal inhospital preparation followed.

It appears that age and sex differences account for many of the significant results obtained on the Palmer Sweat Index. Younger children in the immediate preparation group showed less arousal than older children in this same group at the postoperative assessment $t(22) = 2.50, p < .05$. The immediate preparation group that had standard preparation during their hospital stay revealed less arousal in younger children at the postoperative assessment than in the older children $t(10) = 2.46, p < .05$. Since there were initial prefilm differences in the minimal preparation group when age is evaluated with older children having greater arousal than younger children $t(22) = 2.45, p < .05$, the effect of the post-film assessment $t(22) = 2.67, p < .05$ becomes difficult to interpret. Younger children who viewed the film one week in advance had higher arousal than younger children seeing the film at admission at the postop assessment $t(21) = 2.07, p < .06$.

As for sex differences, the only significant t-test revealed that males in the week in advance group had lower arousal than females immediately after seeing the film $t(10) = 3.55, p < .005$. There were initial prefilm differences in arousal level with blacks in the immediate preparation group having lower arousal than whites $t(22) = 2.64, p < .05$; whereas the reverse trend was noted in the week in advance group with whites having lower scores than blacks $t(22) = 2.85, p < .01$.

Hospital Fears Rating Scale. There was a significant reduction in reported medical concerns across time of measurement $F(3,132) = 3.34$, $p < .02$. The greatest reduction occurred from prefilm to postoperative assessment (Tukey $q = 3.87$). There was also a significant reduction in ratings from prefilm to postfilm $t(46) = 20.47, p < .001$. No effects of time or type of preparation resulted on this measure.

As in previous research employing this scale (Melamed & Siegel, 1975) younger children reported more medical concerns. This difference obtained significance at the postoperative assessment $t(46) = 3.48$, $p < .001$. When the groups were further subdivided by age the younger children in the immediate preparation group showed more medical concerns than older children preoperative $t(22) = 2.38, p < .05$ and postoperative assessments $t(22) = 4.06, p < .001$. The immediate preparation group receiving standard preparation had a significant age effect with younger children reporting more concern than older at preop $t(10) = 2.23, p < .05$ and postop $t(10) = 3.85, p < .005$. In the minimal preparation group at the postoperative assessment younger children had higher medical concerns than older children $t(22) = 2.14, p < .05$. Younger children in the standard preparation group also reported more medical concerns than older children at the postoperative evaluation $t(22) = 2.79, p < .05$.

Black children reported more medical concerns on this measure than whites at all measurement times. These differences, however, were already in effect at the prefilm measurement $t(46) = 2.17, p < .05$ and cannot be attributed to differential effectiveness of the film.

Observer Rating Scale of Anxiety. There was a significant main effect of time of measurement F (3, 132) $= 15.48, p < .001$. Subsequent Tukeys tests revealed that the preoperative mean was significantly lower than prefilm ($q = 6.47$), post-film ($q = 4.97$), and postoperative ($q = 9.37$). The post-film rating was significantly lower than the post-operative rating ($q = 3.19$). The children who came one week in advance of actual hospitalization were rated as significantly more anxious prefilm than those who were observed at the time of admission prior to seeing the film. Group F (1,44) $= 6.51, p < .02$ and Group × Time F (1,44) $= 4.08, p < .05$).

When age effects were examined, older children in Group II had higher ratings of prefilm anxiety when they saw the film in advance than older children who saw it at the time of admission $t(23) = 2.82, p < .01$.

When sex was taken into account the boys in the week in advance group were rated as less anxious than the girls at preadmission $t(22) = 2.51, p < .05$. By preoperative assessment only the minimal preparation condition showed this effect for sex differences with the boys who had seen the film one week in advance being rated as less anxious than the girls of that same group $t(10) = 2.65, p < .05$.

There were no prefilm differences attributed to race. Immediately after viewing the film (postfilm $t(46) = 2.86, p < .01$) whites were rated as significantly less anxious than blacks. This was maintained at the preoperative assessment $t(46) = 2.03, p < .05$.

DISCUSSION

Effectiveness of Filmed Preparation of Children for Surgery

The results provided a partial replication of previous research (Melamed & Siegel, 1975) which showed a reduction of anxiety in children undergoing elective surgery on a variety of behavioral, physiological and self-reported measures after viewing the film *Ethan Has an Operation.* In the current investigation the reduction of self-reported medical concerns and the decrease in the independent observers' ratings of the childrens' anxiety level after viewing the film, preoperatively and at the postoperative assessment, were consistent with the original findings. In addition, children who had seen the film in this study showed a significant reduction on severity of behavior problems from prehospital to posthospital assessment. The degree of chronic anxiety measured on the Childrens Manifest Anxiety Scale had also been reduced significantly after the hospitalization. In fact, children who had seen the film one week in advance of their actual admission were less anxious on this measure at the time of their admission than they had been a week before.

Can the Film Be Shown Even with Minimal Inhospital Preparation?

The lack of significant group differences between children receiving minimal as opposed to more extensive preoperative preparation is supportive of the potency of the film's effectiveness in preparing children for hospitalization and surgery even where high patient/staff ratios do not allow for individual attention. The only significant interactions between time of film preparation and type of inhospital preparation occurred on the Anxiety Scale of the Personality Inventory for Children and the Palmar Sweat Index. These results, until replicated, can only be taken as tentative findings.

On the indicator of Anxiety as reported by the parents, the children viewing the film one week in advance had less anxiety if they also received the standard preoperative preparation in the hospital. If the film was shown at the time of admission, the children who did not receive further preoperative preparation due to assignment to the minimal preparation group, were rated by their mothers as less anxious on the Personality Inventory for Children.

In terms of situational anxiety as assessed by the PSI, the children who had seen the film on the day of admission showed lower arousal when they also had standard preoperative preparation, whereas those who had been shown the film one week in advance of admission came in to the hospital less aroused and showed least overall arousal when only minimal preparation was offered. This would be consistent with previous results (Melamed & Siegel, 1975) that showed that children seeing the film at admissions showed an increase in postfilm arousal followed by a reduction preoperatively. That group combined film viewing and standard preparation. It would be premature to speculate on the effectiveness of seeing the film a week in advance without a control group who came to view an unrelated film one week in advance and then had minimal inhospital preparation.

Is There an Advantage to Having Children Receive Film Preparation One Week in Advance of Their Hospitalization?

This question cannot be addressed without examining the age, sex and racial differences. Although there were no main effects of time of preparation on any of the dependent variables, when age is examined the findings yield several group effects. Unfortunately our counterbalancing resulted in too few older males in the week-in-advance group to include age as a main factor in the repeated measures analysis. The results of the multiple t-tests performed on specific expected results revealed that older children who viewed the film one week in advance had fewer behavior problems after their hospital experience than older children who viewed the film at the time of admission. In addition, mothers reported fewer behavior problems for white children who had seen the film one week in advance than for blacks at the time of admission to the hospital. All children who had been given the opportunity to see the film one week in advance reported less chronic anxiety at the time of admission. Boys in the group prepared by seeing the film 6 to 9 days before hospital admission were rated as less anxious at admission than girls who had been given this opportunity. This lends credence to the idea that the results were more likely due to the effect of the film, rather than the desensitizing effect of coming to the hospital area in advance. The advantage appears specific to observers most similar to the peer model. Efforts had been made to minimize the familiarization effect by having the group receiving film preparation a week in advance come to a research laboratory remote from the children's hospital. It was also noted that all children had been in the reception area of the children's hospital to see the surgeon prior to a decision to operate. These results would appear to support Mellish's (1969) position that age should be an important consideration in deciding when a child should be prepared for imminent surgery. It appears from our results that younger children benefit more from immediate preparation at the time of the actual hospitalization. They showed less Palmar Sweat Index arousal than older children prepared at the same time when the postoperative assessment was evaluated. There was in fact a significant increase in arousal at the postoperative assessment of younger children prepared a week in advance when compared with younger children who saw the film on the day of admission. However, this difference was not noted on other anxiety indicants such as the self-report of medical concerns or the observers' ratings of anxiety.

Is There Any Support for the Notion That Perceived Similarity to the Model Facilitates Extinction of Fear Behaviors?

Previous research cited (Flanders, 1968; Kazdin, 1973; Kornhaber & Schroeder, 1975; and Rosenkrans, 1967) supported the position that imitative behavior increased with similarity of the model to the observer. The current investigation offers further support of these findings. On all situational measures of fears the children resembling the model in sex, race, and age (over 7 yrs.) showed a greater reduction in anxiety.

Boys showed fewer behavior problems than girls. These sex differences remained even when standard preparation was given to the children individually in the hospital. Boys who saw the film one week in advance had less physiological arousal than girls immediately after viewing the film. They were rated less anxious than girls at the time of admission even though both had seen the film.

Racial differences are more difficult to understand because of greater manifest anxiety and more medical concerns reported in black children even at the prefilm assessment. This could be due to cultural bias of our measures or to the fact that many more of the black children were staff patients rather than having their own doctors. The one rather interesting finding supportive of the contention that black children did not identify as well with the white child was that the white children were significantly less anxious as rated by observers than blacks at postfilm and preoperative assessment despite the lack of race differences on this measure at the prefilm assessment.

These results can be taken to support the greater effectiveness of film modeling where perceived similarity to the model is obtained. As Bandura (1969) indicated, this problem may be reduced by the use of multiple models. Although our film has a play room scene which has black and white boys and girls discussing their surgery, the main narrator is a white seven-year-old boy. Future films might make use of several children who represent the characteristics of the major viewers.

REFERENCES

Dimock, H. G. *The child in hospital: A study of his emotional and social well-being.* Philadelphia: Davis, 1960.

Flanders, J. A review of research on imitative behavior. *Psychological Bulletin*, 1968, *69*, 316-337.

Heller, J. A. *The hospitalized child and his family.* Baltimore: The Johns Hopkins Press, 1967.

Johnson, R., & Dabbs, J. M. Enumeration of active sweat glands: A simple physiological indicator of psychological changes. *Nursing Research,* 1967, *16,* 273-276.

Kazdin, A. The effect of model identity and fear-relevant similarity on covert modeling. *Behavior Therapy,* 1974, *5,* 624-635.

Kornhaber, R., & Schroeder, H. Importance of model similarity on extinction of avoidance behavior in children. *Journal of Consulting and Clinical Psychology,* 1975, *43,* 601-607.

Melamed, B. G., & Siegel, L. J. Reduction of anxiety in children facing surgery by modeling. *Journal of Consulting and Clinical Psychology,* 1975, *43,* 511-521.

Mellish, R. W. P. Preparation of a child for hospitalization and surgery. *Pediatric Clinics of North America,* 1969, *16,* 543-553.

Peterson, D. Behavior problems of middle childhood. *Journal of Consulting Psychology,* 1961, *25,* 205-209.

Peterson, D., Becker, W., Shoemaker, D., Luria, Z., & Hellmer, L. Child behavior problems and parental attitudes. *Child Development,* 1961, *32,* 151-162.

Robertson, J. *Young children in hospitals.* New York: Basic Books, 1958.

Rosenkrans, M. Imitation in children as a function of perceived similarity to a social model and vicarious reinforcement. *Journal of Personality and Social Psychology,* 1967, *7,* 307-315.

Scherer, M. W., & Nakamura, C. Y. A fear survey schedule for children (FSS-FC): A factor analytic comparison with manifest anxiety (CMAS). *Behavior Research and Therapy,* 1968, 173-182.

Thomson, M. L., & Sutarman. The identification and enumeration of active sweat glands in man from plastic impressions of the skin. *Transactions of the Royal Society of Tropical Medicine and Hygiene,* 1953, *47,* 412-417.

Vernon, D. T. A., & Bailey, W. C. The use of motion pictures in the psychological preparation of children for induction of anesthesia. *Anesthesiology,* 1974, *40,* 68-72.

Wirt, R. D., & Broen, W. E. *Booklet for the Personality Inventory for Children.* Minneapolis: Authors, 1958.

14

Effect of Mother Presence on Children's Reaction to Aversive Procedures

Edward G. Shaw and Donald K. Routh

University of Iowa

What effect does the mother's presence have on young children's response to stressful medical procedures? The literature on "attachment" of children to their mothers emphasizes that young children, like the young of other species, engage in many behaviors such as crying when the mother leaves which have the effect of maintaining proximity of the mother to the child (Ainsworth, 1964). Attachment theory implies also that the mother's presence helps the child cope more comfortably with novel or frightening experiences, presumably including painful medical procedures. Behavior theory, in contrast, views the infant's crying on mother's departure simply as a learned behavior, reinforced by the mother's intermittent response of returning when the child cries (Gewirtz, 1976). Behavior theory might predict that the child's crying in response to pain would be more likely to be rewarded by effective comforting and would thus be more likely to occur if the mother were present than if she were absent. Thus, at least on the surface, these two theoretical approaches seem to make different predictions about the effect of the mother's presence on young children's crying after medical procedures such as injections.

The statistical analysis and preparation of this manuscript were carried out while the first author was a medical student at Rush Medical College. We are grateful for the assistance of the following persons in carrying out the research: Thomas G. Rosenberger, Peter D. Wallace, Alice Bain, Lyn Kellen, June Twaler, and Karen Wills. Comments on the manuscript by Milton Rosenbaum and by two anonymous reviewers are also appreciated.
Originally published in *Journal of Pediatric Psychology,* 7(1)(1982):33–42.

The research literature on this topic contains few studies and does not permit firm conclusions to be stated. Four decades ago, Shirley and Poyntz (1941) observed that many children went through the experience of spending a day at a health center with little apparent stress, but at the end of the day their "hard won bravery dissolved in tears at seeing their mothers" (p. 277). The first experimental study of this general issue, by Frankl, Shiere, and Fogels (1962) studied children during dental examination and treatment. They found the behavior of young children (41-49 months) to be significantly less negative when the mother was present than when she was absent. Considerable crying and negative behavior by these children were observed at the beginning of the first dental visit, i.e., just after the initial separation from the mother. Thus the results of this study can be readily understood within either attachment or behavior theory frameworks. What is not clear from the data presented is whether the children's specific response to procedures such as injection or local anesthetic was affected by the presence or absence of the mother.

Vernon, Foley, and Schulman (1967) studied the effects of separation from mother on the behavior of children 2 to 5 years old in response to hospital procedures. The mother's presence or absence did not significantly affect the children's response to routine admissions procedures but did affect their behavior during anesthesia induction. Interestingly, the significant effect was not during the first phase of induction, when the mask was placed and held over the child's face, but only the second phase, from 1 minute after the mask was placed until a surgical level of anesthesia was reached. During this so-called excitement phase of anesthesia, the children whose mother was absent were rated as showing more unhappiness, whining, etc., than those whose mother was present. Thus there was an effect of the kind predicted by attachment theory, but only after the child's emotional reactions were somewhat disinhibited by the effects of the anesthesia.

The only other relevant study known to the authors is that of Schwarz (1968), who observed the response of children 3 to 5 years old to a fear stimulus, a mechanical toy gorilla which unexpectedly emerged from a box, beat its chest, and walked toward the child. Children whose mothers were present were judged to express significantly more fear than those who were in the room with an assistant to the experimenter rather than their mother. Since a review of the literature provided an inadequate basis for understanding the effect of mother presence upon children's reaction to aversive procedures, the following two studies were planned, systematically varying mother presence and absence when children received injections in a pediatric office.

METHOD

Subjects

All of the subjects were being seen for routine well-child examinations and immunizations. Though specific information was not collected on demographic variables, this was generally a white, middle-class sample of families. For convenience, Experiment I is referred to as a study of "18-month-olds." Actually, only 14 of the 20 subjects in this experiment were exactly 18 months old, with the others being up to 26 months of age. Ten of the 20 subjects were randomly assigned to the mother-present group and 10 to the mother-absent group (the former group consisted of 6 males and 4 females, with a mean age of 18.9 months; the latter of 7 males and 3 females, with a mean age of 18.5 months).

Experiment 2 is similarly referred to for convenience as a study of "5-year-olds." It included 20 children whose actual age range was from 59 to 67 months. Ten of these subjects were randomly assigned to the mother-present group and 10 to the mother-absent group (the former group consisted of 5 males and 5 females, with a mean age of 62.3 months; the latter of 6 males and 4 females, with a mean age of 60.3 months). The age differences between groups in both experiments were nonsignificant statistically.

The children in the above experiments were those whose mothers gave their consent to their random assignment to one of the two treatment conditions. Some mothers would only consent to their child's participation in research on the condition that they be present during all procedures. This raised the question of whether the children in the two experimental groups, who were allowed to participate unconditionally, were representative of the population of children in the pediatric practice. Therefore, 10 additional children in each of the two age groups whose parents gave only conditional consent were observed under the same procedures as those randomly assigned to the mother-present group. Since statistical analysis showed these "conditional parental consent" subjects to be entirely comparable in their behavior to those randomly assigned to the mother present group, no further mention will be made of them.

Procedure

The studies were conducted in the office of two pediatricians in private practice. The names and addresses of prospective subjects were obtained from the receptionist 3 weeks in advance of the child's regularly scheduled visit. The prospective subjects' parents were then mailed a letter informing them of the nature and procedures of the study. At the pediatrician's office the experimenter explained the study further and inquired whether or not the parent was interested in participating. Parents who agreed to participate were then randomly assigned to either the mother-present or the mother-absent group.

Initially, mothers accompanied their children to the examination room. For 16 of the subjects, two behavior coders were in the examination room for the entire procedure. One of the coders was a senior premedical student and the other a first-year graduate student in clinical psychology. The coders had been trained through the observation of several pilot subjects while the codes were being worked out and refined.

For Experiment 1, the examination procedure included the following seven time intervals, each coded separately: (1) the nurse interviewed the mother while she undressed her child. The nurse then indicated where toys were for the child to play with, and she left the room. (2) The pediatrician entered shortly thereafter, interviewed the mother, and proceeded with the physical examination. The pediatrician then left the room. (3) The nurse returned. At this point mothers in the mother-absent group left the examination room and remained in the waiting room. Mothers in the mother-present group remained in the examination room. (4) The child was then placed on the examination table by the nurse and measured, taken to the scale in the hallway and weighed, and returned to the examination room. (5) With the child on the examination table, the nurse administered the oral polio vaccine. (6) The child was placed in a supine position and, with the parent (in the mother-present group) or one of the behavior coders (in the mother-absent group) holding the child's hands, was given the DPT injection in the thigh by the nurse. (With practice, coders found that when necessary they could carry out their coding of the behavior during the injection immediately after the injection had been given. The interrater reliabilities obtained under these circumstances were at least equal to those reported below.) (7) Children in the mother-present group were immediately picked up by their mothers, while children in the mother-absent group were picked up by the nurse and taken to the waiting room where they were reunited with their mother. The mother and child then returned to the examination room. The children were then dressed by their mothers for their return home.

For Experiment 2, the examination procedure included the following nine time intervals, each coded separately: (1) The nurse interviewed the mother. (2) The nurse then took the child to the hallway to be weighed, and then (3) into a separate room where the child's vision was checked on a standard visual acuity device. Mothers in the mother-present group accompanied their child for the weighing and the eye test. Those in the mother-absent group remained behind in the examination room. The nurse, the child (and the mother in the mother-present group) then returned to the examination room. The nurse indicated where the toys were, and left the room. The events just described, except for the eye test itself, were actually included in scoring interval 2, i.e., scoring interval 3 included only the eye test. (4) The pediatrician entered the examination room, interviewed the mother and child, and proceeded with the physical examination; then he left the room, and (5) the nurse entered again. Mothers in the mother-absent group then left to sit in the waiting room. (6) The nurse then gave the child the oral polio vaccine, and (7) a TB-tine test, involving four tiny prongs which pricked the child's forearm. (8) The child was next placed on the examination table in a supine position. The child's hands were held by the mother if present or by one of the behavior coders, while the tetanus injection was given in the thigh by the nurse. (9) Children in the mother-present group were than assisted in dressing by their mothers, while children in the mother-absent group waited for the nurse to retrieve their mother before dressing to return home.

Measures of Behavior

The behavior of children was evaluated by two methods: Modified Frankl Scale ratings (Frankl et al., 1962) for each separate part of the procedures, and behavioral coding for each part of the procedures. The Frankl rating procedure was modified into the following 5-point scale: 1-definitely positive, pronounced exhibition of overt positive behavior; 2-positive, some exhibition of overt positive behavior; 3-neutral, absence of overt negative or positive behavior; 4-negative, some exhibition of overt negative behavior; and 5-definitely negative, pronounced exhibition of overt negative behavior. The reliability of the modified Frankl Scale was indicated by an interrater correlation coefficient of .90. The two raters agreed perfectly on 73% of these ratings and never disagreed by more than 1 scale point.

The tally sheets used by the behavior coders divided each part of the examination time into 20-second intervals. The coders recorded, for each interval, the presence of each of the following behaviors. The Pearson product-moment correlation coefficient representing the interrater reliability of each behavioral code is given in parentheses after the description of that code.

(a) Fussing, which included all vocal protest behavior short of actual crying ($r = .94$)

(b) Crying and screaming (r = .95)

(c) Laughing and smiling (r = .88)

(d) Talking, or in the case of the subjects in Experiment 1, any apparent verbalizations even when not intelligible to the coder (r = .94)

(e) Playing with toys (r = .99)

(f) Pushing or covering up, which included any physical blocking or pushing away of the pediatrician or nurse during the examination procedure (r = .69)

RESULTS

Our statistical strategy in each experiment was to analyze the Frankl ratings first, analyzing coded behaviors only for those parts of the procedure where examination of the ratings indicated significant group differences.

Experiment 1

Multivariate analysis of variance of the Frankl scale ratings for the seven parts of the examination for the younger subjects indicated significant differences between the mother-present and mother-absent conditions, F (7, 12) = 3.33, p < .05. Follow-up univariate analyses of variance indicated significant differences in the ratings only for Interval 3 (when the mother left in the mother-absent condition), F (1, 18) = 7.14, p < .02, and Interval 6 (when the injection was given), F (1, 18) = 5.00, p < .05. The nature of these differences is indicated in Table I. In the Interval 3 rating, the children in the mother-absent group received a rating suggesting some negative behavior, while children in the mother-present group received a rating on the positive side of neutral. Univariate analysis of variance of the coded behaviors during the Interval 3 coding indicated a significant difference between groups only in the amount of crying, F (1, 18) = 10.76, p < .01.

Table I. Means and Standard Deviations Corresponding to Significant Differences in Frankl Ratings in Experiment 1 (Toddlers)

Part of procedure rated	Mother-present group		Mother-absent	
	Mean	SD	Mean	SD
Mother leaves	2.60[a]	.97	3.90	1.20
Injection	5.00	.00	4.50	.71

[a] A rating of 3 indicates neutral, 4 negative, and 5 definitely negative.

On the average, children in the mother-absent condition cried during 35% of those 20-second intervals (actually, 6 of these 10 children cried at least some), while children in the mother-present group did not cry at all.

On the other hand, Table I shows that in the Interval 6, children in the mother-present group received the maximum possible negative rating, while those in the mother-absent group received a significantly less negative rating. Statistical analysis of the coded behaviors during Interval 6 did not, however, reveal significant differences between the mother-present and mother-absent groups. Descriptively it can be reported that all 10 children in the mother-present group cried at least some while receiving their injections, while only 7 of the 10 in the mother-absent group did so.

Experiment 2

Multivariate analysis variance of the Frankl Scale ratings for the nine parts of the procedure for the older subjects indicated a significant difference between the mother-present and mother-absent groups, $F (9, 10) = 3.76$, p .05. Follow-up univariate analyses of variance indicated significant differences in the ratings for the Interval 8, when the children received their injections, $F (1, 18) = 22.23, p < .001$, and the ninth interval immediately afterwards, $F (1, 18) = 12.27, p < .01$. The nature of these differences is indicated in Table II. In Interval 8, children in the mother-present condition were rated as showing definite negative behavior and those in the mother-absent condition as showing between neutral and some negative behavior. Univariate analyses of variance of the coded behaviors during the Interval 8 indicated a significant difference between groups only in the amount of crying, $F (1, 18) = 10.41, p < .01$. On the average, children in the mother-present condition cried during 64% of the 20-second intervals, while children in the mother-absent condition cried in only 10% of these intervals. To put it another way, 8 of 10 children in the mother-

Table II. Means and Standard Deviations Corresponding to Significant Differences in Frankl Ratings in Experiment 2 (Older Children)

Part of procedure rated	Mother-present group		Mother-absent group	
	Mean	SD	Mean	SD
Injection	4.60[a]	.52	3.50	.53
Afterwards	3.60	1.17	2.15	.58

[a] A rating of 3 indicates neutral, 4 negative, and 5 definitely negative.

present condition cried at least some of the time during Interval 8, while only 1 of the 10 children in the mother-absent condition did so.

In Interval 9, univariate analysis of variance indicated a significant difference between groups only in the amount of fussing, F $(1, 18)$ = 8.87, $p < .01$. On the average, children in the mother-present condition fussed during 40% of the 20-second intervals, while children in the mother-absent condition fussed in only 3% of these intervals. To put it another way, 7 of 10 children in the mother-present group fussed at least some of the time, while only 1 of the 10 in the mother-absent group did so.

DISCUSSION

The toddlers in the mother-absent group in Experiment 1 tended to cry when their mothers left the room, while those in the mother-present group did not. These findings and their specificity to the younger group of children provide a clear example of separation protest, a phenomenon well known to students of attachment such as Ainsworth (1964). The results of some other studies in the literature on children's response to stress may be explainable primarily on the basis of this separation protest effect. One example is the study by Frankl et al. (1962) which found a beneficial effect of parent presence in the dental operatory. It will be recalled that in that study much crying was observed right at the beginning when the mother left, and the significant findings were confined to the younger group of children (age 3 and 4 years).

The main findings of the present study, however, were that when they receive injections, children are rated as showing more negative behavior and cry and fuss longer when their mother is present than when she has been asked to stay in the waiting room. These are, so far as the authors are aware, the first experimental findings supporting the clinical observations of Shirley and Poyntz (1941) many years ago that children "cry longer and more loudly when their mothers are within sight or earshot than when they are absent" (p. 251). The present findings may be explainable at least in part by our deduction from behavioral principles that, given a painful experience, children are more likely to be reinforced by effective comforting when their mother is present than when she is absent. Thus they are more likely to cry under these circumstances.

When our findings are put in context with others in the literature, however, we believe it could be argued that children under stress are actually more emotionally upset in the sense of physiological arousal when their mothers are absent than when they are present. The data of Vernon et al. (1967), for example, suggest that children are more emotionally aroused when mother is absent, but this is only evident when the behavioral expression of the emotional arousal is disinhibited by anesthesia. In our study, with no anesthesia being given, the children were more likely to express their feelings by crying and fussing when mother was there. In other words, the presence of the mother disinhibited the expression of whatever emotional arousal the child was experiencing. This is essentially the same interpretation given by Schwarz (1968) for his data on young children's reaction to a fear stimulus. If this interpretation is correct, attachment theory and behavior theory may not be so far apart as has been thought, each providing but a partial account of the events observed. Future research aimed at unraveling further the effects of the parent's presence or absence on the child's response to stress should carefully distinguish between separation protest and response to stressful events. It should also differentiate emotional arousal as such from factors (such as anesthesia or parent presence) which inhibit or disinhibit its expression.

Formal statistical analysis of age differences, i.e., between subjects in Experiments 1 and 2, was precluded by the many differences in the procedure in the pediatric office in dealing with toddlers as opposed to older children. The main differences between the two age groups as observed in this study seem to be (a) the absence of separation protest in the older children, and (b) the fact that, at least with the mother absent, the older children are considerably less likely to cry when receiving injections than are the toddlers.

All the significant findings of the present study concerned negative behaviors such as crying and fussing, despite the fact that positive behaviors were included in both the ratings and the behavioral observation codes used. It should be commented that positive behaviors certainly occurred. The children, especially the toddlers, spent considerable time playing, talking, and laughing and smiling. In fact, the toddlers seemed to be rather unaware of the likelihood that the visit to the pediatrician's office would include injections. The older children, in contrast, were in many cases quite aware of this possibility and seemed a bit more wary or sober in their general behavior.

IMPLICATIONS

We do not interpret our results to mean that pediatricians should ask mothers to remain in the waiting room while their children are receiving injections. At this time, the most convincing interpretation of our findings is probably that given a minor pain experience, the child may inhibit protest if no parent is present. Conversely, the presence of the mother may disinhibit crying and fussing under such circumstances.

REFERENCES

Ainsworth, M. Patterns of attachment behavior shown by the infant in interaction with his mother. *Merrill-Palmer Quarterly,* 1964, *10,* 51-58.

Frankl, S. N., Shiere, F. R., & Fogels, H. R. Should the parent remain with the child in the dental operatory? *Journal of Dentistry for Children,* 1962, *29,* 152-163.

Gewirtz, J. L. The attachment acquisition process as evidenced in the maternal conditioning of cued infant responding (particularly crying). *Human Development,* 1976, *29,* 143-155.

Schwarz, J. C. Fear and attachment in young children. *Merrill-Palmer Quarterly,* 1968, *14,* 313-322.

Shirley, M., & Poyntz, L. The influence of separation from the mother on children's emotional responses. *Journal of Psychology,* 1941, *12,* 251-282.

Vernon, D. T. A., Foley, J. M., & Schulman, J. L. Effect of mother-child separation and birth order on young children's responses to two potentially stressful experiences. *Journal of Personality and Social Psychology,* 1967, *5,* 162-174.

15

Assessment of Pediatric Pain
An Empirical Perspective

Donald J. Lollar
Atlanta Pediatric Psychology Associates

Stanley J. Smits
Georgia State University

David L. Patterson
Georgia Department of Human Resources

The assessment of pain among children has been a perplexing task. Pain is clearly a personal phenomenon, which confounds many attempts to evaluate it. Even beyond this, assessing perception of pain among children is very complex because of several different factors. First, children's relative inability to communicate has placed them at a disadvantage. Second, our understanding of the actual neurological and physiological mechanisms involved in children's pain has been impaired by both the lack of basic research and these same communication problems. Third, health care providers have highlighted emotional factors as the major component in pain response among children. Eland (Note 1) contends that adequate instruments for assessing children's pain have been virtually nonexistent, thus requiring evaluation to be totally subjective and dependent upon the beliefs, sensitivity, and skills of the individual provider. It is easy to understand this scarcity.

Physical measures of pain among children have been few. Haslam (1969) used a pressure algometer to measure pain thresholds among children. The results from the 150 children, ages 5 to 18, indicated that the

Presented by the senior author at the Pediatric Behavioral Medicine Conference, Ottawa, Ontario, Canada, May 22, 1981.
Originally published in *Journal of Pediatric Psychology,* 7(3)(1982):267–277.

younger the child, the lower the pain threshold. Conversely, the older the child, the higher the threshold at which pain was experienced.

Eland began a series of studies in 1974 to develop instruments to assist in children's communication of pain. From these eight projects, three assessment procedures were developed. Cartoon line drawing of animals in four pain-evoking situations were initially developed and used (Hester, 1979; Eland, Note 2; Ward, Note 3).

Alyea (Note 4) used a similar format but with human facial expressions. The drawings, however, were abandoned due to the lack of continuity among the children's responses. Second, Hester (1979) used four poker chips to allow youngsters to represent the intensity of their pain. Finally, a color spectrum was adapted from Stewart (1977) to assist children in communicating the intensity of their pain. Eland (Note 1) concluded that an eight-color scale was useful in helping children ages 5 to 10 to describe the intensity of their pain experience. Severe pain was most represented by the color red, moderate pain by brown, mild by yellow, and no pain by the color green. The results of the studies indicate that the color scale is an excellent state-specific instrument. Trait measurement with the color scale was not pursued.

Scott (1978) also used illustrative cartoons as a projective instrument to measure children's perceptions of pain. The two situations for the cartoons were similar to the pictures developed much earlier by Petrovitch (1975) for use with adults. The instrument was used to measure perceptions other than pain intensity. "Sensory, cognitive, and affective factors" associated with children's perceptions of pain were assessed. Children, ages 4 to 10, were asked to describe the pain in each of the two cartoons according to (a) color, (b) texture, (c) shape, (d) pattern, and (e) continuous vs. intermittent quality. Although the author concluded that the results could have occurred by chance, it appeared that younger children (4- to 6-year-olds) were, as suggested by Piaget, more synaesthetic, or intuitive, in their perceptions of pain than older children (7- to 9-year-olds). Older children appeared to approximate the Piagetian state of concrete operations in their cognitive associations of pain.

The conceptual framework and prototype for the present study can be traced to the pioneering works of Petrovitch (1957) and Melzack (1961). Petrovitch has observed clinically that "people vary markedly in their perception of, tolerance for, and reaction to painful stimuli" (p. 340). He postulated that an apperceptive test of pain was desirable:

> By the process of identification and projection, the subject may vicariously experience the pain which has befallen the pictured individual and interpret the pictures in accordance with his own predispositions. (p. 342)

The major premise for Petrovitch's approach was that "each individual is predisposed to perceive pain in others in a characteristic and relatively constant manner which stems from his own experiences and reactions regarding pain" (p. 341). This emphasis on the personal-perceptual nature of pain was also espoused by Melzack (1961):

> The psychological evidence strongly supports the view of pain as a perceptual experience whose quality and intensity is influenced by the unique past history of the individual, by the meaning he gives to the pain-producing situation and by his "state of mind" at the moment. (p. 11)

From the clinical experiences of the authors and on the basis of reviewing the literature, it appeared that a more stable trait-related instrument was needed for assessing children's perceptions of pain. Realizing the numerous physiological, emotional, and behavioral variables which constitute "pain," the authors decided the instrument to be developed should focus on children's perceptions and projected responses to generally accepted pain-eliciting stimuli. The Pediatric Pain Inventory (PPI) was developed as a beginning tool with that rationale.

Several clinical observations formed the practical basis for the PPI. First, it was observed that children respond differently to pain according to the setting, i.e., a shot in a doctor's office is seen differently from the pain resulting from falling off a bicycle. Thus, the instrument needed to reflect pain-evoking stimuli from various settings. Second, the emotional component of pain appeared greater for many youngsters that the actual physical component. Third, it was observed that, for many youngsters, the emotional response to the psychosocial conflict is similar to physical pain. Apley (1976), the pioneer in clinical assessment and treatment of pediatric pain, has stated that "the warning light of pain must be understood to switch on irrespective of whether the cause of the disturbance is physical, emotional, or familial" (pp. 384-385). Also, clinically there appeared to be as intense a response to psychosocial pain as to physical pain among physically disabled and chronically ill youngsters. Therefore, the psychosocial "pain" element needed to be incorporated into the instrument. Fourth, the already-referenced concern with children's less developed communication skills required that the instrument be primarily nonverbal.

As mentioned earlier, the conceptual base for the PPI arose from the work of Petrovitch (1957), who hypothesized two primary dimensions of pain perception: intensity and duration. He developed 25 pictures of an individual in various pain-eliciting situations for presentation to adults. In the instrument-construction phase by Petrovitch, these two dimensions were validated. In addition, two other dimensions were posited: self-inflicted vs. other-inflicted, and actual vs. anticipated. Few data were presented to validate or invalidate these aspects of perception, however.

METHOD

Instrumentation

The Pediatric Pain Inventory was developed as a structured projective instrument to collect data on children's perceptions of pain. The situations were intended to incorporate a spectrum of pain-evoking stimuli on both the intensity and duration dimensions. Therefore, some pictures present more intense pain than others, and some of the situations project an image of pain of greater duration. Although the authors were aware that differences exist in acute versus chronic elements, it was concluded that a broad range of situations should be sampled in order to develop a trait-related instrument. Twenty-four pain-evoking situations representing four types of settings were completed. Due to the exploratory nature of the instrument, female pictures were not initially constructed. The line drawings were thus male figures without facial features. The four types of pain selected were (a) medical, (b) recreational, (c) psychosocial, and (d) activities of daily living. These four settings were selected because they represented the settings in which children most often participate and most often experience pain. Six pictures were constructed for each of the four settings to insure sufficient samples for each. Examples of situations in each setting included the following:

Medical (MED). Getting a shot; lying in a hospital bed beside an intravenous bottle; receiving stitches; getting medicine from a nurse; sitting in a wheelchair in a hospital; and having a cast put on in a physician's office.

Psychosocial (PS). Being scolded by a policeman; being laughed at by schoolmates for misspelling a word; striking out in a baseball game; being reprimanded by a teacher; fighting with another child; being excluded from a game.

Recreation (REC). Being hit by a baseball while batting; falling off a skateboard; having a wreck with a bicycle; dropping a bowling ball on foot; being run over by another football player; falling out of a tree.

Activities of Daily Living (ADL). Closing a finger in a door; getting an electric shock; getting stung by bees; cutting hand while peeling fruit; pulling off a Band-Aid; burning hand on a stove.

Subjects

Nursing students were trained to administer the PPI. Protocols were completed on 370 individuals, including 240 children and adolescents, ranging in age from 4 to 19 years, as well as parents of the youngsters. The sample included 213 females and 157 males.

Procedures

The subjects were asked a series of forced-choice demographic questions, requesting information on number of hospitalizations, illnesses of parents, and school attendance in relation to illness. A set procedure was followed, beginning with questions related to (a) responsibility for the situation presented, (b) whether the youngster depicted needed help with the hurt, (c) who would help, and (d) what would be done. Afterward, each individual rated the pictures on intensity and duration of the perceived pain. All interviews were completed individually without others present.

Duration of pain as a construct depends on children's concept of time, of course. Bradley (1947), who studied the development of time concepts in school-age children, found that 5-year-olds are not yet clear about time words, while 6- and 7-year-olds can answer time questions from a personal reference perspective. Children from then on seem to be able to generalize time concepts. The duration question asked how long the hurt would last and included the following categories: seconds, day, week, or longer.

Intensity of pain was measured by a sorting of the 24 pictures in terms of a three-color spectrum rating scale. The colors red, yellow, and green were selected to represent much, some, and little pain. The color associations are consistent with those made by children in Eland's study. The children were then asked to select that intensity group which represented hurt (a) most like that they had experienced, (b) most like what they believed their mother had experienced, and (c) most like what they believed their father had experienced.

Parents were asked to complete all of the inventory as they perceived the situations relating to their child. On the "most like" experiences, in addition, they were asked to choose the group representing situations most like those experienced by their child.

RESULTS AND DISCUSSION

Both reliability and validity coefficients were computed for the PPI. First, internal consistency statistics were computed on both the intensity and duration dimensions for all four types of setting. Table I presents the alpha coefficients. Nunnally (1967) has suggested that modest reliability is sufficient during the initial construction of an instrument. It is clear that

Table I. Internal Consistency (Alpha) Coefficients of the Pediatric Pain Inventory

Setting	Intensity	Duration
Activities of daily living	.57	.62
Psychosocial	.76	.70
Medical	.41	.49
Recreational	.70	.70

Table II. Pain Intensity and Duration Means Across Settings

Variable	Setting			
	ADL	PS	MED	REC
Intensity	13.2	9.8	13.0	13.1
Duration	11.3	11.2	15.9	11.9

three of the four subareas greatly exceeded that level of internal consistency on both dimensions. The medical pain area, while exceeding a .40 reliability, was not as internally consistent. It is hypothesized that this relatively lower internal consistency is attributable to the greater diversity of experience among the subjects in the medical area than in the more common areas dealing with psychosocial, recreational, and ADL events. Overall, the internal consistency was considered good.

Validity was examined in several ways. Initially, the two dimensions of duration and intensity were examined. The very low correlation ($r = .08$) between the total Intensity and total Duration suggested that apparently different dimensions were indeed being measured and that Petrovitch's constructs have discriminant validity.

Second, an analysis of variance was computed to assess differences in levels of pain for the four dimensions. The means corresponding to these analyses are shown in Table II. The means differed significantly both for intensity, $F(3, 1499) = 114.4, p < .0001$, and duration, $F(3, 1447) = 148.9$, $p < .0001$. These results suggest that psychosocial pain is perceived as significantly less intense than the other types of pain experiences. On the duration dimension, the results suggested that medical pain is perceived as lasting longer than the other kinds of pain. These results are taken to suggest the discriminant validity of the different dimensions being assessed.

To address questions of convergent validity, a correlation matrix was computed in which each item was correlated with the total score for each of the four subareas—medical, recreational, psychosocial, and activities of

Table III. Product-Moment Correlations: Intensity

Picture no.	Assigned category	Level loadings			
		ADL	PS	MED	REC
1	ADL	.64	−.09	−.06	.19
4	ADL	.45	−.02	−.07	.12
7	ADL	.42	.01	.04	.20
12	ADL	.51	−.06	.03	.16
17	ADL	.49	.03	−.01	.23
23	ADL	.49	−.17	−.02	.22
2	PS	.14	.15	−.01	.16
6	PS	.04	.52	−.04	−.01
8	PS	−.14	.52	−.07	−.08
16	PS	−.16	.57	−.05	.01
18	PS	−.02	.44	−.02	.03
20	PS	−.08	.59	.02	.05
3	MED	.12	.01	.38	−.02
5	MED	−.13	.00	.46	−.08
9	MED	.01	−.17	.49	−.03
10	MED	−.06	.03	.40	−.06
13	MED	.23	−.09	.33	.14
14	MED	−.26	.05	.48	−.17
11	REC	.25	−.07	−.13	.60
15	REC	.34	−.01	−.15	.55
19	REC	.25	.04	−.03	.61
21	REC	.24	−.07	−.07	.59
22	REC	.05	.04	.06	.56
24	REC	.14	−.03	.03	.52

daily living. Tables III and IV show these results. As can be seen, of the 24 items on the intensity dimension, 23 correlated most highly with the subareas in which they were placed. Only picture #2 on the psychosocial category did not do so. On the duration dimension, all 24 items correlated most highly with the subareas in which they were originally placed. These results suggest that the items were correctly placed in categories.

A final analysis was computed on the intensity and duration dimensions. Principal components factor analysis of the intensity ratings indicated three factors to be distinguishable. These were labeled medical, psychosocial, and activities of daily living. The recreational items seemed to load on the activities of daily living factor. On the factor analysis of the duration ratings, only one factor emerged, suggesting that the duration of pain is perceived in a unitary way across the different settings.

Table IV. Product-Moment Correlations: Duration

Picture no.	Assigned category	Level loadings			
		ADL	PS	MED	REC
1	ADL	.44	.17	.16	.24
4	ADL	.57	.27	.29	.33
7	ADL	.47	.24	.16	.16
12	ADL	.54	.16	.16	.32
17	ADL	.58	.30	.20	.36
23	ADL	.41	.24	.29	.39
2	PS	.30	.39	.25	.25
6	PS	.11	.63	.23	.09
8	PS	.12	.57	.17	.17
16	PS	.28	.63	.22	.30
18	PS	.30	.55	.21	.37
20	PS	.22	.64	.26	.29
3	MED	.27	.19	.46	.27
5	MED	.26	.22	.48	.30
9	MED	.15	.09	.45	.16
10	MED	.24	.28	.44	.27
13	MED	.25	.22	.28	.23
14	MED	.09	.15	.51	.18
11	REC	.23	.17	.16	.49
15	REC	.32	.26	.19	.55
19	REC	.42	.36	.28	.58
21	REC	.30	.24	.24	.61
22	REC	.33	.23	.19	.58
27	REC	.31	.25	.23	.57

The rank ordering of the 24 different pictures on intensity indicated that the picture of the youngster sitting on a "doctor's table" with a bandaged leg corresponded to the most intense pain. The picture of a youngster being given a shot ranked 17th in intensity and 23rd in duration.

As Table V indicates, there was some tendency for children who ranked their own pain experiences as relatively intense to rank their mother's pain experiences in the same way. This relationship was significant, $\chi^2(4) = 9.4$, $p < .05$. However, the relationship between the child's ranking of his or her own pain experiences and those of the father were not significant.

In addition, a significant difference ($p < .01$) was found between how the children perceived their own pain intensity and how adults perceived children's pain intensity, with the adults underestimating the intensity of the children's reactions. Eland and Anderson (1977) have suggested that

Table V. Perceived Intensity of Pain Experiences: Child's
Own Experience and Child's Perception of Mother's
Experience ($N = 267$)

	Child's perception of mother's experience		
Child's own experience	Little	Some	Much
Little	45	30	24
Some	30	40	32
Much	20	19	27

Table VI. Mean Pain Intensity in Different Settings as a Function
of Perceived Level of Own Pain Experience

Self-reported level of pain experience	Setting			
	ADL	PS	MED	REC
Much	12.6	9.0	12.5	13.0
Some	12.9	9.4	13.0	12.8
Little	14.3	10.4	12.9	13.9

adults tend to underestimate children's pain experience, and this suggestion
is supported by the present findings.

Another group of results focused on differences among the four types
of settings as related to demographic data and perceived pain experiences.
Analyses of variance were computed on both the intensity and duration
dimensions. Using the intensity dimension, significant differences were
found according to age for ADL pain and for the total intensity score. Sex
differences were found on the perceptions of medical pain: for females the
mean was 13.1 and for males 12.5, $F(1, 379) = 3.8, p < .05$. The most
significant differences were found when the variable of perceived intensity
of pain experienced was used to classify subjects. Differences were found
among youngsters who described their own pain experiences as being intense, somewhat intense, and not very intense. These differences are shown
in Table VI. They were significant for the Activities of Daily Living scale,
$F(2, 299) = 7.5, p < .001$, and for the Psychosocial scale, $F(2, 299) = 4.6$,
$p < .01$, but not in the Medical setting.

On the duration dimension, fewer significant differences were found.
Age differences were apparent in the Medical settings, $F(11, 367) = 3.3$,
$p < .001$. The trends indicated a general increase in assessment of pain
duration from age 7 through adolescence. However, the 6-year-olds judged
pain as lasting a significantly shorter time than their elders. Perhaps this

relates to the immaturity of time concepts among younger children already mentioned.

Youngsters who described their pain experiences as relatively high perceived Medical pain, but no other types, as lasting significantly longer than that of youngsters describing their own pain as less intense, $F(2, 298) = 3.1$, $p < .05$.

The results of these analyses are provocative in that the intensity with which a youngster describes his/her own pain intensity and duration does influence his/her responses to both pain intensity and duration in different settings. However, these settings are complementary in that intensity is affected in nonmedical settings, while duration is influenced in medical situations. In addition, it is clear that the PPI is measuring differences relating to sex and age.

SUMMARY AND IMPLICATIONS

The Pediatric Pain Inventory, although in its early stages of development, has sufficiently high levels of reliability and validity to warrant its continued development. The data reported here indicate that the constructs of "intensity" and "duration" are both independent and viable factors in the study of children's pain perception. Several provocative results dealing with variations in the perception of medical pain, the possible modeling influence of the pain experienced by a child's mother, discrepancies between child and adult perceptions of the intensity of the child's pain, and the differences in pain perception associated with age and sex, suggest areas for further research.

While these results are preliminary in nature and require extensive replication, they suggest several clinically useful research hypotheses. For example, could mothers be trained as role models to help their children cope more effectively with the pain associated with chronic illnesses and/or disabilities? Could more effective treatment strategies be developed using the child's PPI scores as an indication of his or her reaction to an anticipated surgical intervention? Could the PPI be used in clinical settings to differentiate children with various types of recurrent pain? Information of this nature would be of great utility to practitioners involved in the treatment of pain in pediatric settings.

It is now almost three decades since Livingston (1953) asked the question, "What is pain?" and responded himself by saying it was a surprisingly difficult question to answer because of "subtle blend of physiological and psychological factors" (p. 3). The PPI is a beginning tool, for use with children, designed to address Livingston's question.

REFERENCE NOTES

1. Eland, J. M. *Minimizing pain associated with pre-kindergarten DPT immunization.* Unpublished doctoral dissertation, University of Iowa, 1980.
2. Eland, J. M. *Children's communication of pain.* Unpublished masters thesis, University of Iowa, 1974.
3. Ward, B. *Externally observed pain.* Unpublished masters thesis, University of Kansas, 1975.
4. Alyea, B. C. *Child pain rating after injection preparation.* Unpublished masters thesis, University of Missouri-Columbia, 1978.

REFERENCES

Apley, J. Pain in childhood. *Journal of Psychosomatic Research,* 1976, *20,* 383-389.

Bradley, N. C. The growth of the knowledge of time in children of school age. *British Journal of Psychology,* 1947, *38,* 67-78.

Eland, J. M., & Anderson, J. The experience of pain in children. In A. Jacox (Ed.), *Pain: A sourcebook for nurses and other health care professionals.* Boston: Little, Brown, 1977.

Haslam, D. R. Age and the perception of pain. *Psychonomic Science,* 1969, *15,* 86.

Hester, N. K. The preoperational child's reaction to immunization. *Nursing Research,* 1979, *28,* 250.

Livingston, W. K. *What is pain?* San Francisco: W. H. Freeman, 1953. (*Scientific American* Reprint #407).

Melzack, R. *The perception of pain.* San Francisco: W. H. Freeman, 1961. (*Scientific American* Reprint #457).

Nunnally, J. C. *Psychometric theory.* New York: McGraw-Hill, 1967.

Petrovitch, D. V. Pain apperception test. *Journal of Psychology,* 1957, *44,* 339-346.

Scott, R. "It hurts red": A preliminary study of children's perception of pain. *Perceptual and Motor Skills,* 1978, *47,* 787-791.

Stewart, M. L. Measurement of clinical pain. In A. Jacox (Ed.), *A source book for nurses and other health care professionals.* Boston: Little, Brown, 1977.

16

An Observation Scale for Measuring Children's Distress During Medical Procedures

Charles H. Elliott
Department of Psychiatry, University of New Mexico

Susan M. Jay
Department of Pediatrics, University of Southern California, School of Medicine

Patricia Woody
Childrens Hospital of Los Angeles

The current state-of-the-art in the area of assessing pain and anxiety experienced by children undergoing painful medical procedures remains at a rudimentary level. Early studies in the preparation literature included global Likert-type rating scales of children's distress and cooperative behaviors (Visintainer & Wolfer, 1975; Wolfer & Visintainer, 1979). More recent studies have focused on the development of more objective and operationalized behavioral observation scales which have been used specifically to measure distress in pediatric cancer patients undergoing bone marrow aspirations (BMAs) and lumbar punctures (LPs) (Jay, in press; Jay & Elliott, 1984; Jay, Ozolins, Elliott, & Caldwell, 1983; Katz, Kellerman, & Siegel, 1980; LeBaron & Zeltzer, 1984). For example, Katz et al. (1980) developed the Procedure Behavior Rating Scale (PBRS) which consisted of 13 operationally defined behaviors that were recorded as present or absent during bone marrow as-

This study was supported by a grant from the National Cancer Institute, National Institutes of Health, to Susan Jay and Charles Elliott. We gratefully acknowledge the assistance of Michael Dolgin and Myra Saltoun for data collection, and Lynn Dahlquist for editorial comments.
Originally published in *Journal of Pediatric Psychology, 11*(4)(1987):543–551.

pirations. The PBRS was found to be a reliable instrument and preliminary validity data (i.e., nurse ratings) were also encouraging. LeBaron and Zeltzer (1984) presented additional validity data on an eight-item version of the PBRS which they labeled the Procedure Behavior Check List.

Jay and Elliott (1984) reported on the development of the Observation Scale of Behavioral Distress (OSBD), an 11-item revision of the PBRS which included two methodological refinements of the PBRS: (a) continuous behavioral recording in 15-second intervals, and (b) a weighting score of severity of distress for each behavioral category in the scale. It was hypothesized that these refinements would result in a more highly sensitive and valid measure of children's distress. Rather surprisingly, initial data suggested relatively small, if any, increases in the sensitivity and validity of the OSBD with these revisions. The purpose of the current study was to replicate and expand the original investigation of validity of the OSBD by (a) expanding the sample size with an emphasis on younger children (since they are most in need of intervention for their distress); (b) expanding the range of variables used to assess the validity of the instrument; and (c) once again assessing the effects of methodological refinements that have been made. An additional purpose was to conduct an item analysis of the OSBD for the purpose of further refining and revising the instrument.

METHOD

Subjects

Subjects were a consecutive sample of 55 children with leukemia who entered the study over a 3-year period (1982–1985). The sample included 35 males and 20 females, a ratio that reflects the higher incidence of childhood leukemia in boys than girls. The age range of the patients was 3 to 13 years with a mean of 6.7 years. Seventy-one percent of the subjects were younger than 8 years of age reflecting the higher incidence of childhood leukemia in younger children. The ethnic composition of the sample was as follows: 55% white, 25% Hispanic, 13% black, 7% Asian.

Procedure

All subjects were part of a longitudinal study designed to evaluate the effects of various preprocedure conditions on distress during BMAs (Jay, Elliott, Katz, & Siegel, in press). The children in this study watched 30 minutes of cartoons prior to being observed during their BMA thus giving them a standardized preobservation experience that was considered unlikely to exert a significant effect on the various validity measures.

Assessment

Observational Scale of Behavioral Distress (OSBD).[1] Two major methodological revisions of the PBRS (Katz et al., 1980) were made in developing the OSBD: (a) behaviors are recorded in continuous 15-second intervals within each of three phases of the BMA procedure rather than simple, single event recording of occurrence over an entire phase; and (b) each behavioral category in the OSBD is weighted according to severity. Other revisions of the PBRS included the addition of a category, "nervous behavior," and the combining of several categories. The behavioral categories and their definitions are listed in Table I.

Observation Procedures. An observer watched the bone marrow aspiration and recorded the occurrence of distress-related behaviors during 15-second intervals (indicated on an audiotape played to the observer over headphones). Observers were trained by the second author over a 6- to 8-week period until a minimum criterion of 75% reliability over 6 consecutive BMA procedures was established.

Self-Report Measures of Fear. Children were asked to rate "how scared" they felt about their upcoming BMA, at the beginning of the session. A "faces" scale was used with three faces ranging from a "happy" face indicating "not at all scared," to a "sad" face indicating "very scared."

Self-Report Measures of Pain. A "Pain Thermometer" (Katz et al., 1982) was used to measure children's anticipated and experienced pain. The Pain Thermometer is a graphic depiction of a large thermometer graded on a 0 to 100 scale, with 0 representing "no pain at all" and 100 representing "the worst pain possible." At the beginning of the session, children were asked to rate how much they thought their upcoming BMA would hurt (Pain I), as a measure of anticipated pain. After the BMA, they were asked to rate how much the BMA did hurt as a measure of actual experienced pain (Pain II).

Physiological Measures. Children's heart rate and blood pressure were taken using a Dinamap Model 845 at three points in time: (a) upon arrival to the clinic, but prior to the cartoon viewing; (b) when the child got on

---

[1]The Observation Scale of Behavioral Distress (OSBD) is available from Susan M. Jay and includes information on development, reliability, validity, and scoring procedures.

Table I. Behavioral Definitions of Categories for the Observation Scale of Behavioral Distress

Category	Definition	Examples
Information seeking	Any questions regarding medical procedure	"Is the needle in?"
Cry	Onset of tears and/or low-pitched nonword sounds of more than 1-second duration	
Scream	Loud, nonword, shrill vocal expressions at high pitch intensity	
Physical restraint	Child is physically restrained with noticeable pressure and/or child is exerting bodily force and resistance in response to restraint.	
Verbal resistance	Any intelligible verbal expression of delay, termination, or resistance	"Stop" "I don't want it"
Seeks emotional support	Verbal or nonverbal solicitation of hugs, physical or verbal comfort from parents or staff	"Mama, help me" Pleading to be held
Verbal pain	Any words, phrases, or statements in any tense which refer to pain or discomfort	"Ouch" "My leg hurts" "That hurt"
Flail	Random gross movements of arms, legs, or whole body	Kicking legs; pounding fists
Verbal fear[a]	Any intelligible verbal expression of fear of apprehension	"I'm scared"
Muscular rigidity[a]	Noticeable contraction of observable body part	Clinched fists; gritted teeth; facial contortions. Legs bent tightly upward off R_x table
Nervous behavior[a]	Physical manifestations of anxiety or fear. Consist of repeated, small physical actions	Nail biting; lip chewing

[a] Eliminated after item analysis.

the treatment table, just before the BMA occurred; and (c) 3 to 5 minutes after the BMA.

Nurse Ratings. After the procedure was over, the nurse who assisted the person conducting the BMA was asked to rate the degree of behavioral distress exhibited by the child on a 5-point Likert-type scale, with 1 representing "no distress" and 5 representing "extreme distress."

RESULTS

Reliability

Pearson product-moment correlations analyses conducted between total OSBD scores for two observers for 20% of the procedures yielded an r of .98. In addition, the number of agreements between two observers as to whether or not each of the 11 behaviors occurred within each 15-second interval were divided by the total number of agreements plus disagreements. The mean agreement score obtained was 84%.

Validity

Analyses were conducted to determine the validity of the OSBD and to investigate the effects of continuous interval coding and severity weights on the validity of the OSBD. Therefore, (a) original OSBD scores were correlated with all of the validity measures and (b) the OSBD data were rescored without using the continuous 15-second intervals or the severity weights and these recalculated scores were then also correlated with the validity measures. Thus, rather than scoring behaviors in 15-second intervals, behaviors were rescored merely for occurrence or nonoccurrence over the entire phase, and severity weights were not used.[2]

Table II contains the Pearson product-moment correlation coefficients between the various validity measures and both original and recalculated OSBD scores. The results indicate, when one views the correlations between original OSBD scores and the validity measures, that the OSBD is significantly related to almost all of the measures of distress including Nurse Ratings ($r = .69, p < .0001$), Fear Ratings ($r = .38, p < .01$), Anticipated Pain ($r = .24, p < .05$), Heart Rate I ($r = .38, p < .01$), Heart Rate II ($r = .55, p < .0001$), Heart Rate III ($r = .33, p < .01$), Systolic Blood

---

[2]The interval coding data sheets for the OSBD allows for scoring of behaviors with or without the severity weights and with or without continuous interval recording.

Table II. Correlation Coefficients Between Validity Measures and Original and Recalculated OSBD Scores

Validity measure	Original OSBD scores	Recalculated OSBD scores
Nurse ratings of distress[a]	.69[e]	.55[e]
Fear ratings	.38[c]	.37[c]
Anticipated pain	.24[b]	.26[b]
Experienced pain	.20	.24
Heart rate I	.38[c]	.41[c]
Heart rate II	.55[e]	.47[d]
Heart rate III	.33[c]	.36[c]
Systolic blood pressure I[a]	.32[c]	.04
Diastolic blood pressure I	.32[c]	.21
Systolic blood pressure II[a]	.38[c]	.11
Diastolic blood pressure II[a]	.38[c]	.20
Systolic blood pressure III	−.13	.03
Diastolic blood pressure III	.03	−.04

[a] On these variables, the differences between the two sets of correlation were significant at the .5 level.
[b] $p < .05$.
[c] $p < .01$.
[d] $p < .001$.
[e] $p < .0001$.

Pressure I and II ($r = .32$, $p < .01$ and $r = .38$, $p < .01$, respectively), and Diastolic Blood Pressure II ($r = .38$, $p < .01$). The only measures that were not significantly correlated with original OSBD scores were Experienced Pain and Systolic and Diastolic Blood Pressure III.

Second, the differences between the validity correlation coefficients for the two sets of OSBD scores (original scores with severity weights and interval coding, and recalculated scores without these refinements) were analyzed using an r to z transformation for dependent samples (Glass & Stanley, 1970) to determine whether the continuous interval recording and the severity weights strengthened the validity of the OSBD. The two sets of validity coefficients for Fear Ratings, Anticipated Pain, and Experienced Pain were virtually identical, with no significant differences. Nor were the differences significant between the two sets of correlations for Heart Rate I, II, and III.

By contrast, the correlation between the original OSBD scores and Nurse Ratings ($r = .69$) was higher than the correlation between the recalculated OSBD scores and Nurse Ratings ($r = .55$), and this difference was significant ($z = -2.5$, $p < .05$). Significant differences (favoring the original OSBD scores) also were found between the two sets of correlations for Systolic Blood Pressure I ($z = -2.3$, $p < .05$), Systolic Blood Pressure II ($z = -4.1$, $p < .05$), and Diastolic Blood Pressure II ($z = -2.7$, $p < .05$). The difference between the validity correlations for the original and recalculated OSBD scores were not significant for the other blood pressure measures. Thus the OSBD, when recalculated without interval data and severity weights, yielded distress scores that were significantly correlated with a number of the validity measures, but the validity was not quite as strong as when the original distress scores were used.

Item Analysis

The 11 behavioral categories of the OSBD were subjected to an item analysis in which individual category scores were (a) scored for frequency of occurrence, (b) intercorrelated, and (c) correlated with total OSBD scores. Item analyses were conducted for the total sample and for each age group separately. The purpose of the item analysis was to eliminate any categories that were of very low frequency and those that were not correlated with other behavioral categories or to total OSBD scores.

The criteria for retaining a behavioral category were as follows: (a) category scores had to occur for at least 10% of the subjects, and (b) category scores had to have an item-total correlation coefficient of +.3 or more for the total sample and/or for at least one age group. One exception to these criteria was made for the category Emotional Support because it correlated .28 for the young age group and it was a very high frequency item, that is, it occurred in over half the sample.

Results indicated that 8 of the 11 OSBD categories met the criteria and three were eliminated. Verbal Fear was eliminated because it occurred in only 5% of the total sample and never in children above the age of 6 years. Nervous Behavior was eliminated because it correlated .07 with the total score for the entire sample, −.28 for children aged 4 to 6 years, and −.11 for children aged 7 to 14 years. Muscular Rigidity was eliminated because it correlated −.20 with the total score for the total sample, −.17 for the children aged 4 to 6 years, and −.37 for the children aged 7 to 14 years.

Cronbach's alpha test of internal consistency was conducted before and after elimination of Nervous Behavior, Verbal Fear, and Muscular Rigidity. Results before the categories were eliminated indicated an alpha internal consistency coefficient of .68 and a coefficient of .72 was obtained after the behaviors were eliminated.

DISCUSSION

The results of this study provide support for the reliability and validity of the Observational Scale of Behavioral Distress. The validity of the instrument is supported by significant correlations between OSBD total scores and a wide range of validity measures including fear, anticipated pain, heart rate, and blood pressure at two time periods, and nurse ratings.

OSBD total scores were not correlated with self-reports of actual experienced pain for the total sample. This finding may be due to the fact that the instrument is a better overall measure of anxiety than actual experienced pain sensations. However, since self-reported experienced pain did correlate significantly with OSBD scores of subjects older than 7 ($r = .51$, $p < .05$), it may be, that younger children are simply unable to rate experienced pain with a high degree of reliability.

The effects of the methodological refinements (interval recording and severity weights) appear to be significant in this somewhat larger sample. It should be noted, however, that even when scored without the refinements, the OSBD has reasonably good validity. Since these refinements greatly complicate the task of scoring and training of observers, one must consider the purpose for using the instrument before deciding whether to include the refinements. These findings suggest that the increased sensitivity derived from the refinements is largely restricted to improving the assessment of relationships between OSBD scores and measures with relatively weak predictive power (e.g., nurse ratings and blood pressure). Thus, studies investigating the influence of subtle individual difference variables such as coping styles and parental anxiety may wish to use a maximally sensitive instrument, whereas clinical applications involving the reduction of overall distress may find that the OSBD is sufficient without including the refinements.

The item analysis has allowed the instrument to be reduced to eight items. This reduction from the original 11 items should make observer training somewhat easier and may increase reliability as well. In its present form, the OSBD appears to be a robust scale which is likely to be equally useful for measuring children's distress associated with a variety of other painful medical procedures.

REFERENCES

Glass, G. V., & Stanley, J. C. (1970). *Statistical methods in education and psychology.* Englewood Cliffs, NJ: Prentice-Hall.

Jay, S. M. (in press). Invasive medical procedures. In D. Routh (Ed.), *Handbook of pediatric psychology.* New York: Plenum Press.

Jay, S. M., & Elliott, C. H. (1984). Behavioral observation scales for measuring children's distress: The effects of increased methodological rigor. *Journal of Consulting and Clinical Psychology, 52,* 1106-1107.

Jay, S. M., Elliott, C. H., Katz, E. R., & Siegel, S. E. (in press). Cognitive-behavioral and pharmacologic interventions of children undergoing painful medical procedures. *Journal of Consulting and Clinical Psychology,* in press.

Jay, S. M., Ozolins, M., Elliott, C. H., & Caldwell, S. (1983). Assessment of children's distress during painful medical procedures. *Health Psychology, 2,* 133-147.

Katz, E. R., Kellerman, J., & Siegel, S. E. (1980). Behavioral distress in children undergoing medical procedures: Developmental considerations. *Journal of Consulting and Clinical Psychology, 48,* 356-365.

Katz, E. R., Sharp, B., Kellerman, J., Marston, A. R., Hershman, J. M., & Siegel, S. E. (1982). β-Endorphin immunoreactivity and acute behavioral distress in children with leukemia. *Journal of Nervous and Mental Disease, 170,* 72-77.

LeBaron, S., & Zeltzer, L. (1984). Assessment of acute pain and anxiety in children and adolescents by self-reports, observer reports, and a behavior checklist. *Journal of Consulting and Clinical Psychology, 52,* 690-701.

Visintainer, M. A., & Wolfer, J. A. (1975). Psychological preparation for surgical pediatric patients: The effect on children's and parents' stress responses and adjustments. *Pediatrics, 56,* 187-202.

Wolfer, J. A., & Visintainer, M. A. (1979). Prehospital psychological preparation for tonsillectomy patients: Effects on children's and parents' adjustment. *Pediatrics, 64,* 646-655.

17

Somatization Disorder in Relatives of Children and Adolescents with Functional Abdominal Pain

Donald K. Routh
University of Iowa

Ann R. Ernst
Dubuque, Iowa

This study assessed the relationship between abdominal pain in children and adolescents and somatization disorder, attention deficit disorder, alcoholism, conduct disorder, and antisocial personality in first- and second-degree relatives. Abdominal pain is a highly prevalent problem in childhood. Apley (1975) has estimated that about 1 child in 10 suffers episodes of such pain, and only about 8% of the cases are found to have some clear-cut organic basis. Undoubtedly some abdominal pain results from as yet unidentified organic disease, but much of it is also thought to be of psychological origin.

Pain is one possible manifestation of the somewhat mysterious condition known as hysteria, discussed by medical writers since ancient Egyptian and Greek times (Veith, 1965). The concept of hysteria has been attacked by Slater (1965), who found that frequently upon follow-up, conditions diagnosed as hysteria turned out to be explainable on the basis of organic disease or prodromal manifestations of gross psychopathology such as schizophrenia.

However, a much more rigorous set of criteria have been developed by Purtell, Robins, and Cohen (1951) and subsequent investigators at Washington

Preliminary data for this study were collected as part of a PhD dissertation submitted by the second author to the Graduate College of the University of Iowa. We thank the physicians and staff of Medical Associates, P. C., Dubuque, Iowa, and Louis F. Brown, Robert A. Forsyth, Kathryn C. Gerken, and Dennis C. Harper, for their assistance.
Originally published in *Journal of Pediatric Psychology,* *1*(4)(1984):427–437.

University, St. Louis, for defining a chronic, polysymptomatic form of hysteria known as Briquet's syndrome or, in the DSM III (American Psychiatric Association, 1980), somatization disorder. The prevalence of somatization disorder in adult women is about 1 or 2%; the condition is much rarer in men (Farley, Woodruff, & Guze, 1968; Robins, Purtell, & Cohen, 1952; Woodruff, 1967). Individuals who meet the criteria for this disorder are generally found at follow-up not to have medical diseases or nonhysterical psychopathology explaining their numerous complaints (Perley & Guze, 1962). They present themselves frequently to physicians and often receive unwarranted surgery or other intrusive medical treatments (Cohen, Robins, Purtell, Altmann, & Reid, 1953). Somatization disorder has well-established linkages within the families of affected individuals to some other disorders, namely alcoholism, attention deficit disorder, conduct disorder or antisocial personality, and secondary affective disorder (Arkonac & Guze, 1963; Bibb & Guze, 1972; Cloninger & Guze, 1970a, 1970b, 1975; Guze, 1964; Guze, Woodruff, & Clayton, 1971; Morrison & Stewart, 1971; Robins, 1966; Woerner & Guze, 1968). However, somatization disorder is *not* hypothesized by the St. Louis group to be related to other types of psychopathology, e.g., schizophrenia.

Retrospective study of persons who have somatization disorder suggests that pain, including abdominal pain, is a common symptom (e.g., Purtell et al., 1951) and that the onset of somatic complaints was usually in childhood or adolescence (Coryell & Norten, 1981). So far, however, there have been only a few direct attempts to link somatization disorder to childhood medical problems (e.g., Robins & O'Neal, 1953). There seems to be good reason to suspect that childhood abdominal pain and adult somatization disorder and related conditions are linked. Joyce and Walshe (1980) presented a dramatic case history of a middle-aged woman with somatization disorder including abdominal pain who had been hospitalized more than 36 times and received numerous surgical operations. Her children had 25 hospital admissions for abdominal pain and had themselves received numerous operations, often unwarranted according to the pathologist's report, e.g., three normal appendices removed.

A previous study by Ernst, Routh, and Harper (1984) of the medical charts of children with abdominal pain found that those with functional conditions increased in the number of somatic complaints (up to four or five on the average) as they got older or had pain which was more chronic, while those with organically based pain did not. It makes sense that the adult with somatization disorder and 12 or 14 or more complaints must have begun sometime in childhood with the first one. If criteria can be discovered for early identification of such children perhaps more effective intervention will be possible. Treatment is certainly difficult to contemplate in the adult with chronic, polysymptomatic somatization disorder.

METHOD

Subjects

A group of 40 children and adolescents ranging from 7 to 17 years of age were chosen from the 149 children in the Ernst et al. (1984) study. All had been examined by pediatricians in a multispecialty medical clinic because of a presenting complaint of abdominal pain.

The 20 subjects in the organic group each had medical findings to explain their abdominal pain, and onset of symptoms less than 1 year prior to the medical examination. The most frequent diagnosis was acute appendicitis, but other conditions included gastritis, duodenitis, gastroenteritis, and peptic or duodenal ulcer. Twelve of these subjects were male and eight were female; their ages ranged from 7 to 17 years, with a mean age of 12.90 years (SD 3.09). Their mean social class level (Hollingshead, 1957) was 3.45 or lower middle-class (SD 1.23).

The 20 subjects in the functional group met the criteria of absence of a medical diagnosis explaining their abdominal pain and onset of symptoms more than 1 year prior to the medical examination. Eleven of these subjects were male and nine were female; their ages ranged from 8 to 15 years, with a mean age of 11.75 (SD 1.86). Their mean social class level was 3.40 or lower middle-class (SD 1.10). None of the demographic variables was significantly different for the two groups of subjects.

Procedure

The mothers of the children from both groups were interviewed using a structured interview format, either at home or in a convenient central location other than the medical clinic. The three interviewers were female college graduates over 30 years of age who were given a total of 6 hours of direct instruction in the procedures to be followed. They were blind to the hypotheses of the study and the group membership of the mothers; they knew only that the children had been examined for abdominal pain and that the research was an effort to find out more about these children and the family characteristics that might be related to this symptom.

Recruitment of parents was carried out by sending a letter from the director of the medical clinic followed by a phone call by a clinic staff member. Forty-three mothers were contacted; two declined, and one was dropped because it turned out that her child was adopted.

The interview was developed from the NIMH Diagnostic Interview Schedule (Robins, Helzer, Groughan, Williams, & Spitzer, 1981), the Family History Research Diagnostic Criteria developed by Endicott, Andreasen, and Spitzer (1978), and an interview developed by Dr. Remi Cadoret of the University of Iowa Department of Psychiatry; copies of the complete interview protocol are available (Ernst, 1982), and include detailed criteria for determining the presence of each of the following disorders in first- and second-degree relatives: alcoholism, conduct disorder (children) or antisocial personality (adults), attention deficit disorder with or without hyperactivity, somatization disorder, and schizophrenia (this last disorder was included as a control condition unrelated to the hypotheses of the present research). Since it would require too much space to give all these details here, the criteria used to determine the presence of somatization disorder may serve as an example:

A. A history of physical symptoms of several years' duration beginning before the age of 30.

B. Complaints of at least 10 symptoms for women and 8 for men, from the 37 symptoms listed below. To count a symptom as present it must be reported that the individual was caused by the symptom to take medicine (other than aspirin), alter his or her life pattern, or see a physician. The symptoms are not adequately explained by physical disorder or physical disorder or physical injury, and are not side effects of medication, drugs, or alcohol. The person interviewed need not be convinced that the symptom was actually present, e.g., that the individual actually vomited throughout her entire pregnancy; report of the symptoms by the individual is sufficient.

1. Sickly: Believes that he or she has been sickly for a good part of his or her life.
2. Conversion or pseudoneurological symptoms: (a) difficulty swallowing; (b) loss of voice; (c) deafness; (d) double vision; (e) blurred vision; (f) blindness; (g) fainting or loss of consciousness; (h) memory loss; (i) seizures or convulsions; (j) trouble walking; (k) paralysis or muscle weakness; (l) urinary retention or difficulty urinating.
3. Gastrointestinal symptoms: (a) abdominal pain; (b) nausea; (c) vomiting spells (other than during pregnancy); (d) bloating (gassy); (e) intolerance (e.g., gets sick) to a variety of foods; (f) diarrhea.
4. Female reproductive symptoms: Judged in the individual as occurring more frequently or severely than in most women: (a) painful menstruation; (b) menstrual irregularity; (c) excessive bleeding; (d) severe vomiting throughout pregnancy or causing hospitalization during pregnancy.

5. Psychosexual symptoms: For the major part of the individual's life after opportunities for sexual activity: (a) sexual indifference; (b) lack of pleasure during intercourse; (c) pain during intercourse.
6. Pain: (a) pain in back; (b) pain in joints; (c) pain in extremities; (d) pain in genital area (other than during intercourse); (e) pain on urination; (f) other pain (other than headache).
7. Cardiopulmonary symptoms: (a) shortness of breath; (b) palpitations; (c) chest pain; (d) dizziness.

The family history interview required the mother first to produce a family tree for her child listing all first- and second-degree relatives. First-degree relatives included the child's biological mother, biological father, and full siblings. Second-degree relatives included half-siblings, nieces and nephews, grandparents, and aunts and uncles. After obtaining the family tree, the interviewer went back to the first name or initial of each person in the family and asked a specific set of questions designed to determine if that person met the criteria for each of the disorders noted above.

Interjudge reliability data were obtained by tape recording 12 of the 40 interviews and having a second rater score the mother's responses while listening to the tapes. Both raters agreed on the disorders attributed to 29 of the relatives described on these tapes, and disagreed with respect to the diagnosis of 4 of the relatives; this corresponds to an effective agreement of 88%. This stringent method of computing rater reliability disregards instances of agreement as to nonpresence of disorder, which would have unrealistically inflated the percentage agreement.

At the end of the interview, a copy of the Achenbach (1978a) Child Behavior checklist was completed on the index child or left with the mother to complete concerning the index child and return by mail. As it happened, all 20 mothers of children with organic abdominal pain returned these checklists, but only 15 of the mothers of children with functional pain did so. There was no evident bias in the demographic characteristics of the subset of mothers of children with functional pain who complied with the request to return these questionnaires.

RESULTS

The interviews generated information concerning a total of 644 first- and second-degree relatives, 319 for the children with organic abdominal pain (mean 15.95 per child, *SD* 5.93) and 325 for those with functional pain (mean 16.25 per child, *SD* 4.86). The typical subject had 3 or 4

Table I. Incidence of Specific Disorders Among Relatives of Each Group

Group (total number of relatives)	Attention deficit disorder	Alcoholism	Antisocial or conduct disturbance	Somatization disorder
Organic (n = 319)	11	22	11	1
Functional (n = 325)	20	37	23	14

first-degree relatives and about 12 second-degree relatives. The difference between groups in number of relatives per child was not statistically significant.

Only one relative in the entire sample (and none among the functional group) was found to meet the criteria for schizophrenia, but at least some met criteria for each of the other disorders under consideration. Thus, all disorders identified were pertinent to the hypothesis of the study and could reasonably be combined for purposes of statistical analysis.

The mean number of disorders per relative for each index child was calculated by dividing the number of disorders identified by the number of relatives in the family (it was possible though not common for a given relative to meet criteria for more than one disorder). The mean number of disorders per relative was significantly higher in the functional pain group (mean 0.31, SD 0.28) than in the organic group (mean 0.14, SD 0.14), $t(38) = 2.33, p < .05$.

An alternative way to describe the results was in terms of the proportion of an index child's relatives who met criteria for one or more disorders. The proportion of relatives with one or more disorders was significantly higher in the functional pain group (mean 0.22, SD 0.20) than in the organic group (mean 0.10, SD 0.09), $t(38) = 2.47, p < .05$.

Table I gives the number of relatives identified as having the various disorders for each group of index children. It is evident that, as predicted, the children in the functional pain group had more relatives with attention deficit disorder, alcoholism, antisocial or conduct disturbance, and somatization disorder than children in the organic group. However, statistical analysis indicated a significant difference only in the case of somatization disorder, where the functional group had a mean proportion of 0.04 affected relatives (SD 0.06) and the organic group a mean proportion of 0.01 (SD 0.02), $t(38) = 2.51, p < .05$.

Looking in more detail at these relatives with somatization disorder, it is of interest that for the organic group only 1 child has a relative meeting the criteria (a father) while for the functional pain group 10 of the 20 children had one or more affected relatives (7 mothers, 2 fathers, 3 maternal grandmothers, 1 paternal grandmother, and 1 maternal aunt). One child with functional pain had three such relatives: the mother, the maternal grandmother, and the paternal grandmother. Of the entire group of 15 relatives with somatization disorder, 12, or 80%, were female, a significant departure from an even sex ratio, χ^2 (1, n = 15) = 5.40, p <.05. There was, however, no evident tendency for children of one sex or the other to be more likely to have relatives with somatization disorder.

The children in the functional and organic groups were compared in terms of normalized T scores on the Achenbach Child Behavior checklist for all scales which exist across the different age and sex groups, i.e., on the social competence scales and the broad factors of an Internalizing and Externalizing as well as the scales shown in Figure 1 representing specific kinds of psychopathology. The only significant difference was that the functional group had higher scores on the somatic complaints scale (mean 69.60, SD 8.27) than did the organic group (mean 62.80, SD 9.37), t(33) = 2.27, p <.05.

DISCUSSION

The present results provide additional evidence that there is a link between functional abdominal pain in children and adolescents and Briquet's syndrome or somatization disorder in adulthood. Thus, abdominal pain in a child or adolescent can be a hysterical symptom and is perhaps a harbinger of more such somatic complaints to come. The previous direct evidence for such a linkage consisted mainly of Robins and O'Neal's (1953) findings that 4 of 23 individuals with hysterical symptoms in childhood met criteria for Briquet's syndrome upon adult follow-up, and Ernst et al.'s (1984) report that the number of somatic complaints increases with chronicity in children and adolescents with functional abdominal pain.

The familial nature of somatization disorder and its higher prevalence in females were well known even to Briquet, whose 1859 treatise suggested that persons born to hysterical parents were 12 times as likely to have hysteria as those whose parents were nonhysterical (Mai & Merskey, 1980). Arkonac and Guze (1963) found that there was an increased prevalence of hysteria among the female relatives of index cases suffering from hysteria. Coryell (1980) found that first-degree relatives of Briquet's syndrome probands had significantly more "complicated" medical histories than those of control subjects. Our research extends such findings to child probands presenting with functional abdominal pain.

Our hypothesis that functional abdominal pain in children and adolescents is linked to other conditions in the family such as alcoholism, attention

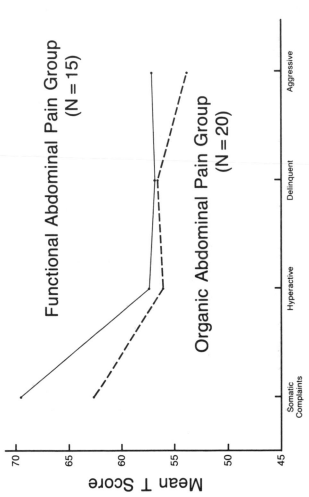

Fig. 1. Mean T scores on the Achenbach Child Behavior checklist scales representing narrow-band factors common to the different age and sex groups.

deficit disorder, and conduct disorder or antisocial personality received some support in that these conditions were all more frequent among their relatives, though not significantly so when the disorders were analyzed one by one. One reason for the weakness of these findings may be the use of the "family history" method, with the child's mother as the only informant. Andreasen, Endicott, Spitzer, and Winokur (1977) suggest that the main defect of this method is significant underreporting of various kinds of psychopathology when compared to the use of the "family study" method—interviewing as many relatives as possible about their own present or past symptomatology. Such underreporting must have been responsible, for example, for our finding only 1 schizophrenic among a sample of over 600 relatives. Another factor possibly important is that many relatives, i.e., siblings, nieces, and nephews, were very young and might be expected to display more psychopathology, such as alcoholism, when older.

Our study did not address the issue of the mechanism underlying the linkage of childhood functional abdominal pain and somatization disorder in relatives. A genetic predisposition to hysteria might be suspected here, but an identification or asocial learning hypothesis would account for the results equally well. Future research, for example, adoption studies, is necessary in order to address this question.

Although the functional pain group was not explicitly selected on the basis of the number of complaints, these children did have a more chronic condition than the organic groups and thus, in line with Ernst et al.'s (1984) findings, would be expected to have more other symptoms. This expectation was confirmed by the findings on the Achenbach Somatic Complaints scale filled out by the mothers: those children with functional pain had higher T scores. The main value of this finding may be as evidence for the criterion-referenced validity of the scale. Achenbach and Edelbrock (1979) report that a somatic complaints factor has emerged from six different behavior checklist studies by four different groups of researchers. Symptoms relevant to abdominal pain such as nausea, pain, and stomach problems are consistently among the items with the highest loadings on Achenbach's Somatic Complaints factor (Achenbach, 1978b; Achenbach & Edelbrock, 1979), and somatic complaints profile patterns have been identified for all age and sex groups except adolescent males (Edelbrock & Achenbach, 1980). However, no previous specific evidence for criterion-referenced validity of the Somatic Complaints scale has evidently been reported.

The clinical implications of these findings suggest that when one is evaluating a child with abdominal pain it may be useful to inquire carefully into the history of the extended family and to determine whether the child has a history of other somatic complaints as well. The Achenbach Child Behavior checklist might assist in this inquiry. Finding a multitude of such complaints or one or more relatives with somatization disorder would increase the likelihood that the abdominal pain represents a hysterical symptom.

REFERENCES

Achenbach, T. M. (1978a). The Child Behavior Profile: I. Boys aged 6-11. *Journal of Consulting and Clinical Psychology, 46,* 478-488.

Achenbach, T. M. (1978b). The classification of child psychopathology: A review and analysis of empirical efforts. *Psychological Bulletin, 85,* 1275-1301.

Achenbach, T. M., & Edelbrock, C. S. (1979). The Child Behavior Profile: II. Boys aged 12-16 and girls aged 6-11 and 12-16. *Journal of Consulting and Clinical Psychology, 47,* 223-233.

American Psychiatric Association. (1980). *Diagnostic and statistical manual of mental disorders* (3rd ed.). Washington, DC: Author.

Andreasen, N. C., Endicott, J., Spitzer, R. L., & Winokur, G. (1977). The family history method using diagnostic criteria. *Archives of General Psychiatry, 34,* 1229-1235.

Apley, J. (1975). *The child with abdominal pain* (2nd ed.). Oxford: Blackwell Scientific Publications.

Arkonac, O., & Guze, S. B. (1963). A family study of hysteria. *New England Journal of Medicine, 268,* 239-242.

Bibb, R. C., & Guze, S. B. (1972). Hysteria (Briquet's syndrome) in a psychiatric hospital: The significance of secondary depression. *American Journal of Psychiatry, 129,* 224-228.

Cloninger, C. R., & Guze, S. B. (1970a). Psychiatric illness and female criminality: The role of sociopathy and hysteria in the antisocial woman. *American Journal of Psychiatry, 127,* 303-311.

Cloninger, C. R., & Guze, S. B. (1970b). Female criminals: Their personal, familial, and social backgrounds. *Archives of General Psychiatry, 23,* 554-558.

Cloninger, C. R., & Guze, S. B. (1975). Hysteria and parental psychiatric illness. *Psychological Medicine, 5,* 27-31.

Cohen, M. E., Robins, E., Purtell, J. J., Altmann, M. W., & Reid, D. E. (1953). Excessive surgery in hysteria. *Journal of the American Medical Association, 151,* 977-986.

Coryell, W. (1980). A blind family history study of Briquet's syndrome: Further validation of the diagnosis. *Archives of General Psychiatry, 37,* 1266-1269.

Coryell, W., & Norten, S. G. (1981). Briquet's syndrome (somatization disorder) and primary depression: Comparison of backgrounds and outcome. *Comprehensive Psychiatry, 22,* 249-256.

Edelbrock, C., & Achenbach, T. M. (1980). A typology of Child Behavior Profile patterns: Distribution and correlates for disturbed children aged 6-16. *Journal of Abnormal Child Psychology, 8,* 441-470.

Endicott, J., Andreasen, N., & Spitzer, R. L. (1978). *Family history research diagnostic criteria* (FH-RDC) 3rd ed. New York: Biometric Research Unit, New York State Psychiatric Institute.

Ernst, A. R. (1982). *The relationship of abdominal pain in children to somatization disorder (Briquet's syndrome) in adults.* Unpublished doctoral dissertation, University of Iowa.

Ernst, A. R., Routh, D. K., & Harper, D. C. (1984). Abdominal pain in children and symptoms of somatization disorder. *Journal of Pediatric Psychology, 9,* 77-86.

Farley, J., Woodruff, R. A., Jr., & Guze, S. B. (1968). The prevalence of hysteria and conversion symptoms. *British Journal of Psychiatry, 114,* 1121-1125.

Guze, S. B. (1964). Conversion symptoms in criminals. *American Journal of Psychiatry, 121,* 580-583.

Guze, S. B., Woodruff, R. A., Jr., & Clayton, P. J. (1971). Hysteria and antisocial behavior: Further evidence of an association. *American Journal of Psychiatry, 127,* 957-960.

Hollingshead, A. B. (1957). *Two-factor index of social position.* Unpublished manuscript. Available from Yale University, New Haven, CT.

Joyce, P. R., & Walshe, J. W. B. (1980). A family with abdominal pain. *New Zealand Medical Journal, 92,* 278-279.

Mai, F. M., & Merskey, H. (1980). Briquet's Treatise on Hysteria: A synopsis and commentary. *Archives of General Psychiatry, 37,* 1401-1405.

Morrison, J. R., & Stewart, M. A. (1971). A family study of the hyperactive child syndrome. *Biological Psychiatry, 3,* 189-195.

Perley, M. J., & Guze, S. B. (1962). Hysteria: The stability and usefulness of clinical criteria. *New England Journal of Medicine, 266,* 421-426.

Purtell, J. J., Robins, E., & Cohen, M. E. (1951). Observations on clinical aspects of hysteria. *Journal of the American Medical Association, 146,* 902-909.

Robins, E., & O'Neal, P. (1953). Clinical features of hysteria in children with note on prognosis. *Nervous Child, 10,* 246-271.

Robins, L. N. (1966). *Deviant children grown up.* Baltimore: Williams & Wilkins.

Robins, L. N., Helzer, J. E., Croughan, J., Williams, J., & Spitzer, R. L. (1981). *NIMH Diagnostic Interview Schedule: Version III.* Rockville, MD: National Institute of Mental Health.

Slater, E. (1965). Diagnosis of "hysteria." *British Medical Journal, 1,* 1395-1399.

Veith, I. (1965). *Hysteria: The history of a disease.* Chicago: University of Chicago Press.

Woerner, P. I., & Guze, S. B. (1968). A family and marital study of hysteria. *British Journal of Psychiatry, 114,* 161-168.

Woodruff, R. A., Jr. (1967). Hysteria: An evaluation of objective diagnostic criteria by the study of women with chronic medical illnesses. *British Journal of Psychiatry, 114,* 115-119.

V

Professional Issues and Training

Diane J. Willis

University of Oklahoma Health Sciences Center

While the United States is recognized as a leader in the world, health care of children in the United States has deteriorated in the 1980s and 90s. Pediatric psychologists, along with other health care professionals, are confronted with illnesses related to societal ills not readily "cured" by antibiotics or a behavioral program. More and more of the children served by pediatric psychologists are part of the "new morbidity" (Haggerty, Roughman, & Pless, 1975); that is, they have health problems related to socioeconomic conditions, poor nutrition, child abuse, sexually transmitted diseases including HIV/AIDS, parental substance abuse, lead poisoning, and so forth.

More children are being born handicapped as a result of toxicity in the intrauterine environment (drugs, alcohol, tobacco use), and prenatal care is still not provided to many mothers of lower socioeconomic status. Teenage pregnancy is at an all-time high, and the incidence of low-birthweight babies continues to increase. Immunizations and other medical technology have decreased the number of organic diseases, but the number of children experiencing psychological, emotional, learning, and chronic health problems has increased at an alarming rate (Baumeister, 1987; Baumeister & Kupstas, 1991; Baumeister, Frank, & Klindworth, 1992). Pediatric psychologists, often practicing in teaching hospitals, must deal now with this new morbidity as they attempt to consult with the poor, minorities, and families at risk of abuse or at risk of failing to provide for the complex needs of their children. Cultural and material changes likely have contributed to changes being seen in children's health and mental health problems (Fuchs & Reklis, 1992). Pediatric psychologists, by the nature of their training and expertise, can contribute to the intervention, prevention, research, and advocacy efforts needed to combat the increase in physical, mental, and emotional problems in children.

Pediatric psychology's early interests focused on developmental issues, assessment, common behavior problems, and behavioral treatment of medically complex problems, such as tracheostomy addiction or noncompliance with a medical regimen. Psychologists in medical settings recognized the need for early intervention in behavioral problems and recognized that parents are a child's first teachers. In recent years, pediatric psychologists, recognizing changes in the health care field and the types of children being served, developed a new statement for the masthead of the *Journal of Pediatric Psychology,* which was printed in 1988, (see Introduction). This new statement encompassed all of the ingredients necessary to combat this new morbidity. As a developing profession of practice and research, a number of important issues arise regarding pediatric psychology's content area, viability, present and future functioning, and its acceptance by those with whom it relates. This section of readings presents articles dealing with this variety of professional issues. Notable in these works are attention to the scientific foundation and the professional practice of pediatric psychology.

TRANSACTING WITH PHYSICIANS

Pediatric psychologists in hospital settings are reliant upon physicians for referrals; the greater the satisfaction pediatricians have with the service, the more referrals are made. In often their first exposure to pediatric practice, pediatric psychology interns must learn the culture and environment of the hospital: physicians refer, consults are made, chart notes are written, and a formal discussion of the patient with the resident or attending physician/nurses takes place. But pediatric psychology trainees learn that service is but one task performed by their supervisors. Training of medical personnel and collaborative research are two other important roles (Stabler, 1979). The economic environment that exists in health care and hospitals across the nation in the 1990s was predicted very accurately by Dennis Drotar's 1983 article presented in this section. Not only did Drotar offer insights in "transacting with physicians," he also pointed out the myths and truths in collaboration between the two professions.

Anticipating trends, given the likelihood of increased future technology and cost-effectiveness pressures, Drotar speculated that psychologists can survive in the new environment if they utilize their strengths in areas of research by being "much more assiduous in evaluating the outcome of our clinical services, consultations, and research, especially in terms of the human 'costs' that are presented or contained through our efforts" (p. 123). Drotar admitted that the future of psychologists in pediatric settings will depend upon their ability to continue to forge an interprofessional relationship with physicians. Psychologists with good research skills can contribute meaningfully to understanding the effects of certain medical conditions or chronic illness, for example, upon peer relations and social functioning (La Greca, 1990), adherence to prescribed medical regimens (La Greca, 1988), and a variety of other conditions.

Professional issues confronting pediatric psychologists, as Drotar states in the article, include the ability to forge good interprofessional relationships but also tend to be economically driven. Cost containment in hospitals forces administrators to cut people and services that do not provide an essential service. The re-medicalization of medical centers, which occurs more often during tight economic periods, can impact on pediatric psychologists, who are often considered allied health staff. Pediatric psychologists who can be reimbursed for their services through insurance or Medicaid and offer essential services to hospitals which are documentable, and who use their research skills to obtain external funding, are in more protected positions. An elaboration beyond Drotar's article is that professional licensure is required in hospitals if one is to consult with patients. Training programs fitting the scientist–practitioner model provide students with the type of research skills, supervised clinical work, and basic graduate courses needed to succeed in the hospital environment. Drotar's article touches on the psychologist–physician relationship, research, and to an extent the economics of the hospital environment, but in the 1990s pediatric psychologists must also be vigilant about insurance-related issues and the ability of the hospital or department to be reimbursed for services rendered.

THE ROLE OF PSYCHOLOGISTS IN PRIVATE PEDIATRIC OFFICE SETTINGS

Carolyn S. Schroeder pioneered a model for pediatric psychology practice in a private pediatric setting. While other psychologists worked in conjunction with pediatricians in their offices, Schroeder more formally established, evaluated, and published articles about such a practice model. Schroeder, Goolsby, and Strangler (1975) described preventive services in a private pediatric practice through an approach that combined service, training, and research. This earliest descriptive article was a prelude to several *Journal of Pediatric Psychology* (*JPP*) articles focusing on psychologists' consultations in private pediatric offices and in pediatric hospitals. It underscored the need for (a) developmentally trained pediatric psychologists, (b) placing emphasis on parent education, and (c) mental health services in centers serving pediatric populations.

Schroeder et al.'s (1975) first article described the services, training, and research agreement worked out between the Division of Disorders of Development and Learning (DDDL) at the University of North Carolina and a private group of pediatricians serving approximately 10,000 children. Services provided in the pediatric office included parent education groups, a Call-In hour, and a Come-In appointment for parents of children whose problems necessitated a face-to-face appointment. No fee was charged parents for this service. In this setting, pediatric residents and psychology trainees, under supervision of the faculty, learned how to consult with parents as they called in and were then offered the opportunity to co-lead parent groups or to consult further with parents during the Come-In appointment times. Schroeder and her colleagues kept records of each call including age of the child and the nature of the child's problem.

Since many parenting education programs emerging in the 1970s focused on single techniques such as Parent Effectiveness Training (PET) or behavior modification, Schroeder et al.'s (1975) article had a threefold message. First, parent training techniques needed to be expanded in response to broad-based concerns and issues with which parents must cope, and they need to be more eclectic. They presented that professionals involved in parent training need to be familiar with community resources and with contributions provided by other disciplines. Second, many concerns parents discuss with the pediatrician involve behavioral and learning issues, concerns that psychologists are best trained to handle. However, this study demonstrated the need to train pediatricians to manage developmental-behavioral problems more effectively. Third, certain problems are more common at certain ages and the need to know normal development is very important. These remain important issues. Two years after Schroeder et al. described their model, Mesibov, Schroeder, and Wesson (1977), in an article included in this section, analyzed the most common pediatric problems expressed by these middle-income parents to pediatric psychologists in a private pediatric office. This analysis found that parental concerns focused mainly on negative behaviors such as tantrums and disobedience, toileting issues, developmental delays, and school and sleep problems. Two years later, Schroeder (1979), in her Presidential Address to the Society of Pediatric Psychology at a meeting of the APA in Toronto, presented further data from the original work described in the 1975 article. In her presidential address, Schroeder described another survey of parental concerns by age of the child and the information source parents use to aid them in child rearing. Schroeder found, for example, that parents of 2-year-old children are more concerned with toileting, sleeping, and eating problems, than with divorce, family or physical complaints. Parents tended to use books as their primary source of information, with their physicians and family/friends ranking second and third. Kanoy and Schroeder (1985), in an article reprinted here, more formally analyzed the results of the suggestions made to parents about common behavior problems in a pediatric primary care office in a five-year follow-up study. They found that the services and predominately behavioral suggestions made to parents were highly rated. However, parents continued to express concerns about their children. Kanoy and Schroeder suggested that parents may need more follow-up help than psychologists or other mental health professionals were then providing.

As a result of Schroeder's early consultation in the private pediatric office, she joined the practice full-time in 1983, establishing her own pediatric psychology and clinical child services within the office of the private pediatricians. Schroeder truly exemplifies the scientist–practitioner model of care in that she systematically gathers and analyzes information obtained from her clinical practice, integrates that knowledge into her practice, and uses it to enhance training of students and advance new information through publications. In 1991, Schroeder and Gordon completed a book titled *Assessment and Treatment of Childhood Problems: A Clinicians' Guide.* One of the chapters of this excellent reference reviews a model for clinical child practice in the pediatric setting (pp. 375–398). In this chapter, Schroeder and Gordon reviewed the pediatric model developed in the 1970s, concluding with a section on the professional and business aspects of practicing in a primary health care setting.

THE ROLE OF PSYCHOLOGISTS IN PEDIATRIC HOSPITAL SETTINGS

A series of articles published by *JPP* focused on consultation in pediatric hospitals (Drotar & Malone, 1982; Singer & Drotar, 1989) and evaluating hospital-based outpatient pediatric psychology services (Charlop, Parrish, Fenton, & Cataldo, 1987) and inpatient consultation services (Olson et al., 1988). Quality of services for children with special health needs according to parental perceptions was also analyzed (Krahn, Eisert, & Fifield, 1990).

Drotar and Malone (1982) described a program of psychological services to infants and reported that coordination between hospital and community-based services posed problems in providing quality services. Coordination often was inconsistent, and community-based programs were ill-prepared to work with infants. The Drotar and Malone article served as a precursor to Public Law 99-457 (which provided for the earlier evaluation and ongoing assessment of the infant and young child), illustrating the need for communities to prepare to deal with infant mental health problems in existence in the 1990s. Drotar and Malone also pointed out that pediatric psychologists, who are well prepared to understand developmental needs of infants, play an important role not only working with infants within the hospital setting, but also serving as advocates to find resources for them in the community.

Reprinted in this section, Olson et al.'s (1988) article described an archival evaluation, covering a period of $4^1/_2$ years, of the types of referrals made to an inpatient pediatric psychology consultation service. This article provided a glimpse of the variety of cases referred to an inpatient consultation service. Children with depression/suicidal attempts were referred most often; however, pediatric psychologists tended to follow the more medically complex patients, and to use community mental health resources for the emotionally distraught patients. Medically complex cases, such as children with a terminal illness, tracheostomy addiction, or severe burns, tended to be followed not only in the hospital but after discharge. Pediatric psychologists are trained to handle almost all of the referrals coming into a consultation service, but this article demonstrated a method of triage that allows the pediatric psychologists time to handle the more complex medically related problems. Olson et al. also describe the nature of the relationship between psychologist, physician, and nurse. A questionnaire developed to evaluate services provided by the pediatric psychology service suggested that the hospital personnel were satisfied, overall, with the consultation/intervention services received, but were more dissatisfied with outpatient follow-up, which necessitated a change in the way the psychologists provided feedback on referrals to the community. Olson et al.'s article further demonstrated the need for psychologists to evaluate the services they do provide and to be open to suggestions/feedback from hospital personnel about the strengths and weaknesses of their consults/recommendations.

Two other related articles published in the *JPP,* but not included in this volume, also illustrate the role of pediatric psychologists in hospital settings. Singer and Drotar's (1989) article on psychological practice in a pediatric rehabilitative hospital indicated the need for good assessment, intervention, and consultation skills with children who may be ventilator dependent, paralyzed, or multiply affected from some type of trauma. Charlop et al. (1987) evaluated referrals to a hospital-based outpatient pediatric psychology service and found that behavioral noncompliance, aggression, and tantrums were the most common referral complaints. This finding is similar to those of Schroeder's in her non-hospital-based private pediatric office.

Aside from the necessity of pediatric psychologists being well trained in child development and knowing how to utilize a variety of skills in training parents to manage common behavior problems presented by their children, psychologists also have been involved in developing written guidelines for pediatric health care providers and parents to use in managing common behavioral problems (Christophersen & Rapoff, 1979). Other parent education techniques reported in *JPP* included teaching mothers through videotape modeling to change their children's behavior (Webster-Stratton, 1981, 1982). In later research, Holden, Lavigne, and Cameron (1990) studied the efficacy of a behaviorally oriented training program for child noncompliance. The mothers in their study were heterogeneous, including different ethnic groups and income levels. Mothers of young children at a lower socioeconomic level and in ethnic minority groups tended to drop out from the program at a higher rate or to take longer in completing the parent training than white, middle-class mothers with older children. Holden et al. (1990) reminded professionals that parent training programs must identify and take into account client characteristics and be prepared to provide additional assistance to selected groups.

The diversity of training guidelines developed by pediatric psychologists is further reflected in research on preparation of young children for surgery. For example, Peterson, Ridley-Johnson, Tracey, and Mullins (1984) compared children who were prepared by a narrative hospital tour to those who received a puppet modeling plus tour procedure and those who received a coping skills plus modeling plus tour procedure. Children exposed to the latter two procedures experienced lower ratings of distress and fewer maladaptive behaviors pre- and postsurgery than those who were in the tour-only group. These training modules can be used by health service providers in any hospital, and they do not require the presence of a psychologist. McFarland and Stanton (1991), following up research by others (Peterson & Ridley-Johnson, 1984; Roberts, Wurtele, Boone, Ginther, & Elkins, 1981), demonstrated the effectiveness of a hospital preparation program in a primary prevention approach. Robinson and Kobayashi (1991) evaluated a hospital-based program for children scheduled for surgery in a secondary prevention approach.

The aforementioned articles all focus on in-hospital programs or services offered by pediatric psychologists and demonstrated what Olson et al. (1988) and Drotar (1983) both stressed: Professionals need to evaluate psychological programs and services in a variety of ways.

PREVENTION OF HEALTH PROBLEMS

The profession of pediatric psychology began to focus attention on prevention issues in the mid-1980's. Michael Roberts (Roberts, 1986a, 1986b;

Roberts & Peterson, 1984) was one of the earliest pediatric psychologists to focus on prevention of psychological and health problems among children and to advocate health promotion in pediatric psychology. Roberts and Peterson (1984) edited a book on the prevention of mental and physical health problems in childhood. Roberts's (1986a) Presidential Address to SPP suggested that the future of children's health care requires psychologists to focus on prevention issues and promotion of health-enhancing lifestyles such as good nutrition, exercise, and the avoidance of smoking.

As associate editor of *JPP,* Roberts guest-edited a special topical issue on health promotion and problem prevention in pediatric psychology. Roberts's (1986b) editorial, reprinted here, provided an overview of the various areas of need for health promotion and prevention and placed the special issue's articles into context. For example, he reported that accidents (automobile, drownings, fires, poisoning) are the leading cause of death among children ages 1 to 14 years. Clearly, pediatric psychologists, who consult with and treat surviving children in the hospital, could add their expertise to prevention efforts. Roberts's thoughtful editorial instructed psychologists on concepts in health promotion and problem prevention and acquainted psychologists with public health models of prevention.

In the special issue of *JPP* on problem prevention and health promotion, the authors reported on such issues as prevention of adolescent alcohol abuse by using educational information and social skills training with an elementary school group (Dielman, Shope, Butchart, & Campanelli, 1986) and focused on the intervention and prevention of sexual abuse (Saslawsky & Wurtele, 1986). Two articles from this special issue were selected for this volume and are reprinted in Section III (Coppens, 1986; Peterson, Mori, & Scissors, 1986). Other pediatric psychologists also began focusing on prevention (e.g., Willis, Holden, & Rosenberg, 1991). Knapp (1991), for example, investigated promotion of children's dental health behavior. Richards, Hendricks, and Roberts (1991) reported on an elementary school curriculum designed to help prevent spinal cord injury. In a behavioral application to primary prevention, Jones, McDonald, Fiore, Arrington, and Randall (1990) taught drug refusal behavior to children. Roberts sensitized others in the pediatric psychology and health community to the issue of prevention, and later issues of *JPP* published numerous articles focusing on prevention.

PEDIATRIC AIDS

Among the new diseases with which pediatric psychologists and other health care professionals must deal, none has more "political and social ramifications" (Olson, Huszti, Mason, & Seibert, 1989, p. 1) than pediatric acquired immunodeficiency syndrome (AIDS). Although pediatric psychologists for years have worked with children with chronic and life-threatening diseases, AIDS presents a new and unique challenge. Olson et al.'s article was selected for this text because of its excellent review of the opportunities and problems confronting psychologists working with this disease, and because it was one of the first comprehensive articles published in *JPP* addressing pediatric AIDS. Olson has also participated in an article on intervention for adolescents with hemophilia (Mason, Olson, Myers, Huszti, & Kenning, 1989).

Olson began her work in pediatric AIDS at Children's Hospital of Oklahoma when children with hemophilia began contracting the disease from blood products. She established a comprehensive prevention program for hemophiliacs who had already contracted the disease. She and her interns held weekend retreats for children, adolescents, and adults with hemophilia and their families to address the prevention or spread of the disease to nonaffected individuals. This work was subsequently published in the *American Psychologist* (Mason, Olson, & Parrish, 1988). Olson was also appointed to the APA's Division 37 (Children, Youth and Family Services) Task Force on Pediatric AIDS; as a result of her contribution to the task force, the book *Children, Adolescents, and AIDS* (Seibert & Olson, 1989) was published by the University of Nebraska's Children and the Law series. This book was one of the first texts regarding AIDS to link public policy, law, medicine, education, prevention, and the needs of children in a single publication.

This devastating illness has mobilized the government to appropriate vast amounts of monies for research to find a "cure or effective prevention." Olson and Mason currently are completing data collection and analysis on a five-year project in which their particular program is one of 15 sites in the country examining children with hemophilia who are HIV positive or negative. Olson is continuing to publish articles on AIDS (Olson, Huszti, & Chaffin, 1992) and has made presentations on her work at the American Psychological Association/APA (1991, 1992) annual convention. She is one of the first pediatric psychologists to make such a substantial contribution to knowledge about pediatric AIDS, especially as contracted by hemophiliacs.

Practitioners and researchers in pediatric psychology have also responded to the challenge of AIDS and its related psychosocial aspects. The *Journal of Pediatric Psychology* has accepted and published a number of articles considering such issues as the impact on adolescents of knowing somebody with AIDS (Zimet et al., 1991), the relationship of parents' and children's attitudes toward persons with AIDS (McElreath & Roberts, 1992), and developmental changes in understanding and attitudes toward HIV and AIDS (Eiser, Eiser, & Lang, 1990; Walsh & Bibace, 1991).

SUMMARY

Through the series of articles published in this section, pediatric psychologists have taught others about the myriad of activities in which pediatric psychologists are engaged. The articles suggest ways of transacting with physicians in a medical setting and demonstrate the types of services psychologists can provide in hospital or in primary care offices within the community. Most of the articles stress the importance of maintaining good interprofessional relationships, evaluating the outcome of treatment or other services provided, and familiarizing oneself with community resources. Pediatric psychologists have forged new programs in the area of prevention and pediatric AIDS and have immersed themselves in training, research, and service activity related to the new morbidity as well as to chronic or complex medical diseases affecting children. In the 1990s this new breed of psychologist must demonstrate his or her value anew given the changing health care environment. Reimbursement to hospitals and departments of psychiatry or pediatrics for services rendered by the psychologist will be an issue which pediatric psychologists must address, and the ability to attract research funds on childrens health/mental health issues will make pediatric psychology a valued profession in hospitals.

The development of the pediatric psychology field has made it a professional subdiscipline with subsequent need to define its character. For example, several articles and chapters have described training backgrounds and affiliations of pediatric psychologists (La Greca, Stone, Drotar, & Maddux, 1988; La Greca, Stone, & Swales, 1989; Roberts, Fanurik, & Elkins, 1988; Routh, 1988). Other work on professional issues has described pediatric psychologists' perceptions of their work settings and functions (Drotar, Sturm, Eckerle, & White, 1993; Stabler & Mesibov, 1984) and predictions of their future activities (Kauffman, Holden, & Walker, 1989; Walker, 1988). More recently, Rae and Worchel (1991) examined the awareness and ethical practices of pediatric psychologists through a survey of SPP members. Attention to these issues and to the continually developing nature of the field as demonstrated in this section is what characterizes it as an empirically and clinically based profession.

ACKNOWLEDGMENTS

The author wishes to thank Brenda Gentry for her patience in typing this section overview. Thanks are also due to Jan L. Culbertson, Ph.D., for her editorial suggestions.

REFERENCES

Baumeister, A. A. (1987). *The new morbidity: Poverty and handicapping conditions in America.* Presentation made at the Institute for Disabilities Studies at the University of Minnesota, Minneapolis.

Baumeister, A. A., Frank, D., Klindworth, L. M. (1992). The new morbidity: A national plan of action. In T. Thompson & S. C. Hupp (Eds.), *Saving children at risk* (pp. 143–177). Newbury Park, CA: Sage.

Baumeister, A. A., & Kupstas, F. (1991). The new morbidity: Implications for prevention and amelioration. In A. Clark & P. Evans (Eds.), *Combatting mental handicap: A multidisciplinary approach* (pp. 46–72). London: A. B. Academic Press.

Charlop, M. H., Parrish, J. M., Fenton, L. R., & Cataldo, M. F. (1987). Evaluation of hospital-based outpatient pediatric psychology services. *Journal of Pediatric Psychology, 12,* 485–518.

Christophersen, E. R., & Rapoff, M. A. (1979). Behavioral problems in children. In G. Scipien, M. Barnard, M. Chard, J. Howe, & P. Phillips (Eds.), *Comprehensive pediatric nursing* (pp. 361–383). New York: McGraw-Hill.

Coppens, N. M. (1986). Cognitive characteristics as predictors of children's understanding of safety and prevention. *Journal of Pediatric Psychology, 11,* 189–202.

Dielman, T. E., Shope, J. T., Butchart, A. T., & Campanelli, P. C. (1986). Prevention of adolescent alcohol misuse: An elementary school program. *Journal of Pediatric Psychology, 11,* 259–282.

Drotar, D. (1983). Transacting with physicians: Fact and fiction. *Journal of Pediatric Psychology, 8,* 117–127.

Drotar D. (Ed.). (1985) *New directions in failure-to-thrive.* New York: Plenum.

Drotar, D., & Malone, C. A. (1982). Psychological consultations on a pediatric infant division. *Journal of Pediatric Psychology, 7,* 23–32.

Drotar, D., Sturm, L., Eckerle, D., & White, S. (1993). Pediatric psychologists' perceptions of their work settings. *Journal of Pediatric Psychology, 18(2).*

Eiser, C., Eiser, J. R., & Lang, J. (1990). How adolescents compare AIDS with other diseases: Implications for prevention. *Journal of Pediatric Psychology, 15,* 97–103.

Fuchs, V. R., & Reklis, D. M. (1992). America's children: Economic perspectives and policy options. *Science, 255,* 41–46.

Haggerty, R. J., Roughman, K. J., & Pless, I. V. (Eds.). (1975). *Child health and the community,* (pp. 94–113). New York: Wiley.

Holden, G. W., Lavigne, V. U., & Cameron, A. (1990). Probing the continuum of effectiveness in parent training: Characteristics of parents and preschoolers. *Journal of Clinical Child Psychology, 19,* 2–8.

Jones, R. T., McDonald, D. W., Fiore, M. F., Arrington, T., & Randall, J. (1990). A primary preventive approach to children's drug refusal behavior: The impact of rehearsal-plus. *Journal of Pediatric Psychology, 15,* 211–223.

Kanoy, K. W., & Schroeder, C. S. (1985). Suggestions to parents about common behavior problems in a pediatric primary care office: Five years of follow-up. *Journal of Pediatric Psychology, 10,* 15–30.

Kaufman, K. L., Holden, E. W., & Walker, C. E. (1989). Future directions in pediatric and clinical child psychology. *Professional Psychology, 20,* 148–152.

Knapp, L. G. (1991). Effects of type of value appealed to and valence of appeal on children's dental health behavior. *Journal of Pediatric Psychology, 16,* 675–686.

Krahn, G., Eiser, D., & Fifield, B. (1990). Obtaining parental perceptions of the quality of services for children with special health needs. *Journal of Pediatric Psychology, 15,* 761–774.

La Greca, A. M. (1988). Adherence to prescribed medical regimens. In D. K. Routh (Ed.), *Handbook of pediatric psychology* (pp. 299–320). New York: Guilford.

La Greca, A. M. (1990). Social consequences of pediatric conditions: Fertile area for future investigation and intervention. *Journal of Pediatric Psychology, 15,* 285–307.

La Greca, A. M., Stone, W. L., Drotar, D., & Maddux, J. E. (1988). Training in pediatric psychology: Survey results and recommendations. *Journal of Pediatric Psychology, 13,* 121–139.

La Greca, A. M., Stone, W. L., & Swales, T. (1989). Pediatric psychology training: An analysis of graduate, internship, and postdoctoral programs. *Journal of Pediatric Psychology, 14,* 103–116.

Mason, P. J., Olson, R. A., Myers, J. G., Huszti, H. C., & Kenning, M. (1989). AIDS and hemophilia: Implications for interventions with families. *Journal of Pediatric Psychology, 14,* 341–355.

Mason, P. J., Olson, R. A., & Parrish, K. L. (1988). AIDS, hemophilia, and prevention efforts within a comprehensive care program. *American Psychologist, 43,* 971–978.

McElreath, L., & Roberts, M. C. (1992). Perceptions of acquired immune deficiency syndrome by children and their parents. *Journal of Pediatric Psychology, 17,* 477–490.

McFarland, P. H., & Stanton, A. L. (1991). Preparation of children for emergency medical care: A primary prevention approach. *Journal of Pediatric Psychology, 16,* 489–504.

Mesibov, G., Schroeder, C. S., & Wesson, L. (1977). Parental concerns about their children. *Journal of Pediatric Psychology, 2,* 13–17.

Olson, R. A., Holden, E. W., Friedman, A., Faust, J., Kenning, M. & Mason, P. J. (1988). Psychological consultation in a children's hospital: An evaluation of services. *Journal of Pediatric Psychology, 13,* 479–492.

Olson, R., Huszti, H., & Chaffin, M. (1992). Children and adolescents with hemophilia. In M. Steuber (Ed.), *Children and AIDS: Clinical issues for psychiatrists* (pp. 69–85). Washington, DC: American Psychiatric Press.

Olson, R. A., Huszti, H. C., Mason, P. J., & Seibert, J. M. (1989). Pediatric AIDS/HIV infection: An emerging challenge to pediatric psychology. *Journal of Pediatric Psychology, 14,* 1–21.

Peterson, L., Mori, L., & Scissors, C. (1986). Mom or dad says I shouldn't: Supervised and unsupervised children's knowledge of their parents' rules for home safety. *Journal of Pediatric Psychology, 11,* 177–188.

Peterson, L., & Ridley-Johnson, R. (1984). Preparation of well children in the classroom: An unexpected contrast between academic lecture and filmed-modeling methods. *Journal of Pediatric Psychology, 9,* 349–361.

Peterson, L., Ridley-Johnson, R., Tracey, K., & Mullins, L. (1984). Developing cost-effective presurgical preparation: A comparative analysis. *Journal of Pediatric Psychology, 9,* 439–455.

Rae, W. A., & Worchel, F. F. (1991). Ethical beliefs and behaviors of pediatric psychologists: A survey. *Journal of Pediatric Psychology, 16,* 727–745.

Richards, J. S., Hendricks, C., & Roberts, M. C. (1991). Prevention of spinal cord injury: An elementary education approach. *Journal of Pediatric Psychology, 16,* 595–609.

Roberts, M. (1986a). The future of children's health care: What do we do? *Journal of Pediatric Psychology, 11,* 3–14.

Roberts, M. (1986b). Health promotion and problem prevention in pediatric psychology: An overview. *Journal of Pediatric Psychology, 11,* 147–161.

Roberts, M. C., Fanurik, D., & Elkins, P. D. (1988). Training the child health psychologist. In P. Karoly (Ed.), *Handbook of child health assessment: Biopsychosocial perspectives* (pp. 611–632). New York: Wiley.

Roberts, M., & Peterson, L. (Eds.). (1984). *Prevention of problems in childhood: Psychological research and applications*. New York: Wiley-Interscience.

Roberts, M. C., Wurtele, S. K., Boone, R. R., Ginther, L., & Elkins, P. (1981). Reduction of medical fears by use of modeling: A preventive application in a general population of children. *Journal of Pediatric Psychology, 6*, 293–300.

Robinson, P. J., & Kobayashi, K. (1991). Development and evaluation of a presurgical preparation program. *Journal of Pediatric Psychology, 16*, 193–212.

Routh, D. K. (1988). A places-rated almanac for pediatric psychology. *Journal of Pediatric Psychology, 13*, 113–119.

Saslawsky, D. A., & Wurtele, S. K. (1986). Educating children about sexual abuse: Implications for pediatric intervention and possible prevention. *Journal of Pediatric Psychology, 11*, 235–245.

Schroeder, C. S. (1979). Psychologists in a private pediatric practice. *Journal of Pediatric Psychology, 4*, 5–18.

Schroeder, C., Goolsby, E., & Strangler, S. (1975). Preventive services in a private pediatric office. *Journal of Clinical Child Psychology, 4*, 32–33.

Schroeder, C. S., & Gordon, B. (1991). Assessment and treatment of childhood problems: A clinician's guide. New York: Guilford Press.

Seibert, J., & Olson, R. A. (1989). *Children, adolescents, and AIDS*. Lincoln: University of Nebraska Press.

Singer, L., & Drotar, D. (1989). Psychological practice in a pediatric rehabilitation hospital. *Journal of Pediatric Psychology, 14*, 479–489.

Stabler, B. (1979). Emerging models of psychologist–pediatrician liaison. *Journal of Pediatric Psychology, 4*, 307–313.

Stabler, B., & Mesibov, G. B. (1984). Role functions of pediatric and health psychologists in health care settings. *Professional Psychology, 15*, 142–151.

Walker, C. E. (1988). The future of pediatric psychology. *Journal of Pediatric Psychology, 13*, 465–478.

Walsh, M. E., & Bibace, R. (1991). Children's conceptions of AIDS: A developmental analysis. *Journal of Pediatric Psychology, 16*, 273–285.

Webster-Stratton, C. (1981). Videotape modeling: A method of parent training. *Journal of Clinical Child Psychology, 10*, 93–98.

Webster-Stratton, C. (1982). Teaching mothers through videotape modeling to change their children's behavior. *Journal of Pediatric Psychology, 7*, 279–294.

Willis, D. J., Holden, E. W., & Rosenberg, M. (Ed.). (1991). *Prevention of child maltreatment: Developmental and ecological perspective*. New York: John Wiley.

Zimet, G. D., Hillier, S. A., Anglin, T. M., Ellick, E. M., Krowchuk, D. P., & Williams, P. (1991). Knowing someone with AIDS: The impact on adolescents. *Journal of Pediatric Psychology, 16*, 287–294.

18

Transacting with Physicians
Fact and Fiction

Dennis Drotar
*Departments of Psychiatry and Pediatrics, Case Western Reserve University
School of Medicine*

Pediatric psychologists share the fact they transact with physicians in a variety of settings and endeavors including clinical services, consultation, and
research. The importance of our interprofessional collaboration with physicians in medical settings centers around shared patient populations, financial resources, and administrative arrangements. Moreover, given the
dominant administrative structures in medical schools and hospitals
(Nathan, Lubin, Matarrazo, & Persely, 1979), physicians have a significant
impact on the professional deployment and career development of psychologists. For this reason, psychologists' ability to maintain professional
resources and integrity in medical settings in an era of expanding technology and accountability may very well depend upon the efficacy of strategies
that are developed to guide professional interactions with physicians. Unfortunately, psychologists in medical settings have not clearly formulated
the premises on which their transactions with physicians are based, recognized the difficult realities of such interprofessional exchange, nor developed programmatic strategies to anticipate and/or remedy problematic
collaboration. Clinical experiences in one major university-based pediatric
referral center (Drotar, Note 1; Drotar, 1976, 1977; Drotar, Benjamin,
Chwast, Litt, & Vajner, 1981) have underscored the stressful realities of
patient care and administrative organization and led to the development

The paper is based on a Presidential Address given to Section 5 of Division 12 (Society of
Pediatric Psychology) at the Annual Meeting of American Psychological Association, August
1982, Washington, D.C. The work described in this paper is supported in part by the National
Institute of Mental Health #30274, and the Cleveland Foundation #82-461-31R.
Originally published in *Journal of Pediatric Psychology*, 8(2)(1983):117–127.

of a conceptual framework which addresses the realistic benefits and problems of interprofessional exchange for professions as well as families

MYTH AND TRUTH IN COLLABORATION

In some respects, the rapid expansion of pediatric psychology in recent years reflects psychologists' successes in creating professional opportunities via interprofessional collaboration. On the other hand, impressive "on line" advances of knowledge and influence in pediatric settings (Salk, 1970; Stabler, 1979; Wright, 1979) may have tempted pediatric psychologists to minimize the complexity of potential problems involved in collaboration and thus assume that collaborative outcomes will be more benign than have generally been experienced with the profession of psychiatry (Albee, 1969). Although pediatric psychology has undergone dramatic expansion in recent years, knotty and as yet unsolved professional dilemmas are posed by the administrative organization of psychologists in pediatric settings, medical authority, and medical concepts of health and illness (Dubos, 1959; Friedson, 1970; Georgeopoulous & Mann, 1979; Mechanic, 1972). Consequently, our professional energies must be devoted to a realistic analysis of the impact of medical culture on professional interaction.

In any collaborative endeavor, each profession makes implicit or explicit assumptions about the impact of their exchanges on their professional development as well as on patients and their families. Descriptions of psychological consultation in pediatric settings (Drotar, 1976) have usually made the following assumptions: (a) collaboration between psychologists and pediatricians can occur without considerable tension or conflict; (b) psychologists can accommodate to almost any medical culture and shape it to suit them; (c) since physicians (pediatricians or psychiatrists) can usually appreciate psychologists' professional interests, it is reasonable for them to wield administrative power that critically affects the development of psychological services, research, and careers; (d) pediatric models of diagnosis and treatment make an important contribution to our understanding of psychosocial problems; (e) rapid growth of medical technology in pediatric settings represents progress that is in the best interest of children and families. Although each of the above statements may be true under certain circumstances, as generalizations they are simplistic myths which not only serve to constrain our professional development but limit our potential as advocates for children and their families in medical settings. Conceptual models of collaboration should replace such generalizations with specific consideration of the tension created by marked differences in professional training backgrounds, work cultures, and clinical perspectives between psychologists and physicians (Tefft & Simeonsson, 1979).

Given the potential for competing claims between professions and families, it is not reasonable to assume that the professional benefits of collaboration inevitably coincide with the needs of children and families. For this reason, interprofessional exchanges concerning research, consultation, or patient care have been well delineated in reports of psychological activities in pediatric settings (Magrab, 1978; Tuma, 1981). On the other hand, exploitive exchanges, e.g., those in which one profession uses another's expertise for its own ends without proper credit, recompense, and/or respect, or where one profession uses its power to limit the influence of another profession, also occur but have not been well delineated, except in preliminary reports (McNett, 1981). Psychologists and pediatricians would concur that optimal interprofessional exchange results in an extension of professional resources for both professions. Although it is tempting to assume that mutually beneficial professional interchanges will always result in demonstrable benefits to children and families, the potential for competing claims between professional and family needs, particularly in an era of rapidly expanding medical technology (Friedson, 1970; Illich, 1975; Knowles, 1977; Mechanic, 1972), is a reality which must also be considered. Professional interactions characterized by apparent benefit to physicians and psychologists, but not to children and families, run counter to our image of ourselves and hence have not been considered in any depth. However, examples of such collaborations include management of children and families according to models of medical or psychological care that are disruptive to family life (Drotar, Malone, & Negray, 1979; Newberger & Bourne, 1978), psychological assessment of children and families for their "suitability" for arduous medical treatments without provision for psychologically supportive care (Drotar, Note 1), or erroneous labeling of a patient's understandable reaction to severe life stress and/or problematic encounters with physicians as a sign of psychological disturbance (Hauser, 1981; Meyer & Mendelson, 1961; Millman, 1982).

THE IMPACT OF CONCEPTUAL MODELS OF PSYCHOSOCIAL PROBLEMS

The danger that health care professionals will become unwitting participants in exchanges that do not do proper justice to the needs of children and families is enhanced by the extraordinary authority granted in our society to physicians to independently define concepts of health, illness, and treatment (Friedson, 1970). Although there is inevitable tension between the incomplete understanding of clinical problems and the pressures on clinicians to apply their knowledge, the zeal to construct models of patient care based on illusions of certainty rather than scientific understanding is particularly strong in medical cultures (Fox, 1979), where patient care demands inevitably require pragmatic solutions of extremely difficult ethical, technical, and human problems long before they are properly understood (Duff & Campbell, 1973; Fox, 1979; Katz & Capron, 1975). In modern pediatric hospitals, one of the most common professional solutions to frustrating and poorly understood psychosocial problems is the premature assumption of concrete, disease-centered labels in which such problems are localized within the child rather than understood in relation to family, community, or school contexts (Hobbs, 1975; Sarason, 1981). Given the remarkable advances in the treatment of infectious disease (Robinson, 1979), the expectation that progress will be based on disease-centered concepts of children's problems is in some sense understandable. Even more than this, disease-oriented models of psychological problems fit with the concreteness of physical diagnostic methods (Foucault, 1975) and extreme reliance on technology (Reiser, 1981) which are part and parcel of medical culture. Unfortunately, since the rules of professional exchange often follow prevailing concepts of clinical practice, conceptual models have tremendous influence on the character of professional collaboration, including the roles of participants, goals of consultation, and psychological research paradigms (Drotar, 1981). The brief history of pediatric psychology is replete with examples of clinical problems that were initially construed as medical conditions for which physicians assumed primary responsibility for management which are now understood as psychosocial problems where the roles of psychologists (or other mental health professionals) have become more primary. For example, hyperactivity was initially thought to be an homogeneous syndrome which was localized within the child and caused by a defect in the brain (Conrad, 1975; Laufer & Denhoff, 1957). In the early 1960s, pediatricians assumed a central role in treatment of hyperactivity via medication. However, in recent years, psychological research has extended earlier concepts of hyperactivity to emphasize the heterogeneity of this condition, the influence of social context (particularly the family) on the expression of this behavior, and the documentation of longer-term treatment outcomes, especially on social-emotional development (Collins, Whaley, & Henker, 1980; Routh, 1980). Another instructive example concerns the history of diagnosis and treatment of environmentally based failure-to-thrive, a condition associated with psychosocial risk which affects infants and is characterized by severe deficits in rate of weight again secondary to environmental (family) stress (Hannaway, 1970; Patton & Gardner, 1963). In pediatric practice, this problem is construed as a syndrome (Vaughn, McKay, & Behrman, 1979) and managed in pediatric hospitals in patterns of care which focus on physical diagnosis and nutritional treatment (Drotar, Malone, Negray, & Dennstedt, 1981). Recent findings from an ongoing clinical outcome study (Drotar et al. 1979; Drotar & Malone, 1982; Drotar, Note 2) have documented the potential utility of a context-sensitive outreach intervention which addresses the family influences which maintain failure to thrive. A parent-centered treatment model which is based upon collaboration with parents with the aim of helping them nurture their infants more effectively appears to have much greater promise in changing the long-term psychosocial risk ordinarily associated with failure to thrive (Drotar, Note 2; Drotar et al., 1979; Drotar, Malone, & Negray, 1980) than traditional hospital-based treatment or foster care which can undermine family integrity (Newberger & Bourne, 1978) and children's psychological development via lengthy parent-child separation (Singer, Drotar, Fagan, Devost, & Lake, in press).

What can these scenarios concerning concept and practice teach us about psychologist–physician transactions? In each instance, the initial concept of a psychosocial problem was focused on deficits in the child but evolved to one in which family and social factors were construed as more prominent. Even more than this, patterns of clinical management and professional collaboration which were based on a strictly medical concept did not result in demonstrable improvements in children's long-term psychosocial outcome. As the conceptual model which guided treatment broadened to consider the family and social context, treatment emphasis changed from something that was "prescribed" or controlled by the care-giver to a primary emphasis on the relationship between professional and family. Finally, the outcomes of treatments based on an understanding of broader social/familial influences appear to be more promising than outcomes of treatments based solely on medical models.

From the standpoint of professional collaboration, one of the most intriguing by-products of such changes involves the evolution of professional roles with respect to clinical management of children's problems. To the extent that conditions like failure-to-thrive reflect predominantly psychosocial and not organic influences, it follows that primary responsibilities for psychosocial management should be undertaken by those professional disciplines who demonstrate understanding of psychosocial factors. For example, responsibilities for the treatment of many psychosocial problems initially resided almost entirely with physicians. However, with the assumption of primary responsibility for psychosocial treatment by other professional disciplines, the pediatrician's role becomes more circumscribed to include (a) early recognition and referral for treatment; (b) assessment of the role of potential organic influences; and (c) monitoring of health and growth in follow-up. This revised allocation of professional responsibilities allows more effective patient care since it limits each profession to what it does best.

ANTICIPATING FUTURE TRENDS

Advances in psychological understanding of pediatric conditions are occurring rapidly. However, even the most cogent of psychological concepts will not have an impact on prevailing patterns of pediatric care without concerted attention to developing strategies of implementation in medical settings. The success of such strategies may very well depend upon the accuracy of understanding of hospital cultural and organizational patterns which inevitably affect the development of any new psychosocial program, especially those that necessitate changes in existing structures (Georgeopoulos & Mann, 1979; Tefft & Simeonsson, 1979). For one thing, physician participation in psychologically oriented treatment programs or comprehensive care requires the kind of sharing of authority with other professions that is often without precedent, either in physician's prior training or in their current work environments (Friedson, 1970). In addition, the implementation of any new psychological treatment, particularly a preventive approach, must address such imposing constraints as patterns of insurance reimbursability that push hospital services in the direction of concrete diseases and technological procedures rather than prevention (Gallagher, 1972; Iscoe, 1981). Despite eloquent pleas from within the profession of medicine to implement more enlightened biopsychosocial models of care and training (Engel, 1977; Haggerty, 1979), there is every reason to expect that future pediatric medicine in many large medical centers will become increasingly specialized, technical, and hence less mindful of human transaction. Unfortunately, the primary focus on technology-based gathering of diagnostic evidence characteristic of medical practice in modern acute care hospitals cannot help but diminish the time and energy for contacts with children and families (Reiser, 1978). Consider the views of one enlightened consumer:

> The modern physician strides forth into the world with a certificate of learning in one hand and a vast array of exotic medication and technological devices in the other. But the humans who look to him for help are fragile, perplexed, and vulnerable. More than anything else they want to know that they matter. The overriding issue before medicine today is one not of proficiency but of humanity. Medical science may change but the need to understand and deal with human beings remain constant. (Cousins, 1981, p. 212)

Given the impact of future technology and cost-effectiveness pressures, the obvious question becomes: How can psychologists not only survive but maintain their professional integrity in medical settings of the future? For one thing, pediatric psychologists have a great deal of work left to do! Thoughtful, realistic solutions to the problems posed by interprofessional collaboration must begin with a clear recognition of the potential dangers of interprofessional exchanges for our profession as well as consumers. Moreover, to best facilitate our professional aims, we should be clear about the assumptions which underlie our conceptual models of diagnosis and service delivery and become much more assiduous in evaluating the outcome of our clinical services, consultation, and research, especially in terms of the human "costs" that are prevented or contained through our efforts. Like their physician counterparts, pediatric psychologists also have their illusions of certainty (Koch, 1981) and often do not put working assumptions of their effectiveness to stringent tests. For example, many pediatric psychologists simply assume that their psychological consultation is effective without subjecting their work to empirical evaluation from the standpoint of potential benefits to pediatricians and/or families. In addition, we assume that our teaching is effective in changing physicians' understanding and/or practice in behavioral or developmental pediatrics but rarely document its effectiveness. Although the design and implementation of such program evaluations are beset by thorny methodological problems and the time pressures inherent in clinical practice, the paucity of empirical descriptions of the impact of psychological services and consultation poses a considerable impediment to the development of our field. Moreover, the failure to test the outcome of our endeavors also results in a loss of critical information that would not only help us allocate our professional resources more effectively but document the effectiveness of our work to cost-conscious administrators. Given the expanding array of choices for clinical work, consultation, training, and research that are now available to pediatric psychologists, it is especially important for us to be realistic about our potential achievements and allocate our professional resources toward specific tasks where we can be most effective. For this reason, we should not blindly assume that we will be equally effective in all endeavors, especially when innovative goals clash with powerful forces in the medical system. For example, given the major emphasis on acute care in pediatric training (Wedgewood, Note 3; *Task Force on Pediatric Education,* 1978) and the pressures of pediatric practice (Bergman, Dassel, & Wedgewood, 1966; Burnett, William, & Olmsted, 1978), improvements in pediatricians' psychological expertise, especially in such areas as communications with family members (Hauser, 1981; Korsch & Morris, 1968; Raimbault, Cachin, Limal, Elincheff, & Rappaport, 1975) are more likely to result from marked structural innovations in training and practice rather than from education in the narrow sense of information exchange.

The future viability and development of psychology in pediatric settings will also depend in our ability to develop realistic ways of working with physicians which recognize and anticipate the consequences of our emerging professional development in medical settings. For example, we might anticipate that as our profession assumes increased responsibility for the design, implementation, funding, and evaluation of psychological services in pediatric settings, some physicians will resent our assumption of leadership and prefer us to function in ways that are more directly helpful to and controlled by them. Yet, we should not seek to be accepted by *all* of our pediatric colleagues, especially when their acceptance constrains our professional responsibilities to families or limits the potential development of innovative service or research programs.

From the standpoint of public health and well-being, the most important consequence of the rapid expansion of pediatric psychology is the access afforded our profession to the health care of large numbers of children and their families. Such access not only provides a base for professional functioning, which is a viable professional alternative to traditional clinical settings (Schofield, 1969), but provides a unique opportunity to contribute to the improvement of children's psychological health in ways that cannot be accomplished by pediatricians alone. For this reason, our profession has a primary responsibility to develop approaches to clinical care and research which change existing patterns of pediatric care to better facilitate the psychological well-being of children and families. The specialty of pediatric psychology has a number of unique strengths which enhance its professional "claims" to a leadership role in the development of services and research concerning children with psychosocial and developmental problems including (among others): (a) understanding of developmental principles; (b) recognition of the salient influences of family, social, and medical systems, on children's development; and (c) the ability to use research methodology to document the efficacy of clinical services and psychosocial outcomes of pediatric populations. I would hope that we would strive to develop these skills in future pediatric psychologists and develop coalitions with colleagues from both within and outside our professional discipline (including physicians) who share these aims. I would also hope that as a profession we will not repeat medicine's isolation from the consumers of services (Knowles, 1977). Wherever possible, we must incorporate the children and families with whom we work into our service programs and outcome evaluations. For this reason, priorities for professional expansion should be set in concert with consumer organizations and systematic documentation of the psychological needs of pediatric populations. Expanding technology (medical and otherwise) which serves to isolate professionals and consumers will turn out to be a poor substitute for professional–consumer relations based on the principles of mutual respect and participation. In whatever ways we can, let us use our expertise in the service of compassionate connections between health care professionals, children, and family members, most especially in hard economic times.

REFERENCE NOTES

1. Drotar, D. *Shared dilemmas of modern medical care.* Paper presented at the meeting of the American Psychological Association, Washington, D.C., September 1976.
2. Drotar, D. *Family-centered preventive intervention in failure to thrive.* Paper presented at meeting of the American Association of Mental Deficiency, Boston, May 1982.
3. Wedgewood, R. J. *The 1970-1971 inventory of pediatric departments: A report and a comparison with the 1966-1967 inventory* (NICHD Order No. PD-135134-3). National Institute of Child Health and Human Development. 1972.

REFERENCES

Albee, G. W. Emerging concepts of mental illness and models of treatment: The psychological point of view. *American Journal of Psychiatry,* 1969, *125,* 42-48.

Bergman, A. B. Dassel, S. W., & Wedgewood, R. J. Time-motion study of practicing pediatricians. *Pediatrics,* 1966, *39,* 254-263.

Burnett, R. D., William, M. K., & Olmsted, R. W. Pediatrics manpower requirement. *Pediatrics,* 1978, *61,* 438-445.

Collins, B. E., Whalen, C. K., & Henker, B. In S. Salzinger, J. Antrobus, & J. Glick (Eds.), *The ecosystem of the "sick child."* New York: Academic Press, 1980.

Conrad, P. The discovery of hyperkinesis: Notes on the medicalization of deviant behavior. *Social Problems,* 1975, *23,* 12-21.

Cousins, N. *Human options.* New York: W. W. Norton, 1981.

Drotar, D. Psychological consultation in a pediatric hospital. *Professional Psychology,* 1976, *9,* 77-83.

Drotar, D. Clinical psychological practice in the pediatric hospital. *Professional Psychology,* 1977, *8,* 72-80.

Drotar, D. Psychological perspectives in chronic childhood illness. *Journal of Psychology,* 1981, *6,* 211-228.

Drotar, D., Benjamin, P., Chwast, R., Litt, C. L., & Vajner, P. The role of the psychologist in pediatric inpatient and outpatient facilities. In J. Tuma (Ed.), *Handbook of pediatric psychology,* New York: Wiley, 1981.

Drotar, D., & Malone, C. A. Family-oriented intervention in failure to thrive. In M. Klaus & M. O. Robertson (Eds.), *Birth interaction and attachment* (Vol. 6). Skillman, N.J.: Johnson & Johnson Pediatric Round Table, 1982.

Drotar, D., Malone, C. A., & Negray, J. Psychosocial intervention with the families of children who fail to thrive. *Child Abuse and Neglect: The International Journal,* 1979, *3,* 927-935.

Drotar, D., Malone, C. A., & Negray, J. Environmentally based failure to thrive and children's intellectual development. *Journal of Clinical Child Psychology,* 1980, *9,* 236-240.

Drotar, D., Malone, C. A. Negray, J., & Dennstedt, M. Psychosocial assessment and care of infants hospitalized for nonorganic failure to thrive. *Journal of Clinical Child Psychology,* 1981, *10,* 63-66.

Dubos, R. *Mirage of health,* New York: Harper & Row, 1959.

Duff, R. S., & Campbell, A. G. M. Moral and ethical dilemmas in the special care nursery. *New England Journal of Medicine,* 1973, *289,* 890-894.

Engel, G. L. The need for a new medical model: A challenge for biomedicine. *Science,* 1977, *196,* 127-136.

Foucault, M. *The birth of the clinic.* New York: Random House, 1975.

Fox, R. *Essays in medical sociology.* New York: Wiley, 1979.

Friedson, E. *Profession of medicine.* New York: Harper and Row, 1970.

Gallagher, E. B. The health enterprise in modern society. *Social Science and Medicine,* 1972, *6,* 619-623.

Georgeopoulous, B. S., & Mann, F. C. The hospital as an organization. In E. G. Jaco (Ed.), *Patients, physicians, and illness.* New York: Macmillan, 1979.

Haggerty, R. J. The Task Force Report. *Pediatrics,* 1979, *63,* 935-937.

Hannaway, P. J. Failure to thrive—A study of 100 infants and children. *Clinical Pediatrics,* 1970, *9,* 96-99.

Hauser, S. T. Physician patient relationships. In E. G. Mishler, L. Amarasingham, S. J. Hauser, R. Liem, S. D. Osherson, & N. E. Waxler (Eds.), *Social contexts of health, illness, and patient care.* New York: Cambridge University Press, 1981.

Hobbs, N. *The futures of children.* San Francisco: Jossey-Bass, 1975.

Illich, I. *Medical nemesis.* New York: Random House, 1975.

Iscoe, I. Conceptual barriers to training for the primary prevention of psychopathology. In J. M. Joffe & G. W. Albee (Eds.), *Prevention through political action and social change.* Hanover, N.H.; University Press of New England, 1981.

Katz, J., & Capron, A. M. *Catastrophic diseases: Who decides what?* New York: Russell Sage, 1975.

Koch, S. The nature and limits of psychological knowledge. *American Psychologist,* 1981, *36,* 257-269.

Knowles, J. H. Doing better and feeling worse: Health in the United States. *Daedalus,* 1977, *106,* 1-7.

Korsch, B. M., and Morris, M. Gaps in doctor-patient communication. Patients' response to medical advice. *New England Journal of Medicine,* 1968, *280,* 535-540.

Laufer, M. W., & Denhoff, E. Hyperkinetic behavior syndrome in children. *Journal of Pediatrics,* 1957, *50,* 463-474.

Magrab, P. R. (Ed.) *Psychological management of pediatric problems (Vol. 1). Early life conditions and chronic disease.* Baltimore: University Park Press, 1978.

McNett, I. *Psychologists in medical settings: APA Monitor,* 1981, *12,* 12-13.

Mechanic, D. *Public expectations and health care.* New York: Wiley, 1972.

Meyer, E., & Mendelson, M. Psychiatric consultations with patients on medical and surgical wards: Patterns and processes. *Psychiatry,* 1961, *24,* 197-205.

Millman, M. The ideology of self care: Blaming the victims of illness. In A. W. Johnson, O. Grusky, & B. H. Raven (Eds.), *Contemporary health services: Social science perspectives.* Boston: Auburn House, 1981.

Nathan, R. G., Lubin, B., Matarazzo, J. D., & Persely, G. W. Psychologists in schools of medicine—1955, 1964, and 1977. *American Psychologist,* 1979, *34,* 622-627.

Newberger, E. H., & Bourne, R. The medicalization and legalization of child abuse. *American Journal of Orthopsychiatry,* 1978, *48,* 593-607.

Patton, R. G., & Gardner, L. I. *Growth failure in maternal deprivation.* Springfield, Ill.: C C Thomas, 1963.

Raimbault, G., Cachin, O., Limal, J. M., Elincheff, C., & Rappaport, L. Aspects of communication between patients and doctors: An analysis of the discourse in medical interviews. *Pediatrics,* 1975, *55,* 401-405.

Reiser, S. J. *Medicine and the reign of technology.* New York: Cambridge University Press, 1978.

Robinson, D. Politics of pediatrics. *Pediatrics,* 1979, *63,* 273-275.

Routh, D. K. Developmental and social aspects of hyperactivity. In C. K. Whalen & B. Henker (Eds.), *Hyperactive children: The social ecology of identification and treatment.* New York: Academic Press, 1980.

Salk, L. Psychologist in a pediatric setting. *Professional Psychology,* 1970, *10,* 395-396.

Sarason, S. B. An asocial psychology and a misdirected clinical psychology. *American Psychologist,* 1981, *36,* 827-836.

Schofield, W. The role of psychology in the delivery of health services. *American Psychologist,* 1969, *24,* 565-584.

Singer, L., Drotar, D., Fagan, J., Devost, L., & Lake, R. The cognitive development of failure to thrive infants: Methodological issues and new approaches. In T. Field (Ed.), *Infants born at risk: Physiologic and sensorimotor processes.* New York: Spectrum, in press.

Stabler, B. Emerging models of psychologist-pediatrician liaison. *Journal of Pediatric Psychology,* 1979, *4,* 307-313.

Task Force on Pediatric Education. *The Future of Pediatric Education.* Evanston, Ill.: American Academy of Pediatrics, 1978.

Tefft, B. M., & Simeonsson, R. J. Psychology and the creation of health care settings. *Professional Psychology,* 1979, *10,* 558-570.

Tuma, J. *Handbook for the practice of pediatric psychology.* New York: Wiley, 1981.

Vaughn, V. C., McKay, R. J., & Behrman, R. E. (Eds.). *Textbook of pediatrics.* New York: Saunders, 1979.

Wright, L. A comprehensive program for mental health and behavioral medicine in a large children's hospital. *Professional Psychology,* 1979, *10,* 458-466.

19

Parental Concerns about Their Children

Gary B. Mesibov, Carolyn S. Schroeder, and Lynn Wesson
University of North Carolina at Chapel Hill

The need for education programs for parents has recently been discussed in a wide variety of places such as The American Academy of Pediatrics (Note 1), the Salvation Army (Cole, Note 2), and the popular media (Brown, 1976). This deep concern of so many people reflects the importance that is attached to this educational need. Presently the need for parent training to help prevent child abuse, mental retardation, and emotional problems as well as to help parents deal with the many unanticipated questions and problems a child presents is being met by the parent education programs that are emerging everywhere (Brown, 1976). Most of these programs instruct parents in single techniques (e.g., behavior modification or PET) and do not systematically emphasize specific issues of concern to a large number of parents. In addition, little thought or attention is being given to unresolved issues such as who should provide this parent education and what should be their training.

In order to broaden the scope of the parent training efforts and address some of these unresolved issues, it seems that we must first ask what problems and questions parents want answered. Most studies to date have defined parental concerns in terms of pediatrician referrals (Korpela, 1973; Smith, Rome, & Freedheim, 1967; Townsend, 1964; Wishingrad, Shulruff, & Sklansky, 1963; Wolfe & Teed, 1967). In other words, the incidence of

The authors would like to thank Ms. Elaine Goolsby and Ms. Sharon Stangler who were instrumental in setting-up and carrying out the Call-in/Come-in service and Drs. Senior, Schaeffer, Conley, and Christian for their continued support in carrying out the training and service in their office. The research was supported in part by U.S. Public Health Service, Maternal and Child Health Project 916 and by Grant HD-03110 from the National Institute of Child Health and Human Development.
Originally published in *Journal of Pediatric Psychology, 11*(1)(1977):13–17.

a specific concern (e.g., toilet training) is defined by how frequently a pediatrician refers a parent with that concern to a psychologist, social worker, or psychiatrist. One problem with this approach is that the judgment of the pediatricians involved might be determining the incidence of specific parental concerns instead of the feelings of the parents themselves.

Chamberlin (1974) has improved upon the pediatrician referral technique for obtaining incidence data on parental concerns by asking parents at well baby check-ups about the kinds of problems they are experiencing and their specific concerns. While valuable, the Chamberlin study depends upon parents' memories and does not identify concerns parents seek help with. The goal of the present study is to build upon the Chamberlin data by recording parental concerns as they occur.

SETTING AND PROCEDURE

The setting for the present study was the preventive parent education services in a private pediatric office as previously described by Schroeder, Goolsby, and Stangler (1975) which includes a Call-In and Come-In service plus evening parent education groups. The service is staffed by pediatric psychologists, social workers, and nurses who are part of a larger interdisciplinary team representing 12 health disciplines that focus on developmental and learning problems. The data for the study are based on the Call-In hour and Come-In appointments. Briefly, the Call-In hour consists of a telephone line in the pediatric office which is open twice weekly for parents to make direct calls on any non-medical problems to the preventive parent education staff. Problems that appear too complex to handle over the telephone are dealt with in a face-to-face Come-In appointment. Complete records concerning the nature of each call and come-in appointment have been kept since the service began in 1973. Although, no doubt, the records are not perfect because of the sometimes frantic activity on very busy days, the records are thought to be relatively complete and certainly representative of the kinds of concerns that parents have brought to the service. The data presented here are based on the first two and one-half years that the program has been in operation. The program's original emphasis was intended to be on the pre-school child, but all calls, regardless of the child's age, were accepted.

RESULTS

In order to analyze the data, 22 categories were developed based on Chamberlin (1974), Korpela (1973) and our own experiences with the Call-

In, Come-In service. These categories were designed to include all of the concerns that parents brought to our service but they represent only one of any number of ways in which this data could be organized.

Table 1 is a list of the categories with an explanation of each one. After developing the list, each parent contact since the start of the service was classified into one or more categories. It was impossible to classify each contact under only one category because many parents had multiple concerns (e.g., sleeping and toileting problems). Reliability was determined by having an independent rater classify a random sample of 100 concerns and the inter-rater reliability coefficient was .84.

Table 2 shows the breakdown of 672 parental concerns by category. These concerns were generated from a total of 428 contacts.

Negative behaviors toward parents like disobeying, having tantrums, and whining account for more of the concerns than any other category (14.58%). Following closely behind negative behaviors are toileting problems (12.65%). With all due respect to Azrin and Foxx (1974), toilet training is still a major concern of parents. It should be noted, however, that a number of the callers have tried the Azrin and Foxx method (with varying success) or wanted more information about it. There were also many parents concerned about developmental delays (10.71%) and school problems (10.71%). This is at least in part a reflection of our local physicians' awareness of these problems and their tendency to refer these patients to us. Sleeping problems (10.12%) ranged all the way from "When should my child give up his morning nap?" to "What can I do for my 14 year old son who has insomnia?" Personal and emotional (personality) problems, a more traditional domain of the clinical child psychologist, accounted for 8.33% of the concerns. This low figure might partially be due to the close proximity of a large hospital with a Psychiatry Outpatient component along with several child psychologists and child psychiatrists in private practice in the local community who might be seeing a large percentage of these cases. The data might also indicate that the demand for services for emotional and personality problems has been over-emphasized. Sibling and peer problems also accounted for 8.33% of the concerns emphasizing parents' need for more information and guidance on interpersonal behavior. Divorce, separation, and problems of single parents accounted for a surprisingly high 6.25% of the concerns. This figure is undoubtedly a reflection of our times. The remainder of the concerns dealt with a wide variety of problems including sex, death, infant management, adoption, and fears.

Table 3 presents the data by age. The program's initial emphasis on pre-school development is reflected in this table. However, in spite of this pre-school emphasis, a considerable number of the concerns involved the 5-10 year old age range (37.36%). The number of questions for this age

Table 1. Definitions of Problem Categories

Problem Category	Definition
Negative behaviors	(Toward parents) — won't listen to parents, doesn't obey, has tantrums, bossy and demanding, cries, whines.
Toileting	Toilet training, soiling, enuresis, encopresis.
Developmental delays	Perceptual motor problems, slow development, school readiness, speech problems (stuttering), overly active.
School problems	Hates school, not doing well in school, reading or math problems, aggression by child toward teacher.
Sleeping problems	Night-time, won't go to bed, naps.
Personality problems	(Emotional) — lacks self-control, no motivation, won't assume responsibility, lies, steals, dependent.
Sibling/peer problems	Won't share, has no friends, aggressive toward peers, siblings fight a lot, sibling rivalry.
Divorce, separation	Who should have custody, appropriate visitation schedule, what should the child be told?
Infant management	Feeding, nursing, post-partum depression, cries all the time (colic).
Family problems	Parents disagree on discipline, mother feels isolated, parents argue a lot, child abuse.
Sex-related problems	Trying on opposite-sexed parent's clothes, no same-sexed friends, lack of sex-appropriate interests.
Food/eating problems	Picky eater, won't eat certain foods, eats too much.
Specific fears	Dogs, dark, trucks.
Specific bad habits	Nail biting, tics, thumb sucking.
Parents' negative feelings toward child	Generally don't like child, get no enjoyment from child.
Physical complaints	Headaches, stomachaches.
Parents' concerns re: school	Is child getting what he needs, does teacher understand child?
Adoption/foster/guardianship	Advice on possible placements, what to tell the child.
Moving	Preparation for new home, problems of adjustment after moving.
Miscellaneous	
Death	Understanding the concept, adjusting to death of someone who was close.
Guidance of talented child	Need for special programs, appropriate stimulation.

Table 2. Frequency and Percentage of Concerns According to Problem

Problem	Frequency	Percentage
Negative behaviors	98	14.58
Toileting	85	12.65
Developmental delays	72	10.71
School problems	72	10.71
Sleeping problems	68	10.12
Personality problems	56	8.33
Sibling/peer problems	56	8.33
Divorce/separation	42	6.25
Infant management	14	2.08
Family problems	17	2.53
Sex-related problems	13	1.93
Food/eating problems	10	1.49
Specific fears	12	1.79
Specific bad habits	10	1.49
Parents' negative feelings toward child	11	1.64
Physical complaints	9	1.34
Parents' concerns re: school	8	1.19
Adoption/foster/guardian	7	1.04
Moving	6	.89
Miscellaneous	2	.29
Death	3	.45
Guidance of talented child	1	.15

Note. Total number of concerns was 672.

Table 3. Frequency and Percentage of Concerns According to Age

Age Range (in years)	Frequency	Percentage
0-1	21	3.13
1-2	68	10.12
2-3	104	15.48
3-4	78	11.61
4-5	81	12.05
5-6	63	9.38
6-7	63	9.38
7-8	50	7.44
8-9	28	4.17
9-10	47	6.99
10-11	21	3.13
11-12	22	3.27
12-13	5	.74
13-14	12	1.79
14-15	8	1.19
15-16	0	0.00
16-17	1	.15

range can be expected to increase now that the evening parent groups, that are another part of the parent training program, have expanded upward through age 9. Although this service was not intended to serve pre-teens or teenagers (age 10 and over), there were still a significant number of concerns about this population as well (10.27%). There are undoubtedly many needs that parents of pre-teens and teenagers have that could be met through parent education services.

In addition to the foregoing analysis, the data were also examined by problem and age combined. Examination of these data revealed some new and interesting aspects of our service. As expected, questions on toileting were primarily for children 4 and under (63.53%), but there were also a number of questions about older children as well. Most of the calls for the older children concerned enuresis. Sleeping problems are evident in the 3-4 year age range (14.71%), giving support to the "waking up at all hours" behavior of the three year old described by Ilg & Ames (1955). This was not as troublesome, however, as the clingy "I don't want to go to bed alone," problems of the 2-3 year old (41.18%). Questions on negative behaviors were dominant during the "terrible twos" but most certainly do not end at age three. A significant percentage of negative behaviors were reported for children beyond age three (65.31%). Developmental delays usually became evident during the pre-school years (45.83%) with the next greatest percentage of developmental problems occurring between the ages 5 and 8 (38.89%). Problems regarding sexual behavior occurred primarily in the 4-5 year age bracket (46.15%), exactly as Freud's oedipal theory (1955) would predict. In addition, several problems were evenly distributed across all ages such as family problems, adoptions, separations, divorce, and interpersonal (sibling and peer) relationships.

Finally the data were analyzed in terms of sex of child and problem. Overall, 383 (60%) of the concerns for which the sex was identified involved boys and 252 (40%) involved girls. Twenty-eight of the concerns were inadequately recorded so that the sex of the child could not be determined, and 9 concerns involved a child of each sex (a boy and girl in a family concerned with divorce or family problems). Assuming that boys and girls are equally distributed in the private pediatric practice that constitutes our sample, parents had significantly more concerns about boys than one would expect by chance (z (635) = 5.04, $p < .01$).

Table 4 presents the data by concerns and sex. Although there was a significant sex difference overall, only 4 of the categories had significantly more concerns about boys than about girls: toileting (z (83) = 2.73, $p < .01$), developmental delays (z (69) = 4.49, $p < .01$), school problems (z (72) = 3.05, $p < .01$), and personality (emotional) problems (z (53) = 2.33, $p < .01$).

Table 4. Frequency and Percentage of Concerns by Sex of Child

Problem	Freq. Male	Percent Male	Freq. Female	Percent Female
Negative behaviors	50	53%	45	47%
Toileting**	54	65%	29	35%
Developmental delays**	53	77%	16	23%
School problems**	49	68%	23	32%
Sleeping problems	38	56%	30	44%
Personality problems**	35	66%	18	34%
Sibling/peer problems	29	58%	21	42%
Divorce/separation	18	55%	15	45%
Infant management	4	31%	9	69%
Family problems	6	55%	5	45%
Sex-related problems	10	77%	3	23%
Food/eating problems	3	30%	7	70%
Specific fears	5	42%	7	58%
Specific bad habits	5	50%	5	50%
Parents' negative feelings toward child	4	40%	6	60%
Physical complaints	5	56%	4	44%
Parents' concerns re: school	5	83%	1	17%
Adoption/foster/guardian	3	43%	4	57%
Moving	3	60%	2	40%
Miscellaneous	1	50%	1	50%
Death	2	67%	1	33%
Guidance of talented child	1	100%	0	0%

**Significant sex difference, $p < .01$.

Although sex differences approached significance for several other categories (i.e., sex-related problems), the small number of concerns in these categories prevented these differences from reaching statistical significance. There were no categories which had significantly more concerns involving girls than boys.

DISCUSSION

The data indicate that certain difficulties (i.e., negative behaviors) and certain ages (i.e., 2-3) are more problematic than others. This suggests that the current emphasis on parent training in specific techniques such as PET or behavior modification (Brown, 1976) should be broadened to include eclectic overviews of certain specific ages and childrearing problems. The particular team answering the questions described in this paper had a distinct advantage of being part of a larger multidisciplinary group. For instance, questions on developmental delays in areas such as language and motor coordination could be most effectively answered with input from communication disorders specialists and physical therapists. Answers to school related problems involved input from the educators, who have considerable knowledge of the types and quality of schools in the community. Of course the questions professionals were faced with in this service are restricted by the population using the service (middle socioeconomic class) and the setting in which the service was offered (private pediatric office). The reporting of questions asked by other groups of parents from a variety of settings would provide important information in developing curriculum for training parent educators.

The fact that 7.29% of concerns involved divorce, separation, adoption and related problems such as visitation schedules, custody arrangements, and guardianship provisions reinforces the notion that the training of parent educators must be broadly based. Children often are not represented in legal divorce proceedings and the fact that child development specialists are now being consulted is important from the children's viewpoint (Williams & Gordon, 1974). Dealing with these problems requires not only an understanding of children's needs, but the ability to work with the hostility that many parents feel toward the spouse who has deserted them. Enabling deserted parents to see that their anger might be interfering with their ability to allow their children to maintain a much needed relationship with the other parent is as important as setting up the most desirable living arrangements for the children in question. Considerable skill and training are also needed to determine a child's understanding of what is happening so that reasonable decisions about the child's involvement in any agreement can be made.

The large number of pre-school and school problems indicates the need for the parent educator to be acquainted with community resources and the potential benefits or hazards they present to children. In addition, if the parent educator is to deal with the significant number of parental questions on sleeping and feeding, he/she needs more than simple exposure to pediatrics in well baby clinics.

In addition to identifying specific training areas, the present study has also provided some interesting information on normal development. The fact that negative behaviors are the most common childrearing problems that come to our attention should come as no surprise to any parent who has had to deal with these behaviors: but the fact that such a high percentage of the so-called "terrible twos" negativism appears well after the third birthday suggests that we might be overemphasizing the concept of negativism as simply a developmental stage (Brazelton, 1974; Ilg & Ames, 1955) and not fully preparing some of our parents for the fact that this might be an ongoing concern.

In regard to toileting problems about 20% of the calls were for children over 5 years of age. Although most of the calls for the older children were for enuresis and encopresis, this is another indication of the prevalence of these problems (Halverstadt, 1976). The high incidence of school problems among pre-school children indicates that we need more information on the effects, both negative and positive, of pre-school programs. These programs might be precipitating as many problems as they hope to solve. The trend for earlier and earlier school placement may not be justified for all children. We also need more information concerning the long-range effects of these earlier demands. The fact that interpersonal and sibling problems occur about equally between ages 1 and 10 is interesting because there is no trend. There does not seem to be any particular age in this range where interpersonal relationships are any more or less problematic although specific issues, of course, vary from age to age.

The overall sex difference should come as no surprise to anyone who has worked with children and noted the higher percentage of boys than girls with problems: however, some might be surprised that our difference wasn't greater. It is also of interest that only 4 of our categories showed significant sex differences, all 4 having more boys than girls. Of the 4 categories with sex differences, 3 of them were in areas with a strong maturational (physical) component (toileting, developmental delays and school problems), suggesting that these differences can be largely attributed to the well-known fact that boys mature more slowly than girls. Boys also had more personality problems (lack of self-control, no motivation, etc.) than girls.

In conclusion, an examination of parental concerns as expressed to child development professionals working in a private pediatric practice reveals a great deal about normal child development as well as parents' needs that should be addressed by parent education training programs. Whether those running these programs require specific academic training or practicum experience is still an open question: however, it seems clear that their training should be eclectic, broad in scope, and multidisciplinary. Furthermore, it is important that those training child development professionals and/or parents be guided by the needs of the parents as expressed in this, as well as a variety of other settings.

REFERENCE NOTES

1. American Academy of Pediatrics. *Statement on parenting.* Unpublished draft, November, 1975.
2. Cole, E. P. *The Salvation Army demonstration in education for parenthood.* Paper presented at the meeting of the Curriculum Materials Producers, Washington, D.C., January, 1976.

REFERENCES

Azrin, N. H., & Foxx, R. M. *Toilet training in less than a day.* New York: Simon and Schuster, 1974.

Brazelton, T. B. *Toddlers and Parents.* USA: Delacorte Press. 1974.

Brown, C. C. It changed my life. *Psychology Today,* November, 1976, 47-57: 109-112.

Chamberlin, R. W. Management of preschool behavior problems. *Pediatric Clinics of North America,* 1974, *21,* 33-47.

Freud, S. *Collected works of Sigmund Freud,* Vol. 10. London: Hogarth Press, 1955.

Halverstadt, D. B. Enuresis. *Journal of Pediatric Psychology,* 1976, *1,* 13-14.

Ilg, F. L., & Ames, L. B. *Child Behavior.* New York: Harper Row, 1955.

Korpela, J. W. Social work assistance in private pediatric practice. *Social Casework,* 1973, *54,* 537-544.

Schroeder, C., Goolsby, E., & Stangler, S. Preventive services in a private pediatric practice. *Journal of Clinical Child Psychology,* 1975, *4,* 32-33.

Smith, E. E., Rome, L. P., & Freedheim, D. K. The clinical psychologist in the pediatric office. *Journal of Pediatrics,* 1967, *71,* 48-51.

Townsend, E. H. The social worker in pediatric practice: An experiment. *American Journal of Diseases of Children,* 1964, *107,* 77-83.

Williams, G. J., & Gordon, S. (Eds.). *Clinical child psychology: Current practices and future perspectives.* New York: Behavioral Publications, 1974.

Wishingrad, L., Shulruff, J. T., & Sklansky, M. A. Role of the social worker in a private practice of pediatrics. *Pediatrics,* 1963, *32,* 125-130.

Wolfe, S.. & Teed, G. A study of the work of a medical social worker in a group medical practice. *Canadian Medical Association Journal,* 1967, *96,* 1407-1416.

20

Suggestions to Parents about Common Behavior Problems in a Pediatric Primary Care Office
Five Years of Follow-Up

Korrel W. Kanoy
Peace College

Carolyn S. Schroeder
University of North Carolina at Chapel Hill

Studies by Clarke-Stewart (1978) and Schroeder and Wool (1979) have shown that the pediatrician is the professional most parents initially contact when they have concerns about their child's development or behavior. How pediatricians have managed these concerns has varied with their perceived role and interest in this area, their skills, and their time limitations. The pediatric psychologist would appear to have much to offer parents and pediatricians in primary health care settings (Wilson, 1964).

The role of psychologists in primary health care settings, however, has been slow to develop, although there are a number of published articles describing various models for this work (Morrison, 1976; Schroeder, 1979; Smith, Rome, & Freedheim, 1967). Providing quality mental health care within the organization of the busy pediatric setting is often difficult given the limited space, lack of privacy, limited time, and expectations of immediate cure (Drotar, Benjamin, Chwast, Litt, & Vajner, 1982; Tefft &

The information in this paper has been presented in part in Schroeder, Gordon, Kanoy, and Routh (1983). This paper describes in greater depth the follow-up procedures given across categories of problems and specific feedback given by parents. Also, we wish to acknowledge grant support from Grant HD-03110 and MCH Project 916 for the second author during the writing of this paper.
Originally published in *Journal of Pediatric Psychology,* 10(1)(1985):15–30.

Simeonsson, 1979). Schroeder and her colleagues developed a model that focuses on early intervention through brief phone consultation and contacts with parents (Mesibov, Schroeder, & Wesson, 1977; Schroeder, 1979; Schroeder, Goolsby, & Stangler, 1975; Schroeder, Gordon, Kanoy, & Routh, 1983). At the time of this study, there was no charge for either telephone or face-to-face contacts. These services are offered in the office of a pediatric-group practice whose patient population is approximately 12,000, ranging in age from birth through adolescence.

From the inception of the services, program evaluation has been important. At the time of each call- or come-in appointment, a log is made with the name and age of the child, the primary presenting problem, relevant demographic information, a list of parents' specific questions or concerns, the staff member's suggestion(s) for each question, the length of the contact, and the staff member's name. The parents are asked at the end of each contact if they can be called in 6 weeks to 1 year to evaluate the effectiveness of the suggestions. The parents are told that they may call back at any time if they have further questions or concerns. Repeated calls regarding the same problem would warrant a referral for more in-depth evaluation/treatment. The types and percentages of concerns that parents had about their children from 1973 to 1982 are shown in Table I.

In general, the intervention approaches used by the staff reflect a behavioral orientation. Suggestions usually focus on environmental changes, punishing or ignoring inappropriate behavior, and rewarding and encouraging appropriate behavior. A key emphasis of the program is to convey information to the parent(s) about appropriate developmental expectations/behaviors so that the parent(s) might understand the child's behavior more thoroughly.

The focus of this article is to describe follow-up evaluations of parents who used the services offered by Schroeder and her colleagues. Mesibov et al. (1977) previously described a follow-up evaluation of parents who used the services from 1973 to 1976. By combining the follow-up evaluation done by Mesibov et al. (1977) with follow-up evaluations done in 1977-1978 and 1979-1980, the total number of cases for specific problems and suggestions is enough to make some recommendations for future work in this area. These follow-up findings are seen as clinically valuable as well as serving as the pilot work for more systematic, controlled research on the relative efficacy and cost-effectiveness of different short-term intervention approaches to common childhood problems.

Several questions can be answered by this follow-up data. First, can short-term cost-effective intervention be offered in a pediatric primary health care setting? Second, what are the most effective suggestions for

Table I. Percentage of Concerns of Parents about Their Children[a]

Rank	Parental concerns	Year			Total (N = 2,008)
		1973-1976 (n = 672)	1976-1979 (n = 724)	1979-1982 (n = 612)	
1	Negative behaviors	15	14	17	15
2	Toileting	13	7	11	10
3	Personality or emotional problems	8	13	9	10
4	School problems	11	8	7	9
5	Sleeping problems	10	6	8	8
6	Developmental delay problems	11	6	5	7
7	Sibling/peer problems	8	8	5	7
8	Divorce/separation problems	6	7	8	7
9	Family problems or concerns	3	5	4	4
10	Infant management	2	3	3	3
11	Specific bad habits	1	3	4	3
12	Specific fears	2	0	3	2
13	Sex-related issues	2	2	2	2
14	Parents' concerns about school	1	3	1	2
15	Physical complaints	1	2	2	2
16	Parents' negative feelings toward child	2	1	2	2
17	Death	0	1	2	1
18	Food/eating problems	1	0	3	1
19	Moving	1	1	1	1
20	Adoption/foster care/guardianship	1	0	1	1
21	Guidance of talented child	1	1	1	1
22	Miscellaneous	1	1	1	1

[a] Data from the 9-year period are blocked in 3-year periods to show stability.

behavioral and developmental problems? Third, do concerns persist at the time of follow-up?

METHODOLOGY

Sample

The sample for the present study consists of all parents who participated in follow-up evaluations during the years 1973-1976, 1977-1978, and 1979-1980 for the following areas of concern: toileting ($n = 54$), sleep ($n = 60$), developmental delays ($n = 21$), negative behaviors ($n = 60$), sibling/peer difficulties ($n = 49$), and personality/emotional problems ($n = 38$).[1] In the 1973-1976 follow-up (Mesibov et al., 1977), slightly more than one-third of the parents eligible for the follow-up participated, primarily because of a long delay in beginning follow-up procedures. For both 1977-1978 and 1979-1980, over 60% of potential subjects participated in the follow-up evaluation. With only rare exceptions, the parents who did not participate could not be located or contacted for follow-up, rather than choosing not to participate.

The sample consisted largely of married and professional individuals. Across the six categories of interest, over 85% of the sample was married, most were professionals (over 65% of fathers and 45% of mothers), and over 60% had two children in the family. In general, parents had slightly more concerns about boys than girls. However, in the areas of toileting and sibling/peer problems, over 70% of the concerns were expressed about boys. Over 90% of the toileting and sleep concerns were expressed about preschool children. Other concerns were distributed evenly between preschool and school-age children.

Procedure

The follow-up evaluations were done between 2 months and 2 years following the time of the original contact, with most of the contacts being

---

[1]Please note that the number of different parents contacted is less than the total for all categories since some parents expressed a concern in more than one category. In addition, follow-up data for developmental delays and personality/emotional problems were collected only in 1977-1978 and 1979-1980.

made within 1 year. Staff members who had not had previous contact with a parent, and graduate or postgraduate level students made the follow-up calls. At the beginning of each call, the parent was given a brief explanation of what the follow-up evaluation would entail. If the parent agreed to participate, the interviewer began a structured interview by asking for any missing demographic information (except for 1973-1976). Next, the parent was asked to recall the reason(s) for the contact as well as the suggestion(s) given. If the parent could not remember, the interviewer told the parent what was recorded on the client's record. It was rare for the parent not to remember the specifics of the concern and the suggestions given. Then, parents were asked to rate on a 1 to 5 scale (with 1 being a low rating and 5 a high rating) the effectiveness of each suggestion. The parents were also asked to rate the service in general and the counselors on a 1 to 5 scale. For the 1977-1978 follow-up calls, parents were asked if they had any current concerns about their child's behavior or development.

RESULTS

Parents' overall evaluations of the service and counselors are contained in Table II. In every area of concern except for developmental delays, at least 88% of the parents thought the service was good. The counselors were rated highly, with 85% of the parents expressing confidence in the counselors across all six areas of concern. Table II also indicates that parents were much more likely to use both the come-in and call-in service when they had concerns about socialization difficulties (about 50% used both services) as opposed to developmental difficulties (less that 30% used both services).

Tables III–VIII contain the types, frequencies, and ratings of each suggestion given to parents in all six areas of concern. In general, parents rated the suggestions for socialization problems higher than those given for developmental problems. About 25% of the suggestions for sleep and toileting difficulties were rated between 4 and 5, whereas about 75% of those for negative behaviors, sibling/peer, and personality/emotional problems were rated between 4 and 5.

Data on the current concerns of parents are contained in Table IX. Some of the original concerns still were evident at follow-up for both developmental and socialization difficulties. Sleep problems persisted the least, at a 21.9% rate, whereas sibling/peer problems persisted the most, at an 83.3% rate.

Table II. Evaluation of Come-In/Call-In Service: 1977-1978 and 1979-1980 Follow-Up Data[a]

Variable	Area of concern					
	Toileting (n = 26)	Sleep (n = 25)	Developmental delays (n = 21)	Sibling/ peer (n = 20)	Negative behaviors (n = 39)	Personality/ emotional (n = 38)
Service used[b]						
Call-in	92	88	81	65	77	47
Come-in	27	28	29	75	54	79
Service evaluation						
Good	88	100	76	95	97	92
Bad	4	0	0	0	3	0
Undecided/mixed	8	0	19	0	0	5
No response	0	0	5	5	0	3
Confidence in counselor						
1 (not confident)	0	0	0	0	0	0
2	0	0	5	0	0	3
3	8	4	5	0	8	5
4	27	20	14	25	18	31
5 (very confident)	61	72	71	70	67	58
No response	4	4	5	5	8	3

[a] All figures are expressed as percentages.
[b] The percentages in this category do not total 100 because some parents used both services.

Table III. Toileting: Effectiveness Ratings for Suggestions for 1973-1976, 1977-1978, and 1979-1980 Follow-Up Data (n = 54 Concerns)

Advice	Mean rating	No. of suggestions
Reward appropriate behaviors like sitting on toilet or successfully eliminating	3.39	33
Do not be overly punitive when child has accidents	3.85	15
Have child clean up when he/she has accidents	3.1	10
Collect data on number, time, and place of accidents	3.28	11
Provide more consistency (e.g., get the child up at night, use training pants, have the child on a schedule)	3.63	11
Referral	5	3

Table IV. Sleep: Effectiveness Ratings for Suggestions for 1973-1976, 1977-1978, and 1979-1980 Follow-Up Data (n = 60 Concerns)

Advice	Mean rating	No. of suggestions
Reward appropriate behaviors with a star or chart	3.64	14
Ignore inappropriate behavior (e.g., let child cry it out)	3.35	19
Rearrange child's schedule	3.56	10
Be supportive and reassuring to child	3.84	12
Story and ritual before bed	4.38	8
Environmental change (e.g., night-light, toys)	3.71	7
Information on what to expect	4.5	2

DISCUSSION

The data clearly support the expectation that effective short-term intervention can be offered within the pediatric primary care setting. The ratings of the service and the counselors reflected the parents' confidence in the intervention. Ratings of the specific suggestions provided evidence that some suggestions, particularly those that focused on specific actions, worked better for short-term intervention.

Table V. Negative Behaviors: Effectiveness Ratings for Suggestions for 1973-1976, 1977-1978, and 1979-1980 Follow-Up Data (*n* = 60 Concerns)

Advice	Mean rating	No. of suggestions
Reward appropriate behavior with stars, or charts	4.57	13
Focus more, in general, on positive behaviors by giving more praise and special time	4.78	21
Punish inappropriate behavior using time out	4.24	23
Ignore inappropriate behavior	3.58	14
Reassurance to parents that behavior represents a normal developmental stage	4.8	10
Parental consistency, environmental changes, and recommended books	3.65	10

Table VI. Sibling/Peer: Effectiveness Ratings for Suggestions for 1973-1976, 1977-1978, and 1979-1980 Follow-Up Data (*n* = 49 Concerns)

Advice	Mean rating	No. of suggestions
Reward positive interactions with other children using a star or chart	4.71	8
Focus more, in general, on positive behaviors by giving more praise and special time	5	2
Punish inappropriate behavior using time out	4.68	14
Leave children alone and allow them to work out their own problems	3.34	7
Reassurance to parents that behavior represents normal developmental stage	4.20	5
Invite friends and structure children's time	4.25	4

Methodological Limitations

Before discussing the effectiveness of specific suggestions, several methodological limitations of the evaluation procedure used need to be addressed. The Come-In/Call-In Service was not designed as an experimental research effort. Everyone who sought help was given it immediately. The sample then is self-selected, and may not be representative of all parents and their children. A second selection bias occurred at the follow-up

Table VII. Developmental Delays: Effectiveness Ratings for Suggestions for 1977-1978 and 1979-1980 Follow-Up Data (n = 21 Concerns)

Advice	Mean rating	No. of suggestions
Focus more, in general, on positive behaviors by giving more praise and special time with parents	2	1
Reassurance to parents about age-appropriate behaviors	4	9
Shape desired behaviors gradually	4.08	6
Information about developmental expectations	3.33	5
Referral for evaluation	4.28[a]	10
Provide more stimulation (e.g. play more with the child, do favorite activities)	5	2

[a] Three of the parents given the referral suggestion did not use it and thus did not rate the suggestion. If a 0 is added as the effectiveness rating for these three parents, the mean score drops to 3.0.

Table VIII. Personality/Emotional: Effectiveness Ratings for Suggestions for 1977-1978 and 1979-1980 Follow-Up Data (n = 38 Concerns)

Advice	Mean rating	No. of suggestions
Reward appropriate behaviors like not whining	4.42	12
Focus more, in general, on positive behaviors by giving more praise and special time	4.37	8
Provide alternative behaviors/activities for the child (structure behavior for the child in positive ways)	4.21	12
Referral	5[a]	7
Information about charting behavior and developmental expectations	2.87	4
Reassurance to parent/encouraging them not to overreact	4.25	10
Have parent talk with/reassure child (e.g., parent reflect child's feelings, give encouragement)	4.37	8

[a] Three of the parents who were given the referral suggestion did not use it. When a 0 rating is added to the ratings of those who did use the suggestion, the mean drops to 2.86.

Korrel W. Kanoy and Carolyn S. Schroeder

Table IX. Current Concerns of Parents Involved in Follow-Up Evaluations by Area of Original Concern: 1977–1978 Follow-Up Data[a]

Current concern	Original concern					
	Toileting	Sleep	Developmental delays	Sibling/peer	Negative behaviors	Personality/emotional
Toileting	58.3	42.9	36.0	8.3	26.8	17.9
Sleep	0	21.9	9.1	16.7	26.8	7.1
Developmental delays	16.7	42.9	40.0	25.0	50.0	46.4
Sibling/peer	41.7	35.7	80.0	83.3	63.5	82.4
Negative behaviors	41.7	71.4	70.6	66.7	75.0	71.4
Personality/emotional	50.0	42.9	40.0	50.0	33.3	53.6

[a]The figures represent the percentage of parents expressing a current concern for any of the six categories of interest. Percentages exceed 100% because parents may have expressed several areas of concern.

evaluations because many of the parents had moved and were not able to be contacted. The fact that follow-up was done at inconsistent time intervals makes the data more difficult to interpret. Follow-up done 2 months after the original contact versus that done 12 months after the original contact may lead to different results. Because of the small sample that would have been created in some categories by adding time as a variable, we cannot be sure what the effect of time was in these data.

In addition, because we did not collect observational data, it is difficult to know whether the parents' or children's behavior changed. Knowing parents' ratings of the suggestions is different from knowing how parents implemented the suggestions. A final difficulty occurred in classifying parental concerns and the sometimes complex intervention techniques. In some cases, categorizing the intervention techniques leads to an oversimplification of what actually occurred.

Even with these difficulties, the information presented is of clinical value because it represents an effort designed primarily for intervention as opposed to research purposes. The information presented here accurately represents the types of concerns parents are likely to report in a pediatric setting and the types of procedures that may be used to deal with such concerns. Consistent patterns in the ratings can be detected and used to improve services within the pediatric setting.

Effectiveness of Specific Suggestions

In comparing suggestions across categories, it is useful to classify suggestions such as those involving (a) taking positive action toward the child, (b) punishing or ignoring inappropriate behaviors, (c) making structural or environmental changes, (d) providing information or support to parents, and (e) referring the case elsewhere. Trends in the ratings across the six areas of concern can be noted more easily using these categories.

Taking Positive Action. Several suggestions involved taking positive action including rewarding appropriate behaviors, focusing more on positive behaviors by giving the child special time with parents, and reassuring or talking with the child. All three of these specific suggestions were rated more highly (between 4 and 5 as opposed to between 2 and 4) when given for a socialization-related concern than when given for a developmental concern. As noted by Schroeder, Gordon, and Hawk (1983), developmental problems such as sleep difficulties may become exhausting for parents. Under such circumstances, parents may find it difficult to focus on positive behaviors or reassure the child in an effective way. Also, parents expressing a developmental concern were encouraged not to be punitive and time-out procedures were not recommended as they were for socialization problems. If punishment procedures are appropriate for a problem (such as time-out for negative behaviors), parents may possibly find the positive suggestions (such as rewarding appropriate behavior) easier to implement and/or more effective. Time-out reduces negative behaviors (Forgatch & Toobert, 1979), perhaps giving parents more opportunities to reinforce positive behaviors, thus increasing positive child behavior.

Punishing or Ignoring Inappropriate Behavior. Punishing inappropriate behaviors by the use of time-out was suggested only for negative behaviors and sibling/peer problems. High ratings by the parents (between 4 and 5) indicated that time-out had been effective. Whenever time-out was suggested, specific instructions were given verbally to the parents regarding how to implement the procedure. The fact that this procedure was taught to parents in a short time using only verbal instructions has important clinical implications. As Forgatch and Toobert (1979) noted, more cost-effective strategies need to be demonstrated as successful in order to help parents deal with "normal" child-rearing concerns.

Ignoring inappropriate behavior was not rated as highly as the timeout procedure. Ignoring was recommended for sleep problems (e.g., letting the child cry it out), negative behaviors (e.g., not responding to threats of noncompliance), and sibling/peer problems (e.g., leaving the children alone to work it out). The average ratings for these three areas of concern were 3.35, 3.58, and 3.34, respectively, indicating that parents thought the advice was moderately helpful. Drabman and Jarvie (1977) noted that implementing a suggestion to ignore has many problems. Unless parents are given specific information about what to expect (i.e., the behavior may become worse before getting better), how to ignore, and how intermittent schedules of reinforcement work, the procedure is likely to fail. In addition, ignoring some behaviors, such as children fighting or a child screaming in bed, is difficult no matter how much parents may know! Although all parents are asked whether they can implement a particular suggestion, it is possible that parents underestimate just how difficult it is to ignore some behaviors.

Making Routine or Environmental Changes. Many of the suggestions involved some type of environmental change such as developing a specific routine, modifying the child's physical environment, or arranging activities and shaping behavior so that the child would be successful. These types of suggestions spanned all six categories, and generally were rated between 3.5 and 4.5 for both socialization and developmental concerns. Researchers have shown that maladaptive child behavior of both a developmental nature (e.g., bed-wetting) and a socialization nature (e.g., noncompliance) can be remedied by teaching parents to rearrange structural aspects of their children's environment (Patterson, Reid, Jones, & Conger, 1975; Reid & Patterson, 1976).

The routine changes suggested for toileting required more effort (e.g., having the child sit on the toilet at particular times, collecting data on accidents) than suggestions for other developmental problems such as sleep, perhaps accounting for the more moderate ratings. For sleep concerns, one particular suggestion, reading a story about the expected bedtime ritual, was seen as very effective. Consequently, a storybook, prepared by Anne Spitznagel (1976), has been used frequently with more recent concerns about sleep problems. For developmental delays, the suggestions to shape behaviors gradually and to provide more stimulation to the child were rated highly but given to only a few parents. High ratings with a larger sample of parents might indicate that parents want to be able to "do something" about their concerns rather than just hoping the child will outgrow the problem.

Environmental changes for socialization problems primarily involved suggestions to the parents to structure time for the child to interact with peers in a positive way. This suggestion was rated highly for sibling/peer problems (4.25) and personality/emotional problems (4.21). Parents were also asked to modify the environment to prevent negative behaviors. This suggestion was rated moderately (3.65), perhaps because it was not as specific as other suggestions for negative behaviors such as time-out and rewarding with stars. Also the fact that this suggestion was not given very frequently may reflect the counselors' belief that this is a difficult suggestion to implement effectively.

Giving Parents Information and Support. Information about appropriate developmental expectations was given as a routine part of the service to all parents. In some cases, this developmental information was particularly highlighted, making it the "suggestion" for how to handle the concern. Only in rare cases did staff focus totally on developmental information; usually they gave parents specific behavioral suggestions to alleviate their concerns. Focusing on developmental information was the major strategy for only two parents whose children had sleep problems. In both cases, providing such information was rated highly. For developmental delays and personality/emotional problems, parents did not rate such information very highly. Perhaps in some situations such information does as much to augment parental concerns as it does to allay them. Although individual differences in the rate of development are very pronounced during the preschool years, such information may not comfort a parent whose child seems to be behind other children of the same age.

Providing reassurance or encouragement to the parents was rated highly for all three areas of socialization difficulties (negative behaviors = 4.8, sibling/peer = 4.20, personality/emotional = 4.25). Although parents reacted very positively to reassurance that negative behaviors may be part of a developmental stage, caution must be exerted not to mislead parents into believing that negative behaviors will be outgrown. Any reassurance given to the parents must be combined with specific suggestions for how to improve the problem behavior, as was done with the parents represented here.

Referring the Problem. Because the Come-In/Call-In Service is designed to provide brief intervention for normal childhood problems, some cases must be referred. Usually referrals are made after two or three contacts with the parent(s) reveal that the problem needs more extensive attention. Even so, 33% of the parents who had been referred did not use the referral suggestion. The lack of follow-through for referrals is a serious problem because these children are probably the most in need of effective treatment. As Forgatch and Toobert (1979) noted, treatment approaches designed to deal with minor problems may provide an effective screening source for more serious problems. The problem of how to ensure further intervention for these more serious problems may be resolved by the second author now providing services full-time in the pediatric office. When parents did follow through with referrals, the suggestion was rated very highly, indicating the effectiveness of the counselors in screening more serious problems.

Current Concerns of Parents

When collecting 1977-1978 follow-up data, parents were read the list of 22 concerns the service handles and asked if they had any current concerns about the child for whom they made the original contact. We realized that by naming the areas of concern, parents would identify more concerns than if they had to generate their own. This strategy was chosen to make the data comparable to a random sample of parents from the pediatric office files who were asked about current concerns for their children (Schroeder & Wool, 1979). Sleep problems were the least persistent (21.9% of the parents reported a continued concern) and sibling/peer problems were the most persistent (83.3% of parents reported a continued concern). Somewhat ironically, the effectiveness of the original suggestions was among the lowest for sleep problems and among the highest for sibling/peer difficulties. Two explanations seem feasible. First, children might outgrow their sleep difficulties, whereas they are unlikely to outgrow sibling/peer problems. Second, long-term studies have indicated that behavioral principles may be implemented effectively over a short time, but may be difficult to maintain over a long time period (Christophersen & Gyulay, 1981; Patterson & Fleishman, 1979). Thus, parents could have implemented the suggestions for sibling/peer problems effectively at one time, but have failed to maintain consistency. If such is the case, then follow-up phone calls to review procedures and check progress may become an essential part of short-term intervention for normal concerns.

CONCLUSION

Forgatch and Toobert (1979) challenged psychologists to demonstrate the effectiveness of programs for training parents to deal with minor concerns about their children. Our results indicate that brief but effective training can be offered within the pediatric primary care setting for both developmental and socialization problems.

With developmental problems, parents are concerned about a skill or ability the child has *failed to acquire* by the age the parents believe is normal. Providing parents with developmental information may augment their concerns unless it is combined with suggestions for specific actions the parents can take. The effectiveness of giving specific suggestions was evident for socialization problems, which are behaviors the child has *acquired that are undesirable*. Suggestions such as time-out and rewarding appropriate behaviors with stars gives parents specific strategies to use.

Even though parents rated most of the suggestions as effective, the number of concerns parents had at the follow-up evaluation should alert psychologists to the need for rigorous follow-up. Parents may not be able to implement suggestions on a consistent basis over a long time and may need more follow-up help than is normally provided. The challenge exists to understand why some concerns persist and to provide effective corrective action.

REFERENCES

Christophersen, E., & Gyulay, J. (1981). Parental compliance with car seat usage. A positive approach with long-term follow-up. *Journal of Pediatric Psychology, 6,* 301-312.

Clarke-Stewart, A. (1978). Popular primers for parents. *American Psychologist, 33,* 359-369.

Drabman, R., & Jarvie, C. (1977). Counseling parents of children with behavior problems: The use of extinction and time-out procedures. *Pediatrics, 59,* 78-85.

Drotar, D., Benjamin, P., Chwast, R., Litt, C., & Vajner, P. (1982). The role of the psychologist in pediatric outpatient and inpatient settings. In J. Tuma (Ed.), *Handbook for the practice of pediatric psychology.* New York: Wiley.

Forgatch, M., & Toobert, D. (1979). A cost-effective, parent training program for use with normal preschool children. *Journal of Pediatric Psychology, 4,* 129-145.

Mesibov, G. B., Schroeder, C. S., & Wesson, L. (1977). Parental concerns about their children. *Journal of Pediatric Psychology, 2,* 13-17.

Morrison, T. L. (1976). The psychologist in the pediatrician's office: One approach to community psychology. *Community Mental Health Journal, 12,* 306-312.

Patterson, G., & Fleishman, M. (1979). Maintenance of treatment effects: Some considerations concerning family systems and follow-up data. *Behavior Therapy, 10,* 168-185.

Patterson, G., Reid, J., Jones, R., & Conger, B. (1975). *A social learning approach to family interventions. I. Families with aggressive children.* Eugene, Oregon: Castalia.

Reid, J., & Patterson, G. (1976). The modification of aggression and stealing behavior of boys in the home setting. In A. Bandura & E. Ribes (Eds.), *Behavior modification: Experimental analyses of aggression and delinquency.* Hillsdale, NJ: Lawrence Erlbaum.

Schroeder, C. S. (1979). Psychologists in a private pediatric practice. *Journal of Pediatric Psychology, 4,* 5-18.

Schroeder, C. S., Goolsby, E., & Stangler, S. (1975). Preventive services in a private pediatric practice. *Journal of Clinical Child Psychology, 4,* 32-33.

Schroeder, C., Gordon, B., & Hawk, B. (1983). Clinical problems of the preschool child. In C. E. Walker & M. C. Roberts (Eds.), *Handbook of clinical child psychology.* New York: Wiley.

Schroeder, C. S., Gordon, B. N., Kanoy, K., & Routh, D. K. (1983). Management of behavior problems in pediatric primary care settings. In M. Wolraich & D. K. Routh (Eds.), *Advances in developmental and behavioral pediatrics* (Vol. 4). Greenwich, CT: JAI Press.

Schroeder, C., & Wool, R. (1979, March). *Parental concerns for children one month to 10 years and the informational sources desired to answer these concerns.* Paper presented at the Southeastern Psychological Association, New Orleans, LA.

Smith, E. E., Rome, L. P., & Freedheim, D. K. (1967). The clinical psychologist in the pediatric office. *Journal of Pediatrics, 71,* 48-51.

Spitznagel, A. (1976). *I'll see you in the morning.* Chapel Hill, NC: Divisions for Disorders of Development and Learning.

Tefft, B. & Simeonsson, R. (1979). Psychology and the creation of health care settings. *Professional Psychology, 10,* 558-570.

Wilson, J. L. (1964). Growth and development of pediatrics. *Journal of Pediatrics, 65,* 984-991.

21

Psychological Consultation in a Children's Hospital
An Evaluation of Services

Roberta A. Olson
University of Oklahoma Health Sciences Center

E. Wayne Holden
Auburn University

Alice Friedman
St. Jude's Children's Hospital

Jan Faust
Stanford Children's Hospital

Mary Kenning
University of Nebraska—Lincoln

Patrick J. Mason
University of Oklahoma Health Sciences Center

Relatively few studies have examined the types of patients seen and services provided by pediatric psychologists in clinical settings. Even fewer studies have provided a program evaluation of these services. Kanoy and Schroeder (1985) examined referrals received from a "Call In/Come In" service from a private pediatric group, whereas Ottinger and Roberts (1980) surveyed referrals from pediatricians to a pediatric psychology practicum. Walker (1979) examined both inpatient and outpatient referrals from a large chil-

Originally published in *Journal of Pediatric Psychology,* *13*(4)(1989):479–492.

dren's hospital. A relatively consistent pattern of results was obtained across the three settings. The most frequent referrals were for negative behaviors, developmental delays, psychosomatic problems, school problems, and toileting problems. Pediatric psychologists in each setting also received a smaller number of referrals for problems associated with acute and chronic medical illnesses and developmental problems in childhood and adolescence.

The specific examination of referral patterns from inpatient medical wards has received limited attention. Inpatient referrals have only been partially represented in one study (Walker, 1979) and the only survey that focused on pediatric psychology services to children on inpatient medical wards was completed 10 years ago (Drotar, 1977). Drotar reported that approximately one-half of the referrals from inpatient medical units were for developmental or intellectual problems associated with medical illness, language disabilities, or deprivation. Referrals for management of chronic illness, adjustment to burns, child abuse, and accidents represented 30% of the referrals. Less than 10% of the referrals were for behavioral or psychiatric problems. A more recent survey (Drotar & Malone, 1982) of pediatric psychology services examined only referrals received for infants and toddlers.

Anecdotal evaluations of medical inpatient services suggest that pediatric psychologists are well integrated into medical settings and that their services are highly valued by other medical personnel (Willoughby, 1978). A documentation of the value of pediatric psychology services was provided by Kanoy and Schroeder (1985) in a 5-year follow-up study of outpatient pediatric psychology services. Evaluations were based on parents' ratings of advice for common childhood problems provided by psychologists through a private pediatric clinic. Parents were most satisfied with advice concerning socialization problems such as negative behaviors, sibling/peer difficulties, and personality/emotional problems. Similar systematic evaluations of pediatric psychology programs serving inpatient medical settings are not currently available in the literature.

Further integration of pediatric psychologists into the health care system is dependent on: a clearer understanding of the roles and functions of psychologists in a health care setting *and* on health care providers perceptions of and satisfaction with these psychological services.

The goals of the present paper are to (a) provide a descriptive archival analysis of 4 1/2 years of pediatric psychology services provided to inpatient medical units within a large tertiary care children's facility and (b) report on the results of an evaluation of pediatric psychology services by health care providers working within that setting.

STUDY 1

Method

The current study was based on records of inpatient consultations provided by a Pediatric Psychology Service associated with a children's hospital from June 1981 through February 1986. The Pediatric Psychology Service was begun in the late 1960s. Records of consults prior to 1981 did not include sufficient data to be included in the study. The Pediatric Psychology Service typically included two predoctoral clinical psychology interns, two postdoctoral fellows, four doctoral level faculty, and two master's level staff. A child psychiatrist was available for medication consultation upon request from the Pediatric Psychology faculty. Psychological consultations were provided to medical and surgical units at a 330-bed tertiary care teaching facility that utilized a team approach to medical care for pediatric patients. The hospital patient population was primarily from central and western Oklahoma.

Referrals were made to the Pediatric Psychology Service from faculty physicians and medical residents who were assigned to the nine different medical services in the hospital. Nurses and social workers, who identified children in need of services, made recommendations to physicians for consultation requests. Data from consultations to outpatient clinics, the Hematology/Oncology service, and the Neonatal Intensive Care Unit were compiled separately and were not included in this survey.

Requests to the Pediatric Psychology Service for consultation were typically made by telephone and information about the referrals were recorded on both individual record forms and in a chronological log book. Information was obtained in the following areas: age and sex of the child, date of referral, response time to referral, status of referral (emergency or routine), referral question, referral source, location of the child in the hospital, title of therapist seeing the child, number of times seen, and discharge disposition. Information about the referral problem consisted of the initial question presented to Pediatric Psychology and did not represent multiple complaints or problems found during the consultation or outpatient follow-up. Data were analyzed by tabulating the frequency of occurrence for each of the above variables.

Results

Demographic Information

A total of 749 hospitalized children were seen for consultation by the Pediatric Psychology Service from June 1981 to February 1986. Of the children seen, 59% were male and 41% were female. Patient ages ranged from birth to 21 years of age with a mean age of 10 and a modal age of 17.

Referring Information

Although patients were referred from all services in the hospital, the majority of consultations were requested by General Pediatrics (40%), Surgery (21%), and Adolescent Medicine (16%). The remaining consultations were evenly distributed across the other hospital services (pulmonary, genetics/endocrinology/metabolic, orthopedics, nursing service, and social service). Consultations were conducted within a teaching hospital that utilized a team approach to medical care with both faculty and resident physicians assigned to each patient. Faculty physicians requested 37% of the referrals, residents requested 57% of the referrals, and the remaining 6% were referred by other hospital staff. The problems for which children were referred are listed in Table I. The most frequent referral categories included depression/suicide attempts, poor adjustment to chronic illness, and behavioral problems. A total of 46% of the referrals were for medically related problems (adjustment to chronic illness, psychosomatic problems, pain control, eating problems, medical noncompliance, enuresis/encopresis, decannulation of tracheostomy, grief/death/dying, and anorexia/bulimia). More males than females were referred across these diagnostic categories.

Table I. Reason for Referral to Pediatric Psychology Service[a]

Reason	Frequency	% of total sample
Depression/suicide attempt	145	19.4
Adjustment to chronic illness	92	12.3
Behavioral problems	69	9.2
Psychosomatic problems	61	8.1
Psychological evaluation	61	8.1
Pain control	57	7.6
Eating problems/failure to thrive	51	6.8
Medical noncompliance	33	4.4
Parent problem	28	3.7
Enuresis/encopresis	20	2.7
Child abuse	20	2.7
Substance abuse	18	2.4
Decannulation of tracheostomy	15	2.0
Grief/death and dying	11	1.5
Anorexia nervosa/bulimia	5	0.6
No referral question/other	63	8.4

[a] Excludes referrals from Hematology/Oncology and Neonatal Intensive Care Services.

In addition, the specific hospital services requesting consultation for these diagnostic categories varied. The majority of the referrals for depression/suicide attempts were from General Pediatrics (40%) and Adolescent Medicine (39%). Referrals for adjustment to chronic illness were primarily from General Pediatrics (38%), Surgery (17%), and Pulmonary (11%). Consultations for behavioral problems were requested most frequently by General Pediatrics (45%) and Surgery (29%).

Consultation Process

The vast majority of patients (76%) were seen by a psychologist on the same day the service received a request for a consultation. Another 17% were seen within 24–48 hours of the request. The remaining children (7%) were seen within 5 days. However, 87% of the referrals for depression/suicide attempts were seen on the same day as the consultation request. Delays in contacting patients were due to requests for services made within the context of an extended hospitalization, requests for services made prior to the child's admission to the hospital, or the inability to contact the child or parent.

Most of the contacts with pediatric patients and their families were brief, with 37% of the sample seen only once. Another 35% were seen two to four times. Children seen more than 10 times accounted for 13% of the sample. These children were referred for problems that required more intensive contact such as decannulation of tracheostomy, pain management for burns, terminal illness, and eating disorders. Typically, teams of therapists including both faculty and trainees were involved in treating these children.

Training

Interns and postdoctoral fellows saw 65% of the consultations. A psychology team including trainees, master's level psychologists, and a faculty member accounted for 20% of the consultations. In addition to supervising trainee cases, faculty maintained sole responsibility for 15% of the referrals. Faculty members were more likely than interns or postdoctoral fellows to make brief contacts with patients. In 75% of the referrals seen by faculty and only 50% of the referrals seen by trainees, one to two contacts were made with the patient.

Depression/suicide attempt was the most frequent referral category seen by interns (19%), postdoctoral fellows (20%), and faculty (24%). The distribution of the remaining consultation time depended upon the level of training of the staff member. For example, adjustment to chronic illness, behavioral problems, pain control, psychosomatic disorders, and eating disorders were the most frequent referral problems that were seen by interns. Pain control, psychosomatic disorders, and eating disorders were the most frequent referral problems seen by postdoctoral fellows. Adjustment to chronic illness and request for psychological evaluation were the most frequent problems referred to faculty members. Team consultations, which included assessment and treatment by more than one staff member, were primarily distributed between decannulation of tracheostomy, behavioral problems, adjustment to chronic illness, eating disorders, depression/suicide attempts, and pain control.

Consultation Follow-Up

Pediatric Psychology continued to treat, on an outpatient basis, 32% of the children seen for inpatient consultations. Referrals to community mental health services for outpatient follow-up were made in 37% of the cases. The remaining 32% did not require or refused follow-up. Of the children followed on an outpatient basis by Pediatric Psychology, the greatest number (21%) were referred for depression or previous suicide attempts. Adjustment to acute and chronic illness accounted for 16% and psychosomatic problems accounted for 10% of the inpatient consultations that were followed on an outpatient basis.

The probability of any one inpatient consultation being followed on an outpatient basis through the pediatric psychology clinic varied as a function of diagnostic category. Clinical cases in which medical illness or somatic symptoms were a primary factor were more likely to be followed. For example, although referrals for grief/death and dying accounted for only 1.5% of all inpatient consultations, 44% of these referrals were seen for outpatient patient treatment. Similarly, 40% of all inpatient referrals for adjustment to chronic illness and 39% of all inpatient referrals for psychosomatic problems were followed on an outpatient basis even though they accounted for 13 and 8% of all inpatient referrals, respectively. Only 33% of depression/suicide attempts were followed as outpatients despite it being the largest diagnostic category overall for which inpatient consultations were requested.

It is interesting to note that faculty members were more likely to follow inpatient consultations on an outpatient basis than trainees. Of the cases seen for inpatient consultation by faculty members, 50% were followed on an outpatient basis; only 30% of trainee consultations received similar outpatient services.

STUDY 2

Method

A 26-item questionnaire was developed by the authors to assess physicians', nurses', and social workers' evaluations of the consultation and liaison services provided by Pediatric Psychology and to examine the relationship among the health care professionals' confidence in detecting psychological problems, satisfaction with the pediatric psychology service, and the likelihood of referring a child to the service.

The questionnaire comprised the four sets of items contained in Table II. The first set of items termed *self-perception* evaluated staff's perceptions of their level of confidence in their own abilities to identify and treat psychological problems, the level of agreement between their perceptions of patients' psychological status and the consultant's feedback, and the number of contacts with the Pediatric Psychology service that they had within the last year. The second set of items evaluated overall *referral patterns* to the Pediatric Psychology service and the likelihood of referral of specific diagnostic categories. The third set of items assessed overall *satisfaction* and satisfaction with specific aspects of the Pediatric Psychology services. The last set of items evaluated the likelihood of future requests for Pediatric Psychology consultation services, the impact of discontinuation of Pediatric Psychology consultation services on patient care, and the percentage of inpatient Pediatric Psychology consultations that should be followed on an outpatient basis.

The questionnaire was distributed to faculty physicians, pediatric residents, nursing staff, and social workers during a general assembly and through intercampus mailings. A total of 170 questionnaires were distributed. Respondents who had not had contact with the Pediatric Psychology service within the last year were instructed to answer only the items evaluating their ability to identify patients in need of psychological services, their ability to provide psychological services, and referral patterns. Respondents were asked to complete the questionnaire and return it through campus mail. All responses were anonymous.

Results

An overall total of 77 (48%) completed questionnaires were returned. The faculty physicians had the highest return rate (52%), followed by the pediatric residents (46%), nursing staff (42%), and finally social workers

Table II. Mean Scores on Questionnaire Items for the Sample Surveyed

Item	Mean	n
Self-perception questions		
Confidence in ability to identify patients in need of psychological services[a]	4.1	74
Confidence in ability to provide psychological counseling to patients[a]	2.9	74
Level of agreement between perceptions of patients and feedback provided from pediatric psychology consultations[a]	3.9	63
No. of cases worked on in the last year for which a pediatric psychology consultation was provided	5.2	73
Referral pattern questions		
% of patients identified with psychological problems who should be referred for services	62%	71
Likelihood of referral of specific diagnostic categories[b]		
Depression/suicide	1.2	73
Psychoses/autism	1.2	72
Child abuse	1.4	72
Drug & alcohol abuse	1.5	69
Death & dying	1.5	71
Psychosomatic disorders	1.5	71
Enuresis/encopresis	1.7	69
School problems	1.7	73
Developmental delay	2.0	71
Pain control	2.1	72
Medical noncompliance	2.3	72
Satisfaction questions[a]		
Overall services	3.6	65
Time between ordering consultation and feedback	3.7	65
Usefulness of feedback	3.7	63
Written feedback	3.6	64
Verbal feedback	3.6	62
Effectiveness of intervention	3.5	58
Outpatient follow-up	3.0	43
Other questions		
Likelihood of future requests for pediatric psychology consultation[a]	4.3	62
Impact of discontinuation of pediatric psychology services on patient care[a]	4.3	64
% of inpatient consultations that should be followed on an outpatient basis by pediatric psychology	67%	55

[a] Item rated on a 1 to 5 Likert-type scale with (1) *not at all*, (3) *somewhat*, and (5) *very*.
[b] Item rated on a 1 to 3 Likert-type scale with (1) *very likely*, (2) *somewhat likely*, and (3) *not at all likely*.

(23%). A review of the last year's consultation requests indicated a total of 32 faculty physicians and 52 resident physicians requested inpatient psychological services. Therefore a total of 84 physicians were eligible to respond to all sections of the questionnaire. A response rate for this group was 84% for faculty physicians and 60% for resident physicians. A recent reduction in social workers employed by the hospital indicated five of these social workers were not involved in inpatient services and two social workers were assigned to hematology/oncology or neonatal units which were not included in this survey. The social workers responses were not included in subsequent data analyses due to the small number of subjects eligible to participate.

Responses from a total of 74 questionnaires were analyzed to assess staff's perceptions. On eight of the questionnaires only the items evaluating ability to identify patients in need of psychological services, ability to provide psychological services, and referral patterns were completed. These subjects had not had contact with the Pediatric Psychology consultation and liaison service within the last year.

A one-way MANOVA was computed on all completed questionnaires (57) to evaluate differences between the responses of faculty physicians, pediatric residents, and nurses across the self-perception items and referral pattern items. The overall results indicated significant differences between the three groups of respondents, Pillai's trace $= .87$, $F(32, 80) = 1.94$, $p < .01$. Investigations of the subsequent univariate F tests revealed only three significant effects. The amount of contact that respondents had with the consultation and liaison service during the last year was significantly different, $F(2, 54) = 8.5$, $p < .001$. Faculty physicians reported contact with a greater number of cases ($M = 6.3$) for which a consultation was provided than pediatric residents ($M = 4.8$). Differences were also found between nurses ($M = 6.4$) and pediatric residents but not between nurses and faculty physicians. The second significant effect was found on the question evaluating the likelihood of referral of death and dying cases for consultations, $F(2, 54) = 4.02$, $p < .02$. Nurses ($M = 1.0$) were more likely to refer death and dying cases to pediatric psychology than faculty physicians ($M = 1.6$) or pediatric residents ($M = 1.6$). There was also a significant effect for ability to identify patients in need of psychological services. Faculty physicians' ratings of their ability to identify pediatric patients in need of psychological services ($M = 4.4$) was greater, $F(2, 54) = 4.3$, $p < .02$, than pediatric residents' ratings ($M = 4.2$) and nurses' ratings ($M = 3.9$). It is important to note that Cochran's test for homogeneity of variance failed to demonstrate that the homogeneity of variance assumption was violated across all three variables for which a significant univariate difference was found.

Since 13 of the 16 dependent variables were not significantly different in a one-way analysis of variance, the groups were combined and the mean scores were calculated for individual items. Mean scores for all questionnaire items and the number of subjects responding to each item are contained in Table II. Staff members were relatively confident in their ability to identify patients in need of psychological services, but were less confident in their ability to provide psychological services to identified patients. Agreement between staff's perceptions of the patients' psychological problems and consultation feedback was rated as relatively high. In addition, the majority of patients identified appeared to have a high likelihood of referral for services. Ratings of the likelihood of referral of specific diagnostic categories, however, revealed variation in referral rates depending upon the problem encountered. As can be seen from Table II, more traditional psychological problems received higher likelihood ratings then those considered to be within the behavioral medicine area. These differences were not statistically significant.

Examination of mean scores on items evaluating level of satisfaction with specific aspects of consultation and liaison services indicated that the sample was relatively satisfied with the services provided. The lowest level of satisfaction was with outpatient follow-up. It is interesting to note, however, that only 43 subjects (58%) responded to this item. This result contrasts strongly with the respondents indicating that 67% of patients seen for inpatient consultation should be followed on an outpatient basis by Pediatric Psychology. Additional results revealed a strong interest in future requests for pediatric psychology consultations in that the respondents perceived that discontinuation of Pediatric Psychology Consultation Services would have a strong negative impact on patient care.

To evaluate the relationship between self-perception and satisfaction variables a canonical correlational analysis was computed. The first set of variables in the analysis included items evaluating the ability to identify patients in need of psychology services, the ability to provide psychological services to those patients, and the level of agreement between the respondents' perceptions of patients' psychological problems and the consultants' feedback. The second set of items included all of the satisfaction variables in the questionnaire except for the item evaluating outpatient follow-up. This item was excluded from the analysis due to the low number of subjects electing to respond. The analysis was based on responses from a total of 58 subjects due to missing data on several items.

The relationship between the two sets of variables was highly significant, canonical correlation = .71, $F(18, 139) = 2.6$, $p < .001$. The magnitude of the correlation indicated that approximately 50% of the variance was shared between the two sets of variables. The standardized canonical

Table III. Correlations Between Level of Agreement With Consultation Feedback and Satisfaction Items[a]

Satisfaction item	Pearson r
General satisfaction	.60
Reaction time satisfaction	.46
Usefulness of feedback	.60
Written feedback satisfaction	.32
Verbal feedback satisfaction	.58
Effectiveness	.47

[a] Based on the responses of 58 subjects. All correlation coefficients are significant beyond the .001 level.

coefficients for the first set of variables were −.08 for the ability to identify patients in need of psychological services, −.16 for the ability to provide psychological services to those patients, and .99 for the level of agreement between the perceptions of the respondent and psychological consultant's feedback.

Pearson product-moment correlation coefficients were computed between the individual variables included in the analysis. No significant correlation coefficients were found between the six satisfaction items and the respondents' level of confidence in their ability to identify patients in need of psychological services, or their level of confidence in their ability to provide psychological services to those patients. All six satisfaction items were correlated significantly beyond the .001 level with the respondents' rating of their agreement between their perceptions of the patients' psychological status and the feedback provided by the consultant. These correlation coefficients are reported in Table III.

DISCUSSION

The present study examined the role of pediatric psychologists in a single children's hospital. Thus, conclusions drawn from this study about the role of pediatric psychologists are limited. A second limitation is the lack of preexisting psychometric data on the evaluation questionnaire. Additional data are being collected to evaluate the psychometric properties of the evaluation questionnaire.

Results of the present study suggest that the Pediatric Psychology consultation service is characterized by brief, timely interventions for referral problems ranging from those traditionally seen by child clinical psychologists, such as behavior problems, to those specific to a medical population, such as pain control during painful medical treatments. It is noteworthy that the largest single category of referrals was for patients with depression/suicide attempt. Such a referral would not be unusual at a community mental health center. However, unlike a traditional setting, the patient was typically seen the day the referral was received by the department. The psychologist's role was generally limited to one or two brief contacts. Decisions about intervention and disposition were made quickly while the child was hospitalized. Most children were seen fewer than four times and were referred for outpatient counseling to a community mental health center.

Referral problems unique to medical settings represented almost one-half of all referrals and they accounted for a proportionally larger percentage of psychologists' time. Comparisons to past inpatient and outpatient Pediatric Psychology Services indicated larger percentages of referrals are for medically related consult requests. Children referred for problems such as pain management, tracheostomy decannulation, and terminal illness were followed on an almost daily basis during extended hospitalizations. A larger portion of these children were followed after discharge through the Pediatric Psychology Service than children referred for more traditional psychological problems. The differential follow-up of these children may reflect the staff's confidence that children with more traditional problems could be followed and treated at a mental health center in the community, whereas the pediatric psychology service had unique skills for handling the problems related to medical illness.

The nature of the relationship between psychologist, physician, and nurse depended on the specific referral problem. When the nature of the problem was similar to that seen traditionally by outpatient psychologists (depression) the psychologists' contact with the patient was brief. The recommendations were made to the medical staff and the child was referred to an outpatient mental health facility. The physician retained the major responsibility for the child. This relationship fits the "indirect psychological consultation model" described by Roberts (1986). When referral problems were directly related to medical problems such as pain management or feeding disorders, the pediatric psychologist worked with the physician in a "team collaboration model" (Roberts, 1986). Whether working in a collaborative or consultant role, one factor in determining the health care professionals' level of satisfaction and probability of future consults appeared to be dependent upon an appropriate and timely response to the referral concerns.

Overall medical and nursing staff were satisfied with the Pediatric Psychology Services. The level of medical/nursing staff satisfaction appears strongly related to mutual diagnostic agreement between referring physician/nurse and pediatric psychology. When a physician or nurse made a referral, this represented a concern about the child. When the psychologist addressed this problem, through verbal and written feedback as well as therapeutic intervention, the medical personnel's initial concern was validated. Physicians are involved in the process of differential diagnosis (Drotar, 1976), and the pediatric psychologist is consulted in this diagnostic process once medical disorders are ruled out (Walker, 1978). As a result, the psychologists' feedback often verifies the physician's suspected differential diagnostic hypotheses. This diagnostic affirmation appears to lead to a positive valence the physician attributes to the psychologist. This process fits Byrne's (1971) attitude similarity attraction paradigm which states that the attraction between two or more people is a positive effect of the degree to which they share similar attitudes. As a result, the physician's and psychologist's similar diagnostic beliefs appear to heighten the physician's positive regard for pediatric psychological services. This positive valence for pediatric psychology services is further evident in the consultation/liaison satisfaction scores obtained from staff as well as their continued interest in making future pediatric psychology consultation requests. Additionally, staff noted a negative impact on patient care if pediatric psychological services were discontinued.

Interestingly, compared to all other factors, the medical/nursing staff was least satisfied by the follow-up provided by psychologists. While the percentage of patients the medical staff suggested pediatric psychology follow (67%) far exceeds the number actually followed by the service, it is congruent with the number of children who either were followed by the Pediatric Psychology Service or referred to an appropriate outpatient facility. Therefore, the staff's relative dissatisfaction with the outpatient follow-up may have reflected inadequate written and verbal feedback provided from the pediatric psychology staff to the medical staff about the disposition of the patient. As a result, the psychology service has instituted new guidelines for hospital chart notes and letters to physicians outlining the plans for follow-up services for all inpatient consults. An evaluation of this procedure and possible effects on general satisfaction will be assessed.

This survey has helped to identify the varying roles of pediatric psychologists in a single hospital setting. Further research is needed to evaluate the roles of the pediatric psychologist in other inpatient hospital settings. In addition to the data that were gathered, variables that need to be evaluated in the future include the number of inpatient hospital days prior to the request for a psychological consultation, the DSM-III diagnosis, and the number of repeated hospitalizations for individuals receiving psychological services (i.e., noncompliance with medications, failure to thrive). Computer entries for each consultation would greatly enhance the ability to quickly obtain data needed for descriptive studies of a patient population.

A further analysis of the factors associated with physicians'/nurses' evaluation of these services is also needed. A brief confidential evaluation of psychological services could be sent to each referring physician and primary nurse on a monthly basis. A more timely evaluation of services could help to pinpoint possible problems and allow for changes to be made in the service.

In times of rising medical costs, research must begin to evaluate the long-term impact of inpatient hospital-based psychological interventions. There is an increased need to identify and document cost-effective psychological interventions that reduce future hospitalizations and medical costs for chronically ill children and their families.

REFERENCES

Byrne, D. (1971). *The attraction paradigm.* New York: Academic Press.

Drotar, D. (1976). Psychological consultation in a pediatric hospital. *Professional Psychology, 7,* 77-83.

Drotar, D. (1977). Clinical psychological practice in the pediatric hospital. *Professional Psychology, 10,* 72-80.

Drotar, D., & Malone, C. A. (1982). Psychological consultation on a pediatric infant division. *Journal of Pediatric Psychology, 7,* 23-32.

Kanoy, K. W., & Schroeder, C. S. (1985). Suggestions to parents about common behavior problems in a pediatric primary care office: Five year follow-up. *Journal of Pediatric Psychology, 10,* 15-30.

Ottinger, D. R., & Roberts, M. C. (1980). A university-based predoctoral practicum in pediatric psychology. *Professional Psychology, 11,* 707-712.

Roberts, M. C. (1986). *Pediatric psychology: Psychological interventions and strategies for pediatric problems.* New York: Pergamon.

Walker, C. E. (1979). Behavioral intervention in a pediatric setting. In J. R. McNamara (Ed.), *Behavioral approaches to medicine: Application and analysis* (pp. 227-266). New York: Plenum Press.

Willoughby, R. H. (1978). Pediatric psychologist as "polyglot": or training students to communicate clearly in a multidisciplinary world. *Journal of Clinical Child Psychology, 7,* 55-57.

22

Health Promotion and Problem Prevention in Pediatric Psychology
An Overview

Michael C. Roberts

The University of Alabama

Pediatric psychologists have long been concerned with the healthy development of children in both physical and psychological growth. In practice, most professional attention has been given to the treatment of existing physical and psychological problems so that children can regain the normal developmental pathways. However, throughout its existence pediatric psychology has maintained a basic orientation toward enhancing the status of healthy children, taking action to avoid the development of problems, and identifying problems early enough to minimize their potential negative outcomes (Peterson & Roberts, in press; Roberts & Peterson, 1984a). These concepts are generally labeled *promotion* and *prevention*.

The purpose of any special issue of this *Journal of Pediatric Psychology* is to draw attention to a topic in order to reflect the progress being made and stimulate further work in the area. Pediatric psychologists recently have begun making notable contributions to the promotion of children's physical health and to the prevention of problems in childhood. Thus, this issue highlights these activities, and we hope it will catalyze more research and applications.

In general, health promotion refers to improving an individual's health-enhancing life-style and to intervening with the environment for population-wide improvement. Health promotion efforts improve the quality of life for both the child and the later adult. Training to assume responsibility for health behaviors early in life may lead to lifelong positive

The author thanks Lizette Peterson and James E. Maddux, for their review and feedback of an earlier draft of this paper.
Originally published in *Journal of Pediatric Psychology, 11*(2)(1986):147–161.

habits. This involves both avoiding hazards (e.g., not playing in the street
in childhood and safe pedestrian behavior in the elderly) and adopting positive behaviors (e.g., exercise, healthy diet).

The concept of problem prevention intertwines with health promotion
by removing various hazards to healthy development where possible and
by intervening early to reduce further trauma when problems arise. These
activities in pediatric psychology include the application of psychology to
the prevention or early remediation of psychological disorders as well as
the prevention of physical problems such as injuries and illness in childhood
(Roberts & Peterson, 1984a). Thus, promotion/prevention in childhood involves two goals: (a) improving the well-being of children while they are
children, and (b) improving the later health status of the child as an adult
(Maddux, Roberts, Sledden, & Wright, 1986). The poem by Dorsel (in this
issue of the *JPP*) clearly portrays this orientation.

The *Journal of Pediatric Psychology* has published a number of articles over the years on prevention and promotion topics. Not surprisingly,
given the pediatric setting and mental health interests of pediatric psychologists, prevention of anxiety and stress due to medical or dental procedures has been the most prominent topic. Other topics have included
dental hygiene such as dental flossing, children's use of car safety devices
to prevent injury and death, early interventions with high risk children,
nutrition training to prevent obesity, and parent education for teen-age
mothers to promote their child's development and to prevent unwanted
pregnancies. Some papers have studied the characteristics of children and
their environments related to injuries and insults such as lead ingestion.
Thus, the topic of prevention/promotion in pediatric psychology is not
new to the Journal, but a renewed emphasis is demonstrated through the
articles in this issue.

AREAS OF NEED FOR PROMOTION AND PREVENTION

Promotion and prevention are concepts critical to both the future of
children and pediatric psychologists' roles as health care professionals for
children (Roberts, 1986). The importance of promotion/prevention becomes clearest when considering data that outline the problems afflicting
young people and the causes of death in this age group. Butler, Starfield,
and Stenmark (1984) note that only 2% of the child population at any one
time is afflicted by major medical problems (e.g., cancer, cerebral palsy,
diabetes). Contrasting data are available from *The Surgeon General's Report
on Health Promotion and Disease Prevention* (Califano, 1979a). For children,

ages 1 to 14 years, the leading cause of death is the category of "accidents," with motor vehicle collisions the single greatest factor.[1] Other accidents include drownings, falls, fires, and poisoning.

The remaining causes of death in children are at much lower rates (cancer, birth defects, influenza/pneumonia). For adolescents and young adults (ages 15–24 years), the leading causes of death are motor vehicle collisions and homicides, with other accidents and suicides also at significantly high rates (all combined to about three-fourths of all deaths). Cancer and heart disease are substantially lower morbidity factors. Additional health threats for this age group are misuse of alcohol and drugs, sexually transmitted diseases, and unwanted pregnancies. For adults (ages 24–65 years), deaths are due primarily to cardiovascular disease (one-third of all deaths) and cancer. Over the life-span, clear relationships exist between these causes of death and human behavior such as exercise, smoking, diet, and coping with stress (Koop, 1983; Matarazzo, 1982). These epidemiological data indicate areas of substantial professional concern for those with the knowledge and methodology to enhance the welfare of children and facilitate their development into adulthood.

Psychology and other disciplines (notably medicine and public health) are increasing their investigations and development of effective strategies for promoting health and preventing problems. For psychology, Matarazzo (1980, 1982) has advanced the concept of "behavioral health" to cover this area with extensions to "pediatric behavioral health" utilizing a developmental perspective (Maddux et al., 1986; Roberts, Maddux, & Wright, 1984).

The papers in this special issue can be considered through several perspectives. Additionally, there are important issues relevant to any work in promotion/prevention. This overview of the concepts and research is neither comprehensive nor exhaustive. But, then, the entirety of this Journal issue really represents only a sampling of what is available to learn and do.

---

[1]The term "accidents" is put in quotation marks here to reflect that the category was used in most of these analyses. However, it is important to note that childhood injuries are not just random, unavoidable, or inexplicable events based on chance. Although the term accidents is used more in the literature and vernacular, recent preference is given to the term "nonintentional injuries" to convey the attitude that most accidents are preventable and not merely capricious events. Strictly speaking, "prevention of accidents" would refer to the avoidance of an event such as a car collision, not to the prevention of injuries in the collision. Many preventive efforts are targeted toward preventing injuries to the child (e.g., increasing children's use of car safety seats), not to preventing the actual event (e.g., the collision).

CONCEPTS IN HEALTH PROMOTION AND PROBLEM PREVENTION

Active Versus Passive Interventions

Public health workers frequently differentiate between active and passive interventions, primarily in reference to prevention. Active prevention requires repeated action by individuals, such as wearing motorcycle helmets, brushing teeth daily, putting on seat belts, exercising, and maintaining a proper diet. Protective benefit is achieved only by those individuals performing the action. Passive prevention, on the other hand, requires minimal or no action regardless of any personal action, for example, fluoride in the water, flame retardants in children's sleepwear, and environmental improvements for health and safety. Often effective and comprehensive intervention efforts rely on combinations of passive and active strategies. For example, passive changes that promote health include reducing sodium and fat content in prepared foods, with additional benefit to preventing heart disease realized through individuals' changes in exercise and diet. Inflatable air bags for cars as a passive intervention would result in savings of lives and reduced injuries, but active use of safety seats and seat belts would still be needed for maximal protection in side collisions and roll-overs and to potentiate the air bag's benefits. Fluoridated water is a passive strategy for preventing dental caries, whereas active teeth brushing and flossing are necessary for maximal reduction of caries and for prevention of periodontal problems. These examples demonstrate the necessity and utility of combining passive and active strategies for optimal health promotion and problem prevention. In addition, there are passive strategies that must be reactivated continually. For example, replacing the child-proof caps on a poison container or closing a gate across a stairway limits the need for continuous adult vigilance, but are required if these environmental aids are to achieve any safety benefits. Finally, there are areas in which no environmental aids yet exist (e.g., care when bathing a child to prevent drowning), so continually active strategies are necessary.

Individual Versus Population Approaches

Pediatric psychology and health psychology generally emphasize intervention with individuals and their behavioral life-styles. The individual life-style approach underlies the three major health reports in North America. The Surgeon General's report, *Healthy People,* based its recommendations on the assumption that individual life-styles are the most significant obstacles to health improvement (Califano, 1979a). Similarly, the Canadian health document, *A New Perspective on the Health of Canadians,* espoused the view that moderating the individual's self-imposed risks in his or her life-style should be the major approach to health policy (Lalonde, 1974). Specifically oriented to children's health needs, the U.S. Select Panel for the Promotion of Child Health issued its report, *Better Health for Our Children* (Harris, 1981), with considerable emphasis on the philosophy that "the health of children and youth is significantly affected by their own behavior and by the behavior of others, particularly their parents and peers" (p. 103). All three reports acknowledged environmental contributions to health hazards but at a lower level than individual life-styles.

The underlying philosophy of these reports is readily understandable and acceptable to most pediatric and health psychologists since many psychologically based interventions follow the philosophy of changing individual life-styles and behaviors. For example, Roberts, Elkins, and Royal (1984) proposed a model of targeting prevention programs at individuals to improve child health. The first target is the care-giver of the child who is encouraged to change (a) the care-giver's own unsafe behavior (e.g., to stop speeding, not to drink and drive), (b) the care-giver's behavior on behalf of the child (e.g., to seek well-child health care, to provide nutritious meals), and (c) the care-giver's behavior to modify the child's behavior (e.g., teaching dental hygiene, teaching habits of buckling up in seat belts). The second target is the child himself or herself to take personal responsibility for healthier behaviors and life-style (e.g., buckling up, exercising, refraining from smoking). These types of programs and targets require individuals to change personal behaviors, and they rely on active promotion/prevention efforts.

Public health specialists, on the other hand, propose that better interventions are those that are applicable to community-wide populations. They argue that social engineering or structural changes are necessary to achieve better health throughout the population (Baker, 1981; Robertson, 1983). These structural changes are typically passive interventions, as noted earlier, that are directed not at the individual but at aspects of the environment that are particularly hazardous or impede healthy development. Williams (1982), for example, notes the successful control of infectious diseases that were the leading causes of death before passive, environmental changes were instituted for water purification, milk pasteurization, sanitation improvements, and immunization. Public health interventions often take the form of regulation, legislation, and environmental change because these methods can affect more people positively at one time than individually based interventions. Thus, public health proponents have been active in passage of state laws requiring use of safety seats for children (now in all 50 states) and in advocating safety belt laws for adults (now in 17 states). An even better approach to car safety, in this view, however, would be the implementation of air bags in all cars to provide fairly effective protection to all front seat passengers (Robertson, 1983). Additional structural changes for car safety include improvements in cars and roads. Many population-oriented interventions are passive prevention strategies. Other such interventions with successful outcomes include requiring security bars on windows on upper levels of buildings to prevent falls by children (Spiegel & Lindaman, 1977), changing automatic thermostats on hot water heaters to prevent scalds (Harris, 1981), and requiring childproof caps on products harmful to children (Walton, 1982). A slightly different population-wide health approach is illustrated by the requirement that all children must be fully immunized before school entry. Such requirements have resulted in 95% compliance (McGinnis, 1985).

Psychologists are likely to be most comfortable with active interventions, but the intuitive and objective benefits of passive interventions should not be ignored or neglected. For most health problems, multilevel, multifaceted approaches are needed. The approach of making the environment safer through structural passive intervention is important but is insufficient in many situations. Similarly, singular, active prevention efforts also are limited. In all likelihood, multilevel and multifaceted prevention and promotion strategies have maximum benefits if they combine passive and active interventions targeted at populations *and* individuals (Singer & Krantz, 1982; Williams, 1982). Peterson, Mori, and Farmer (in press) argue that if environmental modifications are proven effective (not just presumed to be), then they are the logical intervention. However, they note that for the majority of health risk areas environmental interventions may not be possible or effective. Psychologists can be most helpful in contributing to these most difficult problem areas.

Developmental Perspective

Since its inception, pediatric psychology has recognized the value of understanding developmental processes. As applied to health promotion and problem prevention, the developmental perspective has been useful in determining (a) when during the life-span intervention and prevention services are most needed and for what kinds of problems, (b) when these services should be offered to maximize their efficacy and acceptance by the child and those responsible for the child, and (c) what types of services might be most effective (Roberts, Elkins, & Royal, 1984; Roberts,

Maddux, & Wright, 1984). In many ways, these determinations can be assisted by epidemiological studies of problems and groups across the life-span (Zuckerman & Duby, 1985). For example, in assuming the developmental perspective, one can see that certain periods of high risk indicate when particular interventions may be most needed and effective. For example, for children under 1 year of age, falls constitute the largest cause of injuries, with choking and drowning close in frequency. Additionally, most nonintentional poisonings occur among children 1 to 4 years old. Many child pedestrian injuries occur during the ages 5 to 9 years. Recreational equipment is involved in many injuries for ages 6 to 11 years. While epidemiology contributes these actuarial data, the developmental perspective contributed by psychology also notes, for example, during the first year of life, the normal child squirms and rolls, places things in the mouth, and is helpless in water. These normal aspects of development indicate when and how prevention programs should be implemented. Many other analyses and examples would also demonstrate the worth of the developmental perspective in approaching promotion/prevention. Several papers in this issue demonstrate the developmental perspective and contribute valuable information for understanding negative and positive health situations. Huba, Newcomb, and Bentler describe adolescent drug use and adverse reactions relationships. Coppen's article demonstrates the relationship of cognitive development and causal reasoning to children's understanding of safety and prevention. Matheny reports on a longitudinal study examining injury liability and characteristics of toddlers' mothers and home environment. Peterson, Mori, and Scissors examine children's understanding of home safety in comparison to their parent's rules.

Pediatric medicine has always held a prevention perspective, often more than other medical specialties. Pediatricians have stressed regular check-ups for children (well-child visits), a series of disease inoculations, and health counseling. Anticipatory guidance, in particular, utilizes the knowledge base in child development to anticipate the abilities typically emerging at different ages (Zuckerman & Duby, 1985). As the child ages, the parents are told to expect certain events and behavior; they then are prepared for any increased health hazards posed by the developing abilities. For example, given the normal behavior exhibited by children in the first year noted above, the pediatrician providing anticipatory guidance would instruct the parents in preventive measures such as not leaving the child alone on a table or in a tub of water, and child-proofing the house by removing small objects and placing harmful materials out of reach. For another example, as the child gets larger and outgrows the infant car safety seat, the pediatrician would recommend a child safety seat and then a booster seat. Other examples of anticipatory guidance include preparatory information on potential changes in sleeping, eating, teething, and reactions to immunizations. The American Academy of Pediatrics instituted a project called "The Injury Prevention Program" (TIPP) which involves physician-administered safety surveys, pediatric counseling, and one-page handouts in developmental sequences on topics of car injuries, falls, burns, choking, drowning, and poisoning. Zuckerman and Duby (1985) outline potential topics of anticipatory guidance based on a developmental context. They suggest, for example, the pediatrician discuss water temperatures at 2 months, infant walkers at 4 months, electric sockets and cords at 6 months, and so on, up to substance abuse and CPR instruction in late school age. Cameron and Rice in this issue empirically examine the utility of anticipatory guidance and find that temperament-based anticipatory guidance can be successful for preventive mental health interventions.

Well-child visits also are typical times for other health promotion activities. During regularly scheduled office appointments, the pediatrician and staff can provide information on nutritional care of infants and children, dental care, parenting skills, and toilet training. Screening procedures as preventive measures for a variety of health problems have become well-established in pediatrics such as the test for the metabolic disorder of phenylketonuria. Screening for vision and hearing problems, lead poisoning, and anemia also can take place in well-child visits so that preventive interventions can be implemented early.

The pediatrician-based program to provide childhood immunizations against diseases probably best illustrates the benefits of preventive medicine (Butler et al., 1984). In terms of cost–benefit comparisons, for example, the measles vaccination program over an 8-year period cost $180 million but saved $1.3 billion in long- and short-term care by medicine and rehabilitation (Witte & Axnick, 1975). Vaccination has resulted in the eradication of smallpox and significant reductions in incidence of measles, mumps, pertussis, tetanus, polio, rubella, and diphtheria (Califano, 1979a). Intensive public health and pediatric initiatives to increase immunizations have been important factors in these achievements.

Health education constitutes another preventive medicine/public health intervention. However, its record of achievement is not well documented, even though health education is most often utilized as an initial step in health promotion (Cataldo et al., 1986; Robertson, 1983). Educational programs have targeted parents and children with mixed results: Programs with global health goals generally show fewer effective outcomes, while programs targeted to specific health habits and behaviors do better (Bass, Mehta, Ostrovsky, & Halperin, 1985; Roberts, Maddux, & Wright,

1984). Additionally, research tends to show that individual, behaviorally based training programs appear to be more effective in changing behavior than many media based campaigns (Peterson & Mori, 1985).

Developmentally based programs tend to do better as well. For example, Parcel, Tiernan, Nader, and Gottlob (1979) developed a health education program for kindergarten children with the goals of (a) identifying feelings regarding being well or ill and how to communicate them to caregivers, (b) identifying sources for help regarding health problems, and (c) identifying procedures for obtaining help. Another health educational effort for older children, the "Know Your Body" programs fostered healthier lifestyles and changed risk factors of chronic disease (Williams, Carter, Arnold, & Wynder, 1979). Other health education programs have been directed at increasing knowledge with goals to prevent onset of smoking (Evans et al., 1979), reduce drug and alcohol misuse (McAlister, Perry, Killen, Slinkard, & Maccoby, 1980), and prevent sexual abuse (Wolfe, MacPherson, Blount, & Wolfe, 1986). Unfortunately, thus far, in many cases, these types of programs either measure only information acquisition, not behavior change, or fail to demonstrate behavioral improvements.

Health education is one technique in particular need of additional psychological input and research. An analysis of the failures of some health education programs would reveal that basic psychological principles and knowledge of human behavior were overlooked in designing many efforts (Matarazzo, 1980). All too often health education results in increased knowledge but little behavior change because the programs usually target only knowledge increase. The research literature appears to indicate that, in order to achieve behavioral improvements, it is not enough merely to put information forward in various modalities (e.g., physician counseling, media presentations); additional behavior techniques are needed to promote change based on the acquired health information (Cataldo et al., 1986).

Motivating Behavior Change

A number of effective techniques for promoting healthier and safer behavior derive from psychological research. Roberts, Elkins, and Royal (1984) outlined the use of persuasive fear appeals, rewards and punishments, prompting, and modeling. These techniques are often combined in tackling a variety of health and safety problems. Persuasive appeals are used frequently as a method of initially exposing parents and children to the negative effects or threats of some behavior. In this way, educational goals may be achieved, and the behaviors may then change to avoid the feared consequences. Thus, information is provided through various media on such problems as cigarette smoking, home fires, seat belt use, alcohol use and driving. Sometimes these messages are sufficient to change behavior more or less permanently. However, the efficacy of these fear appeals, as with health education generally, has not yet been definitively established. More research is clearly needed in this application of psychological techniques.

Increasingly, health promotion programs are relying on positive messages and techniques, emphasizing the rewards, internal and external, of changing to certain behaviors. For example, Christophersen and Gyulay (1981) proposed a positive approach to increasing parental use of safety seats for their children. In their procedure, they instruct parents in how to make car riding more enjoyable for both parents and the child in the seat. The improved behavior of the child then becomes rewarding to the parents. No mention is made to the parents about the negative aspects (death or injury) of nonsecured children in accidents; they note only the positive behavioral improvement. Trieber (1986) extended this positive protocol approach combining it with fear appeal messages in an effective program.

External rewards often are used to increase the frequency of health-related behaviors. In order to increase parents' use of child safety seats with young children, in our programs, for example, we have given rewards to parents or to the children upon arrival at day care centers or schools when the children were safely buckled up (Roberts & Fanurik, in press; Roberts & Layfield, in press; Roberts & Turner, 1986). Other similar programs using contingent rewards have obtained positive behavior change such as for parents to bring in their children for immunizations and dental examinations (e.g., Yokley & Glenwick, 1984) and for dental hygiene (e.g., Claerhout & Lutzker, 1981).

Other psychological approaches to health promotion combine several behavioral techniques. For example, systematic programs have been designed to teach children emergency actions in home fires and identifying emergency situations (e.g., Jones, Kazdin, & Haney, 1981). Hillman, Jones, and Farmer, in this issue, expand on training of fire emergency skills. Other researchers have trained children how to cross streets properly (e.g., Yeaton & Bailey, 1978). Peterson (1984a, 1984b) has developed a "Safe at Home" program to train children who are at home without direct adult supervision. Similar behaviorally based and fairly intensive programs have developed for preventing obesity through nutrition education (e.g., Epstein, Wing, Steranchak, Dickson, & Michelson, 1980) and for preventing physical and sexual abuse of children (e.g., Poche, Brouwer, & Swearingen, 1981; Wolfe et al., 1986). In this issue, Saslawsky and Wurtele demonstrate this type of promotion/prevention program by educating children about sexual abuse, while Dielman, Shope, Butchart, and Campanelli describe an alcohol misuse prevention program in elementary schools.

Literature Resources

A number of useful resources has developed to describe the field of health promotion and prevention, many with particular relevance for psychologists. As noted earlier, there are several documents prepared by federal agencies and commissions related to health. These include: *Healthy People* and *Background Papers* (Califano, 1979a, 1979b); *Promoting Health/ Preventing Disease: Objectives for the Nation* (Harris, 1980); *Better Health for Our Children: A National Strategy* (Harris, 1981); *Developing Childhood Injury Prevention Programs* (Department of Health and Human Services, 1983). These are outstanding resources for a wealth of ideas and facts on a variety of health and safety issues.

Several journals now publish promotion/prevention articles. The *Journal of Primary Prevention* (published by Human Sciences Press and sponsored by the Vermont Conference on the Primary Prevention of Psychopathology) publishes four issues a year with a range of prevention articles on mental health and physical health problems. Recent topics have included prevention of cigarette smoking with youth, early intervention models, preventing drug abuse, stress management, preventing alcohol abuse, and preventing child maltreatment. The *Prevention in Human Services* series published by Haworth Press has covered special topics such as early intervention programs for infants, strategies for needs assessment in prevention, and innovations in prevention. Many articles are relevant to the health promotion area. Several journals publish some articles on this topic along with other topics (e.g., *Health Psychology, Health Education Quarterly, American Journal of Public Health, Journal of Applied Behavior Analysis, Journal of Clinical Child Psychology*). The *Journal of Consulting and Clinical Psychology* recently published a special series of papers on prevention of childhood disorders (Peterson, 1985) and the *Journal of Social Issues* is preparing a special issue on "Children's Injuries, Prevention, and Public Policy" (Roberts & Brooks, in press). Of course, the *Journal of Pediatric Psychology* will continue to publish related articles in its general issues.

Several books have been published on promotion and prevention. Many of these are examined in this issue's Book Review section. For the special issue, we selected recently published volumes in behavioral health and pediatric psychology with several specifically on health promotion and problem prevention. In addition, the Journal has reviewed several relevant books over the last three years (e.g., Baum & Singer, 1982; Coates, Peterson, & Perry, 1982; Felner, Jason, Moritsugu, & Farber, 1983; Moss, Hess, & Swift, 1982). In total, these books are valuable resources for work in this field and provide exposure to alternative and stimulating ideas. The Journal will continue to search for and review books that contribute to this aspect of pediatric psychology.

A "Primary Prevention Program Clearinghouse" has been set up to enhance communication among prevention professionals. The Clearinghouse publishes abstracts in the *Journal of Primary Prevention* on prevention programs and sells copies of longer program descriptions through the Psychology Department of the University of Vermont. The Office of Disease Prevention and Health Promotion supports the National Health Information Clearinghouse (P.O. Box 1133, Washington, DC 20013-1133) which disseminates material on this topic as do the *DHHS Prevention Abstracts* and *DHHS Prevention Activities Calendar* (McGinnis, 1985).

THIS SPECIAL ISSUE ON PROMOTION AND PREVENTION

The articles in this issue illustrate what can and should be done to promote the health of children and prevent injury, death, and disease. These papers demonstrate approaches that are useful for the specific topics targeted and that can be modified to apply to other problems. The authors did excellent jobs of conceptualizing and conducting research studies in this cutting edge of pediatric psychology. Yet, flaws can still be seen in this research. We should let these be points for continued development and improvement. I hope readers will say to themselves, "I can do better by . . ." and then do it. These papers depict steps of different sizes in finding the best strategies for prevention and promotion. Some are beginnings of programmatic research, others are further along in development and implementation. All of these lead us to the definitive cliche in science and psychology: "More research needs to be done."[2]

The papers were submitted in response to a widely publicized announcement of the impending special issue. All submissions were reviewed

---

[2]There are other issues confronting the psychologist working in this area often posed by interdisciplinary antagonisms. These include disputes over appropriate approaches to studying the injury problem through epidemiology and the host–agent–environment model or behavioral analysis of parent and child behaviors within sets of environmental conditions. Additional distinctions are often drawn over correctness of terminology and programming based on primary, secondary, or tertiary prevention (Roberts & Peterson, 1984b).

in the standard referee process of the Journal. We owe considerable thanks to Editor Gerald Koocher for efficient management of the increased rate of manuscript submission and to the many reviewers utilized in this process. These papers consider a variety of topics within the promotion/prevention area—ranging from the global health issue to the specific targeted problem. They illustrate a variety of conceptual approaches and methodologies.

Opportunities

There are several topics not contained in this issue that should be significant contributions to promotion/prevention by pediatric psychology. These include analyses and programs for major mental and physical health problems posed by smoking, immunization, medical procedures, nutrition, dental hygiene, among many others. These are important problem areas based on morbidity and mortality rates. Along with the topics covered by articles in this issue, these additional topics might be considered prime areas for behavioral health work, especially by pediatric psychologists. The Journal remains a publication outlet interested in such papers. We hope this issue stimulates researchers and programmers to work further in the area of promotion/prevention.

REFERENCES

Baker, S. P. (1981). Childhood injuries: The community approach to prevention. *Journal of Public Health Policy, 2*, 235-246.

Bass, J. L., Mehta, K. A., Ostrovsky, M., & Halperin, S. F. (1985). Injuries to adolescents and young adults. In J. J. Alpert & B. Guyer (Eds.), *The pediatric clinics of North America: Injuries and injury prevention* (pp. 233-242). Philadelphia: W. B. Saunders.

Baum, A., & Singer, J. E. (Eds.). (1982). *Handbook of psychology and health:* Vol. 2. *Issues in child health and adolescent health.* Hillsdale, NJ: Lawrence Erlbaum.

Butler, J. A., Starfield, B., & Stenmark, S. (1984). Child health policy. In H. W. Stevenson & A. E. Siegel (Eds.), *Child development research and public policy* (pp. 110-188). Chicago: University of Chicago Press.

Califano, J. A., Jr. (1979a). *Healthy people: The Surgeon General's report on health promotion and disease prevention.* Washington, DC: U.S. Government Printing Office.

Califano, J. A., Jr. (1979b). *Healthy People: Background papers.* Washington, DC: U.S. Government Printing Office.

Cataldo, M. F., Dershewitz, R. A., Wilson, M., Christophersen, E. R., Finney, J. W., Fawcett, S. B., & Seekins, T. (1986). Childhood injury control. In N. A. Krasnegor, J. D. Arasteh, & M. F. Cataldo (Eds.), *Child health behavior: A behavioral pediatrics perspective* (pp. 217-253). New York: Wiley-Interscience.

Christophersen, E. R., & Gyulay, J. (1981). Parental compliance with car seat usage: A positive approach with long-term follow-up. *Journal of Pediatric Psychology, 6*, 301-312.

Claerhout, S., & Lutzker, J. R. (1981). Increasing children's self-initiated compliance to dental regimens. *Behavior Therapy, 12,* 165-178.

Coates, T., Peterson, A., & Perry, C. (Eds.). (1982). *Promoting adolescent health: A dialogue on research and practice.* New York: Academic Press.

Department of Health and Human Services: Division of Maternal and Child Health. (1983). *Developing childhood injury prevention programs: An administrative guide for State Maternal and Child Health (Title V) Programs.* Washington, DC: Author.

Epstein, L. H., Wing, R. R., Steranchak, L., Dickson, B., & Michelson, J. (1980). Comparison of family-based behavior modification and nutrition education for childhood obesity. *Journal of Pediatric Psychology, 5,* 25-36.

Evans, R. I., Rozelle, R. M., Mittlemark, M. B., Hansen, W. B., Bane, A. L., & Havis, J. (1978). Deterring the onset of smoking in children: Knowledge of immediate physiological effects and coping with peer pressure, media pressure, and parent modeling. *Journal of Applied Social Psychology, 8,* 126-135.

Felner, R. D., Jason, L. A., Moritsugu, J. N., & Farber, S. S. (Eds.). (1983). *Preventive psychology: Theory, research, and practice.* New York: Pergamon Press.

Harris, P. R. (1980). *Promoting health/preventing disease: Objectives for the nation.* Washington, DC: U.S. Government Printing Office.

Harris, P. R. (1981). *Better health for our children: A national strategy.* Washington, DC: U.S. Government Printing Office.

Jones, R. T., Kazdin, A. E., & Haney, J. I. (1981). Social validation and training of emergency fire safety skills for potential injury prevention and life saving. *Journal of Applied Behavior Analysis, 14,* 249-260.

Koop, C. E. (1983). Perspectives on future health care. *Health Psychology, 2,* 303-312.

Lalonde, M. (1974). *A new perspective on the health of Canadians: A working document.* Ottawa: Ministry of Health and Welfare.

Maddux, J. E., Roberts, M. C., Sledden, E. A., & Wright, L. (1986). Developmental issues in child health psychology. *American Psychologist, 41,* 25-34.

Matarazzo, J. D. (1980). Behavioral health and behavioral medicine: Frontiers for a new health psychology. *American Psychologist, 35,* 807-817.

Matarazzo, J. D. (1982). Behavioral health's challenge to academic, scientific, and professional psychology. *American Psychologist, 37,* 1-14.

McAlister, A., Perry, C., Killen, J., Slinkard, L. A., & Maccoby, N. (1980). Pilot study of smoking, alcohol, and drug abuse prevention. *American Journal of Public Health, 70,* 719-721.

McGinnis, J. M. (1985). Recent history of federal initiatives in prevention policy. *American Psychologist, 40,* 205-212.

Moss, H. A., Hess, R., & Swift, C. (Eds.). (1982). *Early intervention programs for infants.* New York: Haworth Press.

Parcel, G. S., Tiernan, K., Nader, P. R., & Gottlob, D. (1979). Health education for kindergarten children. *Journal of School Health, 49,* 129-131.

Peterson, L. (1984a). The "Safe-at-Home" game: Training comprehensive safety skills in latch-key children. *Behavior Modification, 18,* 474-494.

Peterson, L. (1984b). Teaching home safety and survival skills to latch-key children: A comparison of two manuals and methods. *Journal of Applied Behavior Analysis, 17,* 279-293.

Peterson, L. (Ed.). (1985). Special series: Primary prevention of childhood disorders. *Journal of Consulting and Clinical Psychology, 53,* 575-646.

Peterson, L., & Mori, L. (1985). Prevention of child injury: An overview of targets, methods, and tactics for psychologists. *Journal of Consulting and Clinical Psychology, 53,* 586-595.

Peterson, L., Mori, L., & Farmer, J. (in press). Microanalytic assessment of injury situations: A complement to epidemiological injury prevention approaches. *Journal of Social Issues.*

Peterson, L., & Roberts, M. C. (in press). Community intervention and prevention. In H. C. Quay & J. S. Werry (Eds.), *Psychopathological disorders of childhood* (3rd ed.). New York: Wiley.

Poche, C., Brouwer, R., & Swearingen, M. (1981). Teaching self-protection to young children. *Journal of Applied Behavior Analysis, 14,* 169-176.

Roberts, M. C. (1986). The future of children's health care: What do we do? *Journal of Pediatric Psychology, 11*(1), 3-14.

Roberts, M. C., & Broadbent, M. (1985). *Preschoolers and car passenger safety: Increasing usage with indigenous staff.* Manuscript submitted for publication.

Roberts, M. C., & Brooks, P. (Eds.). (in press). Topical Issue: Children's injuries, prevention, and public policy. *Journal of Social Issues.*

Roberts, M. C., Elkins, P. D., & Royal, G. P. (1984). Psychological applications to the prevention of accidents and illness. In M. C. Roberts & L. Peterson (Eds.), *Prevention of problems in childhood: Psychological research and applications* (pp. 173-199). New York: Wiley-Interscience.

Roberts, M. C., & Fanurik, D. (in press). Rewarding elementary school children for their use of safety belts. *Health Psychology.*

Roberts, M. C., & Layfield, D. A. (in press). Promoting child passenger safety: A comparison of two positive approaches. *Journal of Pediatric Psychology.*

Roberts, M. C., Maddux, J. E., & Wright, L. (1984). The developmental perspective in behavioral health. In J. D. Matarazzo, N. E. Miller, S. M. Weiss, J. A. Herd, & S. M. Weiss (Eds.), *Behavioral health: A handbook of health enhancement and disease prevention* (pp. 56-68). New York: Wiley-Interscience.

Roberts, M. C., & Peterson, L. (Eds.). (1984a). *Prevention of problems in childhood: Psychological research and applications.* New York: Wiley-Interscience.

Roberts, M. C., & Peterson, L. (1984b). Prevention models: Theoretical and practical implications. In M. C. Roberts & L. Peterson (Eds.), *Prevention of problems in childhood: Psychological research and applications* (pp. 1-39). New York: Wiley-Interscience.

Roberts, M. C., & Turner, D. S. (1986). Rewarding parents for their children's use of safety seats. *Journal of Pediatric Psychology, 11*(1), 25-36.

Robertson, L. S. (1983). *Injuries: Causes, control strategies, and public policy.* Lexington, MA: Lexington Books.

Singer, J. E., & Krantz, D. S. (1982). Perspectives on the interface between psychology and public health. *American Psychologist, 37,* 955-960.

Spiegel, C. N., & Lindaman, F. C. (1977). Children can't fly: A program to prevent childhood morbidity and mortality from window falls. *American Journal of Public Health, 67,* 1143-1147.

Treiber, F. A. (1986). A comparison of the positive and negative consequences approaches upon car restraint usage. *Journal of Pediatric Psychology, 11*(1), 15-24.

Walton, W. W. (1982). An evaluation of the poison prevention packaging act. *Pediatrics, 69,* 363-370.

Williams, A. F. (1982). Passive and active measures for controlling disease and injury: The role of health psychologists. *Health Psychology, 1,* 81-91.

Williams, C. L., Carter, B. J., Arnolds, C. B., & Wynder, E. L. (1979). Chronic disease risk factors among children: The "Know Your Body" study. *Journal of Chronic Disease, 32,* 505-513.

Witte, J. J., & Axnick, N. W. (1975). The benefits from ten years of measles immunization in the United States. *Public Health Reports, 90,* 205-207.

Wolfe, D. A., MacPherson, T., Blount, R., & Wolfe, V. V. (1986). Evaluation of a brief in-
    tervention for educating school children in awareness of physical and sexual abuse. *Child
    Abuse & Neglect, 10,* 85-92.
Yeaton, W. H., & Bailey, J. S. (1978). Teaching pedestrian safety skills to young children:
    An analysis and one-year follow up. *Journal of Applied Behavior Analysis, 11,* 315-329.
Yokley, J. M., & Glenwick, D. S. (1984). Increasing the immunization of preschool children:
    An evaluation of applied community interventions. *Journal of Applied Behavior Analysis,
    17,* 313-325.
Zuckerman, B. S., & Duby, J. (1985). Developmental approach to injury prevention. In J. J.
    Alpert & B. Guyer (Eds.), *The Pediatric clinics of North America: Injuries and injury pre-
    vention* (pp. 17-29). Philadelphia: W. B. Saunders.

23

Pediatric AIDS/HIV Infection
An Emerging Challenge to Pediatric Psychology

Roberta A. Olson

Department of Psychiatry and Behavioral Sciences, University of Oklahoma Health Sciences Center

Heather C. Huszti and Patrick J. Mason

Department of Pediatrics and Department of Psychiatry and Behavioral Sciences, University of Oklahoma Health Sciences Center

Jeffrey M. Seibert

Mailman Center for Child Development, University of Miami School of Medicine

Pediatric acquired immunodeficiency syndrome (AIDS) is a disease with social and political ramifications that affect both research and psychotherapy with children and families. This paper examines selected clinical and ethical issues psychologists may encounter in research or psychotherapy with children, adolescents, or parents who are positive for the human immunodeficiency virus (HIV) antibody or have AIDS. A brief overview of AIDS-related research and future directions is presented with particular relevance to pediatric psychology.

THE DISEASE PROCESS

In order to understand the complex issues of AIDS it is helpful first to understand the disease process and the modes of transmission. AIDS is presently thought to be caused by HIV. This virus directly attacks and weakens the immune system thereby allowing opportunistic infections to invade the body (Jaret, 1986; Norman, 1985). HIV appears to directly infect

Originally published in *Journal of Pediatric Psychology,* *14*(1)(1989):1–21.

the T4, or helper T-cells. In a normally functioning immune system the T4 cells are alerted to the presence of a foreign element, such as a virus, and activate "killer T-cells." The killer T-cells multiply, attack, and destroy the foreign virus. As the virus is destroyed suppressor T-cells (T8) signal the system that the virus is gone and the production of killer T-cells is stopped. When HIV enters a helper T-cell it uses its own genetic code to program the host cell into producing additional viruses. Thus, the cells that HIV destroys are those that are designed to recognize the presence of foreign elements and signal the activation of the immune system's defenses. With the destruction of the helper T-cells, multiple infections can enter the body without the activation of the immune system.

HIV TESTING

Two common diagnostic tests used to detect the presence of antibodies to HIV are the enzyme-linked immunosorbent assay (ELISA) and the Western Blot. When both tests are used, the combined false-positive rate is estimated to be 1 in 100 (Centers for Disease Control, 1987a). It may take as long as 6 months, or in rare cases even longer, for the host body to produce enough HIV antibodies for either of the two tests to detect their presence (Ranki, Valle, & Krohn, 1987). The HIV antibodies produced by the body do not offer protection from developing symptoms of AIDS. Antibody-positive ELISA and Western Blot test results indicate that the person has been exposed to the virus and can transmit the virus to others, which is currently believed to be a lifelong condition. Individuals who are HIV antibody positive do not necessarily have AIDS and many are healthy in all other respects. Others experience some physical symptoms and are classified as having AIDS-related complex (ARC). AIDS is a syndrome that is diagnosed by the presence of certain opportunistic infections or characteristic neurological or wasting syndromes (Centers for Disease Control, 1987b; Council of State & Territorial Epidemiologists, 1987).

TRANSMISSION

Fortunately, the AIDS virus is not highly virulent, therefore, many people who come into contact with HIV do not become infected (Friedland & Klein, 1987). The virus is transmitted in three ways: (a) through the direct transfer of HIV-infected seminal or vaginal fluids, (b) through blood contact with HIV-infected blood (such as through the sharing of needles or syringes), or (c) perinatally from an infected mother to her developing child (Friedland & Klein, 1987). Long-term research has repeatedly found that HIV is not transmitted through household contacts (Berthier et al., 1986; Friedland et al., 1986; Mann et al., 1986) or by insects such as mosquitoes (Castro et al., 1987). Effective blood donor screening has virtually eliminated the risk of acquiring HIV infection through contaminated transfusions (Friedland & Klein, 1987).

The highest risk groups for pediatric AIDS differ from adult high-risk groups. The majority of pediatric AIDS cases (72%) are due to perinatal transmission from high-risk mothers (Centers for Disease Control, 1988). Women at highest risk to be infected with HIV are those who use intravenous drugs, or are the sexual partners of IV drug users, bisexual males, or hemophiliacs. Women from countries where AIDS is primarily spread heterosexually, such as African and Caribbean countries, are also at increased risk. The majority of AIDS cases in older adolescents, 17-24 years old, are due to homosexual transmission (Hein, 1988).

It is inappropriate to focus solely on high-risk groups when discussing the HIV transmission because it is not group membership but rather engaging in high-risk behaviors that places an individual at risk. If the focus is predominately on high-risk groups, then individuals who do not consider themselves to be members of these groups but engage in high-risk behaviors may not acknowledge their personal susceptibility to contracting HIV. However, because different types of high-risk behaviors are prevalent in particular groups, there is some utility in considering high-risk groups for prevention programs .

PREVENTION

Health Belief Model

Researchers have explored a number of variables that might predict individual's performance of a variety of preventive health behaviors. One of the most prominent models of the performance of preventive health behaviors is the Health Belief Model (HBM) (Rosenstock, 1966). This model suggests that people are most likely to practice preventive behaviors if they feel susceptible to the disease, that the disease will have serious consequences if contracted, that preventive behaviors are both possible to perform and offer effective protection, and if some warning event occurs that serves to motivate the performance of preventive behaviors (Chen & Land, 1986). Additionally, there is a negative correlation between the number of perceived barriers and the probability that a preventive behavior will be performed. Previous research on the elements of the HBM that are associated with the performance of preventive behaviors has supported the utility of some elements but not of others. Of particular interest for AIDS prevention programs, a number of studies have found little association between the perception of a disease's seriousness and the performance of preventive behaviors (Chen & Land, 1986; Maddux & Rogers, 1983; Simon & Das, 1984). Ironically, the cornerstone of many preventive programs is the detailed descriptions of the seriousness of the disease.

Past research on the HBM has yielded contradictory results, and prospective studies have often failed to show a strong predictive value for the proposed HBM elements on the subsequent performance of preventive health behaviors (Chen & Land, 1986). However, the HBM can be useful to consider in the construction and evaluation of prevention programs. By using a theory-based framework, more cohesive programs can be developed and evaluated. By reviewing previous literature on the outcome of various health prevention programs, more effective programs can be developed and valuable time can be saved by not using elements that have previously proven to be ineffective.

Risk Groups

Each different high-risk group presents its own unique challenges for the health educator. The factors that support the continued practice of high-risk behaviors can be different for each risk group. Therefore, interventions that are successful with one group may not be effective with other groups. The existing social structure of the risk group that reinforces or maintains participation in risk behaviors needs to be understood and interventions must be implemented within the existing social context. To develop the most effective prevention programs, collaboration with individuals already knowledgeable about the risk group's social structure are necessary. Unique issues for groups at risk to contribute to pediatric AIDS are briefly reviewed.

Women At Risk For HIV Infection

Two major groups of women are at the greatest risk for HIV infection and, subsequently, giving birth to an HIV-infected child: women who use intravenous drugs, and the sexual partners of HIV antibody-positive men who use intravenous drugs. The majority of women at highest risk for HIV infection are black and Hispanic minorities which represent 72% of women with AIDS (Centers for Disease Control, 1988). This incidence rate is 10 times greater among Black and Hispanic women than among white, non-Hispanic women (Friedland & Klein, 1987). Many women may not realize their own high risk for HIV infection, because they do not use drugs themselves and sexual partners often do not admit to IV drug use. Many male drug users have sexual partners who are not IV drug users themselves (Des Jarlais, Chamberland, Yancovitz, Weinberg, & Friedman, 1984). Female IV drug users and sexual partners of IV drug users may be difficult to reach because they do not belong to any preexisting social networks that could be utilized to provide prevention education. The majority of IV drug users choose not to participate in drug rehabilitation programs (Huszti & Chitwood, in press). Innovative methods are being used to increase participation in drug treatment centers, such as distributing, to inner-city neighborhoods, coupons that are redeemable for detoxification and treatment (Jackson & Rotkiewicz, 1987).

Many factors combine to decrease the likelihood that the females at greatest risk for AIDS will practice preventive behaviors. Many women from socially and culturally disadvantaged backgrounds do not believe that they have enough control over their lives to effectively use preventive health behaviors (Huszti & Chitwood, in press). Additionally, in the social context of IV drug use, needle sharing is a social behavior that can indicate friendship and trust (Friedman, Des Jarlais, & Sotheran, 1986). Women who use IV drugs are often dependent on males for their drug supply and are consequently reluctant to ask their partners to use preventive sexual and drug use behaviors for fear of losing their drug supply (Huszti & Chitwood, in press).

Some preventive programs designed to reach the women at highest risk have begun to be implemented. Several programs have used peer counselors to go into neighborhoods heavily populated by IV drug users. These counselors distribute information about risk reduction behaviors, information about drug treatment programs, and in some cases, bottles of bleach to clean needles and syringes. Evaluations of these programs indicate increased knowledge and a decrease in both high-risk drug use and sexual behaviors (McAuliffe et al., 1987; Watters, 1987). However, these programs appear to be more effective in reducing high-risk drug behaviors than in modifying risky sexual behaviors (McAuliffe et al., 1987).

The sexual behavior changes that are necessary to prevent the spread of AIDS can be particularly difficult to make. Although high-risk groups have slowly begun to modify their high-risk sexual behaviors, a large percentage of individuals have not made significant changes (Martin, 1987; McKusick, Horstman, & Coates, 1985). In developing prevention programs, one should keep in mind the difference between reducing the practice of high-risk behaviors and increasing the practice of preventive behaviors. Different types of programs appear to affect these areas differently. Primarily informational prevention programs appear to encourage participants to decrease their high-risk behavior but have little affect on the use of alternative safer behaviors, such as the use of condoms (Quadland, Shattls, Schuman, Jacobs, & D'Eramo, 1988). Programs that make the use of safer sexual behaviors erotic (Quadland et al., 1988) or socially appealing within the context of a relationship (Solomon & DeJong, 1986) appear to increase the use of condoms and other safer sexual behaviors but have little effect on decreasing risky behaviors. Prevention programs may need to use several types of approaches both to decrease the practice of high-risk sexual behaviors and to encourage the performance of safer alternative sexual behaviors (Huszti & Chitwood, in press).

Women from countries where AIDS is primarily heterosexually transmitted also present difficult issues. Cultural and language barriers often make these women distrustful of available social services. Due to language barriers, messages about the risk of transmitting HIV to unborn children may not be understood. Additionally, cultural values often stress the importance of bearing children. The recommendation to delay pregnancy, if HIV antibody positive, is often in direct conflict with cultural pressures (Seibert, Garcia, Kaplan, & Septimus, in press). The use of peer counselors, who understand the cultural demands and language barriers, may lead to more effective prevention programs.

Adolescents

Adolescents represent a potential risk group because of the sexual and drug experimentation that often occurs at this age. The typical cognitive processing of adolescents only serves to increase the likelihood that they will ignore warnings of personal risk. Adolescents often believe that they are personally invulnerable to negative consequences (Elkind, 1967). Melton (1987) suggested that, due to their age, adolescents are unlikely to have directly experienced negative consequences from risky health behaviors. Peers, who assume great importance during adolescence, often subtly or blatantly encourage participation in sexual or drug-use behaviors. These factors make it particularly difficult for prevention programs to be successful. There has been a call for AIDS education to be instituted in schools to prevent adolescents' participation in high-risk behaviors (Koop, 1986).

Recent evaluations of AIDS prevention programs for adolescents suggest that these programs do increase knowledge about AIDS (DiClemente et al., 1987; Huszti, Clopton, & Mason, 1988; Miller & Downer,

1987). However, these programs have not resulted in any long-lasting changes in students' attitudes toward practicing preventive behaviors (Huszti et al., 1988). Although the initial data suggest that educational programs are not sufficient to encourage the practice of preventive behaviors, firm conclusions cannot be drawn until data about actual sexual behaviors are collected.

Past prevention programs, which only provided information about the disease, did not have long-term effects on promoting prevention behaviors. Recent smoking and pregnancy prevention programs (Allerd et al., 1985; Casswell, Brasch, Gilmore, & Silva, 1985; Chen & Land, 1986) that emphasize the acquisition of the skills needed to implement preventive behaviors have had some promising results (Herz, Reis, & Barbera-Stein, 1986; Schnike, Blythe, & Gilchrist, 1981; Schnike, Gilchrist, Schilling, Snow, & Bobo, 1986). These programs typically required 12 to 16 sessions. Similar programs on AIDS prevention need to teach adolescents how to assertively communicate with potential or current sexual partners and how to use appropriate problem-solving skills, so that adolescents either abstain from sexual intercourse or insist that condoms be used. Issues of schools' limited resources and time restraints must be balanced with the importance of conducting prevention programs that can increase the use of preventive behaviors. If extended prevention programs are instituted in schools then time must be allotted for teacher training, teacher updating, and class time for prevention programs and booster sessions. This commitment will result in less time being devoted to other education endeavors.

Additionally, the adolescents at highest risk to contract HIV (runaways, prostitutes, and habitual IV drugs users) may not be accessible through a traditional school setting. Innovative methods to reach these groups, such as the use of peer counselors and programs at runaway shelters, must be developed. Sensitive approaches to prevention programs for male homosexual adolescents must also be developed (Hein, 1988).

Persons With Hemophilia

Approximately 92% of males with severe Factor VIII hemophilia, a genetic sex-linked bleeding disorder, have been exposed to HIV through the use of HIV-infected factor concentrate (Stehr-Green, Holman, Jason, & Evatt, 1988). Factor concentrate is made from pooled plasma and is used by hemophiliacs to control bleeding episodes. Currently, this product is heat-treated, which appears to have eliminated the further transmission of HIV (Centers for Disease Control, 1987a). However, those individuals with hemophilia who are HIV-positive can infect their sexual partners, who can then infect their unborn children.

For the hemophilia population, as with any group, changing and maintaining new sexual behaviors can be difficult. A particularly important issue for men with hemophilia is to be "normal." Because of the potential threat of bleeding, many types of physical activities are restricted. Sexual behaviors have traditionally been one of the few activities where male hemophiliac patients have been equal to the nonhemophiliac population. Placing new restrictions on their established or emerging sexual behaviors seems overwhelming. Because the majority of hemophiliacs receive medical treatment through special comprehensive hemophilia centers, this network is used as a framework within which prevention programs have been conducted. Hemophilia treatment centers have also instituted a variety of HIV transmission prevention programs into their health care delivery. Prevention efforts have concentrated on helping sexually active hemophiliacs practice safer sex guidelines and recommending that couples delay pregnancies. Additionally, the national patient organization, the National Hemophilia Foundation, has prepared and distributed a number of informational pamphlets about HIV infection to the patient population. The effectiveness of these programs is currently being assessed. Many of the components found useful in these programs might be useful in prevention programs for other high-risk groups, depending upon the factors that maintain the risk behaviors in those groups. For a thorough review of prevention programs for hemophiliacs, please see Mason, Olson, and Parish (1988).

Evaluation

A critical component of any prevention program is an evaluation of its effectiveness. Past evaluations have suggested that many prevention programs do not achieve their goals (Chen & Land, 1986). Because prevention remains the only means presently to control the further spread of AIDS, it is essential to use programs that have proven effective. Past research has shown that knowledge and attitudes do not reliably predict behaviors. Therefore, assessment of the practice of high-risk and preventive behaviors both before and after prevention programs is needed. It is difficult to assess issues such as sexual and drug-use behaviors. Self-reports are often biased by socially desirable responses. Although it may appear to be a formidable task to construct reliable and valid measures, their development must be pursued in order to effectively evaluate prevention efforts. Innovative methods of measurement need to be pursued, such as monitoring the rate of sexually transmitted diseases in, or condom sales to, groups that have received educational programs.

Psychologists and public health officials must work together to develop, implement, and interpret evaluations of prevention programs.

CLINICAL ISSUES

Psychotherapy with children that are HIV antibody positive or have AIDS and their families presents a series of difficult clinical issues. Psychologists, in the last decade, have had considerable experience working with children that have been diagnosed with a life-threatening or terminal illness. Research and clinical experiences indicate that children as young as 4 or 5 years old begin to conceptualize death as a process involving physical harm (White, Elsom, & Prawat, 1978). By the age of 10 or 11, children who have been diagnosed with cancer understand death as permanent, universal, and with a total cessation of all bodily sensations (Easson, 1981). Children, even when protected from a diagnosis or the gravity of their disease, often understand that they have a life-threatening illness (Schowalter, 1974; Wachter, 1971). Psychologists working with pediatric cancer patients generally have recommended that children be told at the time of diagnosis the name of their disease and the types of medical treatments they will undergo (Koocher, 1980). When treatment is no longer effective and the child is terminally ill, many health professionals and oncologists have recommended that the child be informed of his or her status (Nitschke et al., 1982).

When a child is HIV-positive, or is dying of AIDS, the pediatric psychologist faces a dilemma. Therapeutic goals in working with a child and family typically focus on honest and open communication in which the family has the opportunity to discuss the illness, grieve the pending loss of child, and reassure the child that he or she will not be alone, in pain, or forgotten. Many parents do not want their child to be informed of his or her HIV antibody-positive test or a diagnosis of AIDS. The parental decision to protect the child from the illness is based on several realistic concerns. Because of public fear and misinformation, families with a child that is HIV-positive or has AIDS face potential abandonment by extended family or friends, loss of housing, and loss of employment (Seibert et al., in press). The fear of social rejection often prevents families from dealing openly with the reality that their child may suffer repeated illness and die.

Psychologists may also face the dilemma of what are the child's rights to know his or her diagnosis and medical status as opposed to the parents' rights to withhold diagnostic information to protect the child and family from adverse consequences. Psychologists can share with parents the past research and clinical experience that indicates the school-age child can understand and learn to cope with a potentially life-threatening illness. Psychologists are also aware of the potential emotional distress that can occur when a child realizes that he or she has an extremely serious illness that the family will not discuss. If the parents choose to disclose a diagnosis of HIV-positive status or AIDS to the child, psychologists do not know at what age a child can keep his or her diagnosis a secret from friends, teachers, or extended family; nor is it known what the psychological effects of this demand would be on a child. The social stigma of HIV infection and AIDS creates significant and unnecessary stress on the family and health care worker. Psychologists must focus on both short- and long-term goals. Short-term goals include helping the family to cope with a potentially terminally ill child. Long-term goals for psychologists include participation in creating public education programs that provide accurate information about AIDS and methods of changing public attitudes and beliefs that lead to compassion instead of fear.

PUBLIC EDUCATION

Unlike other potentially fatal diseases, AIDS and HIV infection carry a very negative social stigma. AIDS elicits negative and fearful attitudes from high school students (Huszti et al., 1988), adults (Dawson, Cynamon, & Fitti, 1987), medical students and residents (Kelly, St. Lawrence, Smith, Hood, & Cook, 1987a, 1987b; Link, Feingold, Charap, Freeman, & Shelov, 1988), and physicians (Loewy, 1986). Before HIV was discovered, AIDS was referred to as the "gay disease." As a result, negative attitudes towards homosexuality often become intertwined with attitudes towards AIDS. Instead of compassion towards individuals with HIV infection, many people believe these individuals somehow deserve their fate.

A second explanation for negative public reactions to HIV-positive individuals is a fear of contagion through casual contact. Accordingly, accurate information about the transmission of HIV should be associated with positive attitudes towards infected individuals. Some support for this assumption can be found in a study that revealed modest negative correlations between knowledge about AIDS and fear of AIDS patients among samples of the general public in San Francisco, New York, and London (Temoshok, Sweet, & Zich, 1988). A recent study of the effects of AIDS education with high school students found a modest correlation between increased knowledge about AIDS and increased positive attitudes towards AIDS patients (Huszti, 1987). Positive attitudes declined, however, at a 1-month follow-up. Additional "booster" sessions may be necessary to maintain increased positive attitudes.

Psychologists are uniquely suited to work on issues of attitudinal change. Social psychology has amassed an impressive body of literature on prejudice (Allport, 1954), attribution theory (Jones & Harris, 1967; Kelly, 1967), and attitude change (Ajzen & Fishbein, 1980; Bem, 1972; Festinger, 1957; Petty & Cacioppo, 1981). These studies have led to a better understanding and possible interventions for issues such as racial or sexual discrimination. Based on past research, psychologists can provide theoretically and methodologically sound proposals for changing public attitudes' toward individuals who are HIV antibody-positive or have AIDS.

PEDIATRIC AIDS RESEARCH

Confidentiality

Confidentiality cannot be guaranteed when doing research in pediatric groups with HIV infection. There are legally sanctioned encroachments on research confidentiality including state child abuse and neglect laws. Many mothers of perinatally infected infants are also infected with HIV as a result of IV drug use or sexual contact with IV drug users or bisexual males. These mothers, as a result of HIV infection of the central nervous system or continued drug use, may experience cognitive deficits and provide inadequate care for their infected child. In addition, some states now require mandatory reporting of all HIV antibody-positive individuals. Research that follows high-risk individuals over time may be required to reveal their names to state health departments if they seroconvert to HIV. The researcher may apply to the federal government to obtain certificates of confidentiality that prevent the disclosure of confidential records even when subpoenaed by the court (American Psychological Association, 1985). Applications for certificates of confidentiality are not difficult to complete, but they may require an extensive period of time between application and approval. Gray and Melton (1985) have suggested the certificates may not be effective in the preservation of confidentiality of children with AIDS and their families.

Informed Consent

A second problem encountered in HIV research is obtaining clear, informed consent from research participants. Informed consent must alert the families to risks surrounding possible breaches of confidentiality; it must contain the assurance of continued medical and psychological support regardless of participation; and it must allow for the right to withdraw from the research at any time (American Psychological Association, 1985). Many of the perinatally infected children are born to women who are not involved with social agencies or the traditional health care system. Adolescents at risk for HIV infection through IV drug use are predominantly low income Blacks and Hispanics. In order to design informed consent and appropriate investigational research materials that are sensitive to the concerns of these individuals requires input from representatives of each of these groups.

Attainment and continued retention of proper consent for children to participate in research can become very complicated. As more HIV-infected children become wards of the state and custody shifts from parents to foster parents there will be a need for ongoing verification of consent. In addition, obtaining a continued valid informed consent for a long-term study may be difficult when participants or their parents demonstrate reduced competence due to HIV neurologic involvement or continued drug use.

NEUROPSYCHOLOGICAL EFFECTS

Various neurological symptoms have been found in as many as 60–70% of pediatric AIDS patients (Price et al., 1988). Initially the neuropsychological impairments observed in adult AIDS patients were attributed to depression secondary to the diagnosis of AIDS or to the effects of the multiple opportunistic infections commonly found in AIDS patients. After autopsies revealed HIV in brain cells, it was realized that the virus can directly infect the brain and cause neurological impairments (Price et al., 1988). Early neurologic symptoms of HIV infection can include headaches, encephalitis, aseptic meningitis, ataxia, dementia, loss of developmental milestones, or general developmental delays (Epstein et al., 1986; Price et al., 1988). The cortical changes observed in children with AIDS appear to differ from the changes typically observed in adults. In children with AIDS, cortical atrophy appears more severe than in adults. Children also exhibit calcification of the basal ganglia (Scott, Buck, Letterman, Bloom, & Parks, 1984). The degree and rate of neurological impairment can vary widely in children. Some children display rapid deterioration in developmental milestones, whereas other children evidence a slow decline in motor or cognitive skills. The various factors that contribute to these differences are unclear but may be related to the child's age at symptom onset and the length of time the child has been diagnosed with AIDS (Scott et al., 1984). Further research is necessary to determine what factors contribute to an increased progression of symptoms. A multisite study will soon begin to investigate the long-term neuropsychological effects of HIV infection in children with hemophilia. Children who are HIV-positive will be compared with those who are seronegative. Concurrent Magnetic Resonance Imaging and EEGs will also be performed to evaluate for organic brain changes. This type of research is extremely important in determining the long-term neurological effects of HIV infection.

Subtle neurological changes can be the first symptom of HIV infection (Price et al., 1988). Clinicians who work with developmentally delayed infants and children need to be sensitive to the possibility that HIV infection may be causing unexplained neurological impairment. Improvements in the medical management of infections in perinatally infected children has led to increased life expectancy. Through the use of developmental and neuropsychological testing clinicians can help to define the relative strengths and weakness of HIV-infected children who display neurological symptoms. Psychologists can help school personnel and caretakers of the child understand what tasks the child is capable of performing successfully. These caretakers also need to understand that the child's neurological deficits can be progressive. In addition to direct neurologic infection, other factors can contribute to developmental changes in HIV-infected children. Many pediatric AIDS patients come from environments that are deprived. Factors associated with developmental delays, such as maternal drug use, disabilities as a result of poor prenatal care, neglect or abuse, multiple infections, social isolation, repeated hospitalizations, and poor nutrition may also serve to exacerbate preexisting neurological deficits. Further research is necessary to determine the relative effects of each of these factors.

PSYCHONEUROIMMUNOLOGY

Currently, not all individuals infected with HIV develop clinical AIDS. One study of adults found annual conversion rates of approximately 7% (Moss et al., 1988). The proportion of HIV-infected adults and children who eventually develop AIDS is unknown and it is unclear what cofactors may hasten or retard the development of AIDS. A wide variety of factors have been proposed, including diet, repeated exposure to the virus, multiple infections, social support, continued drug use, and health habits (Coates, Temoshok, & Mandel, 1984; Weber et al., 1986). Eventually a variety of factors may be found to be associated with the development of AIDS in individuals who are HIV antibody positive.

Recent research into the effects of stress on immune system functioning suggests that psychosocial factors can have an effect on immune system functioning in normal subjects. A limited number of well-controlled studies have found associations between stressful events, such as medical school exams, and various indicators of immunosuppression (Kiecolt-Glaser et al., 1986). Although the potential detrimental effects of stress on the immune system is of interest for HIV-infected individuals, of greater importance is the possibility that stress reduction techniques can improve immune functioning. In one study, medical students were randomly assigned to a relaxation training group or to a control group prior to written exams (Kiecolt-Glaser et al., 1986). Although group membership was not a significant predictor of immune system functioning, the frequency of practicing relaxation techniques was a significant predictor. The students who frequently practiced the relaxation techniques had a higher percentage of helper/inducer T-lymphocytes. This finding is of particular interest. It is the decrease of helper T-lymphocytes (T4) that allows the development of opportunistic infections in HIV-infected individuals. These initial studies suggest the value of exploring the effects of stress and using stress reduction techniques with HIV-infected individuals. It is possible that teaching HIV-infected persons stress-reduction techniques may help to improve or maintain their immune system functioning as well as to help them have some sense of control over their illness. With these potential benefits, psychoneuroimmunologic research may be a critical area in the study of AIDS.

ETHICAL ISSUES

AIDS presents numerous ethical dilemmas for the psychologist. Two of the most difficult issues concern the psychologist's duty to warn and to protect the individual's rights to confidentiality. In the landmark case of *Tarasoff v. Regent's of the University of California* (1976) the California Supreme Court ruled that when a patient presents a serious danger to another, the therapist "bears a duty to exercise reasonable care to protect the foreseeable victim of that danger" (Tarasoff II, 1976, 551 P. 2d at 3:45). In a more recent case, *Currie v. United States* (1986) the North Carolina court indicated that therapists have a duty to warn all foreseeable victims. The duty to protect all possible victims may require the therapists to commit the patient to an inpatient psychiatric hospital. In each of the above cases the patient indicated a plan to harm a specific person or persons.

In the case of an HIV-infected adolescent the psychologist is presented with an extremely difficult situation. If an HIV-positive adolescent indicates that he is sexually active and does not plan to use condoms, is the psychologist required to break confidentiality and warn the sexual partner? An important factor in this decision is the evaluation of the potential risk of this patient's behavior. Hearst and Hulley (1988) have estimated the risk of spreading HIV to an uninfected sexual partner is 1 in 500 for a single unprotected heterosexual encounter. The estimated risk of HIV infection rises to 2 in 3 for 500 unprotected sexual encounters with the same partner. The psychologist is placed in the position of assessing how frequently the HIV-infected adolescent plans to engage in unprotected sexual activity that exposes a partner to infected semen or vaginal fluids. There is no clear definition of what constitutes an imminent or serious danger that requires the therapist to warn the sexual partner.

A more typical scenario that a psychologist may encounter is that, after counseling the adolescent about the prevention of HIV infection, the adolescent makes a commitment to using condoms in all future sexual encounters. Assessment of risks to the sexual partner include the effectiveness of condoms and the relative risk of infection. The failure rate of condoms is estimated to be approximately 10% (Williams, 1986). The estimated risk of infecting a partner is 1 in 500,000 for a single protected heterosexual encounter. The risk rises to 1 in 1,100 after 500 protected heterosexual encounters with a single partner (Hearst & Hulley, 1988). Given the extremely low estimated probability of risk of infection, the psychologist may feel there is no need to warn a sexual partner of the potential risk of contracting a fatal disease providing the adolescent consistently uses condoms and spermicide. An additional factor to consider is the probability of the adolescent consistently using condoms. There are no data that examine HIV-positive adolescents' use of condoms. However, a study of sexually active adolescents indicated that most adolescents knew that condoms prevent sexually transmitted disease and place a high value on their use. Yet the majority of adolescents failed to use condoms consistently (Kegeles, Adler, & Irwin, 1988). These findings are consistent with previous literature that indicates a tenuous relationship between knowledge, attitudes, and behavior.

When counseling HIV-positive adolescents, psychologists may choose to evaluate the potential harm and benefits of breaking confidentiality and informing the sexual partner of the potential risk of infection. Weighing the potential benefits and harm incurred by breaking confidentiality may include the probability that the adolescent will drop out of psychotherapy and form relationships with new sexual partners. If the psychologist chooses to maintain confidentiality there could be a continued focus on responsible and caring sexual behavior within an intimate relationship. The APA ethical guidelines concerning AIDS (American Psychological Association, 1985) focused solely on research issues and failed to address the process of deciding when, and under what circumstances, it is appropriate to break confidentiality in a therapeutic relationship. The issues raised by HIV-positive adolescents present difficult ethical decisions for the psychologists as a group. Psychologists need to educate themselves concerning biomedical ethics and decision making in order to develop appropriate ethical guidelines for counseling HIV antibody-positive individuals.

AIDS-EPIDEMIOLOGICAL PROJECTIONS

The number of diagnosed cases of AIDS changes daily. A review of the past progression of the disease and the current statistics suggests that the number of pediatric AIDS patients will continue to grow. Currently, approximately 77% of the CDC-reported pediatric AIDS (birth to 13 years) are as a result of perinatal transmission. Contaminated blood or blood products account for 20% of the pediatric cases (Centers for Disease Control, 1988). All donated blood is now being screened for HIV antibodies and blood coagulation products used by the hemophiliac patients are heat-treated to destroy undetected virus. Because of these blood precautions, the primary mode of HIV infection to preadolescents will be as a result of perinatal transmission. Unfortunately, the number of perinatally infected cases has only increased over time. A sample study of infants born in Massachusetts indicated that 1 in every 476 births were to HIV-positive mothers (Hoff et al., 1988). The authors estimated that from 1,670 to 4,860 HIV-infected children are now born each year in the U.S. The National Academy of Sciences (1986) projected that for every CDC-defined pediatric AIDS case there are four other children with other forms of HIV infection. By 1991 there will be an estimated 3,000 cumulative cases of pediatric AIDS and 10,000 additional children that will be HIV positive. As physicians continue to learn about the effects of HIV more effective treatments will be found, leading to increased lifespans of HIV-infected children. This increase in patients suggests that increasing numbers of psychologists will come into contact with pediatric AIDS cases.

Currently, adolescents represent less than 1% of all AIDS cases. HIV testing of military recruits indicates that 1.5% of 17- to 19-year-olds are HIV positive (Centers for Disease Control, 1986a). However, voluntary recruits for the military are not a random sample of the U.S. adolescent population and probably underrepresent IV drug users and homosexual or bisexual males in this age range. Examination of adolescent sexual behaviors, sexually transmitted diseases, and IV drug use suggests this group may be at higher risk for AIDS than the statistics indicate. The number of adolescents affected by AIDS may be low because the AIDS virus often lies dormant for 5 or more years after the initial infection and before symptoms of AIDS appear. The age group of 20- to 30-year-olds, represents 21% of all AIDS cases, and it is likely that a number of these individuals were infected when they were adolescents.

FUTURE DIRECTIONS FOR RESEARCH

Many education and prevention strategies have been suggested and some have been put into practice. For instance, the Surgeon General mailed AIDS information packets to every American household in June 1988 (Koop & Centers for Disease Control, 1988). An evaluation of a British mailing suggested that although knowledge about AIDS increased, there was no change in preventive behaviors (Sherr & Green, 1987). The results of this study reinforce the need to consider past literature before instituting new and expensive prevention programs. Prevention programs should be evaluated for their effectiveness in decreasing individuals' high-risk behaviors. Findings from research on the prevention of the spread of AIDS can offer unique opportunities for psychologists to learn about how to change attitudes and behaviors of individuals at risk for AIDS as well as changing public perception of the disease. These findings would also contribute to psychologists' ability to design better health promotion and disease prevention strategies for other populations at risk for other preventable diseases.

There are other areas that need further research. For example, as better treatments are found, more of the perinatally infected children will attend school. Initial studies have indicated that HIV can cause neurologic deficits. Educators and parents will need to understand the special needs of these children due to their immune system and neurological deficits. Additionally, stress and depression may play a part in the progression of the illness. Therefore, studies in psychoneuroimmunology may help to establish possible links between psychological variables and physical illness which would lead to possible preventive intervention strategies.

Researchers and clinicians who work with individuals that are HIV antibody positive or have AIDS have a number of ethical and legal dilemmas. Psychologists can use this opportunity to examine and clarify the process of how to reach difficult decisions concerning confidentiality and duty to warn. Consultation between biomedical ethicists, lawyers, representatives of community organizations, persons with AIDS or HIV infection, and psychologists can help to solve the many ethical and legal problems that are presented in working with individuals with a potentially fatal disease.

REFERENCES

Allerd, C. A., Clark, D. S., Nowacek, G. A., Short, J. G., Cox, D. J., & Ayers, C. R. (1985). Measures of knowledge and attitudes toward preventive cardiology. *Journal of Medical Education, 60,* 314-319.

Allport, G. W. (1954). *The nature of prejudice.* Reading, MA: Addison-Wesley.

Ajzen, I., & Fisbein, M. (1980). *Understanding attitudes and predicting social behavior.* Englewood Cliffs, NJ: Prentice Hall.

American Psychological Association. (1985). Ethical issues in psychological research on AIDS. *Issues in Scientific Psychology.* Washington, DC: Author.

Bem, D. J. (1972). Self-perception theory. *Advances in Experimental Social Psychology, 6,* 1-62.

Berthier, A., Chamaret, S., Fauchet, R., Fonlupt, J., Genetet, N., Gueguen, M., Pommerevil, M., Ruffault, A., & Montagnier, L. (1986). Transmissibility of human immunodeficiency virus in haemophilic and nonhaemophilic children living in a private school in France. *Lancet, 2,* 598-601.

Casswell, S., Brasch, P., Gilmore, L., & Silva, P. (1985). Children's attitudes to alcohol and awareness of alcohol-related problems. *British Journal of Addiction, 34,* 191-194.

Castro, K. G., Lieb, S., Calisher, C., Witte, J., Jaffe, H. W., & The Field Study Group. (1987, June). *AIDS and HIV infection, Belle Glade, Florida.* Paper presented at the 3rd International Conference on AIDS, Washington, DC.

Centers for Disease Control. (1986). Human T-lymphotropic virus type III/lymphadenopathy-associated virus antibody prevalence in U.S. military recruit applicants. *Morbidity and Mortality Weekly Report, 35,* 421-425.

Centers for Disease Control. (1987a). Public health service guidelines for counseling and antibody testing to prevent HIV infection and AIDS. *Morbidity and Mortality Weekly Report, 36,* 509-515.

Centers for Disease Control. (1987b). U.S. Department of Health and Human Services: Revising the CDC surveillance case definition for Acquired Immunodeficiency Syndrome. *Morbidity and Mortality Weekly Report, 36*(Suppl. No. IS), 35-55.

Centers for Disease Control. (1988). AIDS profile update. *The AIDS Record, 2,* 11.

Chen, M., & Land, K. C. (1986). Testing the health belief model: LISREL analysis of alternative models of causal relationships between health beliefs and preventive dental behavior. *Social Psychology Quarterly, 49,* 45-60.

Coates, T. J., Temoshok, L., & Mandel, J. (1984). Psychosocial research is essential to understanding and treating AIDS. *American Psychologist, 39,* 1309-1314.

Council of State & Territorial Epidemiologists. (1987). A revision of the CDC surveillance case definition for Acquired Immunodeficiency Syndrome. *Morbidity and Mortality Weekly Report, 36,* 35-155.

Currie v. United States, 644F. Supp. 1074 (M.D.N.C. 1986).

Dawson, D. A., Cynamon, M., & Fitti, J. E. (1987). AIDS knowledge and attitudes: Provisional data from the national health interview survey. *Advancedata, 146,* 1-10.

Des Jarlais, D. C., Chamberland, M. E., Yancovitz, S. R., Weinberg, P., & Friedman, S. R. (1984). Heterosexual partners: A large risk groups for AIDS. *Lancet, 2,* 1346-1347.

DiClemente, R. J., Pies, C. A., Stoller, E. J., Haskin, J., Oliva, G. E., & Rutherford, G. W. (1987, June). *Evaluation of a school-based AIDS education curricula in San Francisco.* Paper presented at the 3rd International AIDS Conference, Washington, DC.

Easson, W. M. (1981). The *dying child: The management of the child or adolescent who is dying* (2nd ed.). Springfield, IL: Charles C. Thomas.

Elkind, D. (1967). Egocentrism in adolescence. *Child Development, 38,* 1025-1034.

Epstein, L. G., Sharer, L. R., Oleske, J. M., Connor, E. M., Goudsmit, J., Bagdon, L., Robert-Gurof, M., & Koenigsberger, M. R. (1986). Neurologic manifestations of human immunodeficiency virus infection in children. *Pediatrics, 78,* 678-687.

Festinger, L. (1957). *A theory of cognitive dissonance.* Stanford, CA: Stanford University Press.

Friedland, G. H., & Klein, R. S. (1987). Transmission of the human immunodeficiency virus. *New England Journal of Medicine, 317,* 1125-1135.

Friedland, G., Saltzman, B., Kahl, P., Lesser, M., Mayers, M., Feiner, C., & Klein, R. (1986). Reply. *New England Journal of Medicine, 315,* 258-259.

Friedman, S. R., Des Jarlais, D. C., & Sotheran, J. L. (1986). AIDS health education for intravenous drug users. *Health Education Quarterly, 13,* 383-393.

Gray, J. N., & Melton, G. B. (1985). The law and ethics of psychosocial research on AIDS. *Nebraska Law Review, 64*(4), 637-688.

Hearst, N., & Hulley, S. B. (1988). Preventing the heterosexual spread of AIDS: Are we giving outpatients the best advice? *Journal of the American Medical Association, 259,* 2428-2432.

Hein, K. (1988, March). *AIDS in adolescence: Exploring the challenge.* Paper presented at the National Invitational Conference on AIDS and Adolescence, New York, NY.

Herz, E. J., Reis, J. S., & Barbera-Stein, L. (1986). Family life education for young teens: An assessment of three interventions. *Health Education Quarterly, 13,* 201-221.

Hoff, R., Berardi, V. P., Weiblen, B. J., Mahoney-Trout, L., Mitchell, M. L., & Grady, G. F. (1988). Seroprevalence of human immunodeficiency virus among childbearing women. *New England Journal of Medicine, 318,* 525-530.

Huszti, H . C. (1987). *The effects of educational programs on adolescents' knowledge and attitudes about Acquired Immunodeficiency Syndrome (AIDS).* Unpublished dissertation, Texas Tech University.

Huszti, H., & Chitwood, D. (in press). Pediatric AIDS risk reduction. In J. Seibert (Ed.), *Pediatric AIDS,* Lincoln: University of Nebraska Press.

Huszti, H. C., Clopton, J. R., & Mason, P. J. (1988). *Effects of an AIDS educational program on adolescents' knowledge and attitudes.* Paper submitted for review.

Jackson, J., & Rotkiewicz, L. (1987, June). *A coupon program: AIDS education and drug treatment.* Paper presented at the 3rd International Conference on AIDS, Washington, DC.

Jaret, P. (1986). Our immune system: The wars within. *National Geographic, 169,* 702-735.

Jones, E. E., & Harris, V. A. (1967). The attribution of attitudes. *Journal of Experimental Social Psychology, 3,* 1-24.

Kegeles, S. M., Adler, N. E., & Irwin, C. E. (1988). Sexually active adolescents and condoms: Changes over one year in knowledge, attitudes and use. *American Journal of Public Health, 78,* 460-461.

Kelly, H. H. (1967). Attribution theory in social psychology. In D. Levine (Ed.), *Nebraska symposium on motivation* (Vol. 15). Lincoln: University of Nebraska Press.

Kelly, J. A., St. Lawrence, J. S., Smith, S., Hood, H. V., & Cool, D. J. (1987a). Medical students' attitudes toward AIDS and homosexual patients. *Journal of Medical Education, 62,* 549-556.

Kelly, J. A., St. Lawrence, J. S., Smith, S., Hood, H. V., & Cook, D. J. (1987b). Stigmatization of AIDS patients by physicians. *American Journal of Public Health, 77*(7), 789-791.

Kiecolt-Glaser, J. K., Glaser, R., Strain, E. C., Stout, J. C., Tarr, K. L., Holliday, J. E., & Speicher, C. E. (1986). Modulation of cellular immunity in medical students. *Journal of Behavioral Medicine, 9*(6), 5-21.

Koocher, G. P. (1980). Initial consultations with the pediatric cancer patient. In J. Kellerman (Ed.), *Psychological aspects of childhood cancer* (pp. 231-237). Springfield, IL: Charles C. Thomas.

Koop, C. E. (1986). *Surgeon General's report on acquired immune deficiency syndrome.* Washington, DC: U.S. Department of Health and Human Services.

Koop, C. E., & The Centers for Disease Control. (1988). *Understanding AIDS* (DHHS Publication No. (CDC) HHS-88-8404). Washington, DC: U.S. Government Printing Office.

Link, R. N., Feingold, A. R., Charap, M. H., Freeman, K., & Shelov, S. P. (1988). Concerns of medical and pediatric house officers about acquiring AIDS from their patients. *American Journal of Public Health, 78,* 455-459.

Loewy, E. H. (1986). AIDS and the physician's fear of contagion. *Chest, 89,* 325-326.

Maddux, J. E., & Rogers, R. W. (1983). Protection motivation and self-efficacy: A revised theory of fear appeals and attitude change. *Journal of Experimental Social Psychology, 19,* 469-479.

Mann, J. M., Quinn, T. C., Francis, H., Nzilambi, N., Bosenge, N., Bila, K., McCormick, J. B., Ruti, K., Asilia, P. K., & Curran, J. (1986). Prevalence of HTLV-III/LAV in household contacts of patients with confirmed AIDS and controls in Kinshasa, Zaire. *Journal of the American Medical Association, 256,* 721-724.

Martin, J. L., (1987). The impact of AIDS on gay male sexual behavior patterns in New York City. *American Journal of Public Health, 77,* 578-581.

Mason, P. J., Olson, R. A., & Parish, K. L. (1988). AIDS, hemophilia, and prevention efforts within a comprehensive care program. *American Psychologists, 43(11),* 971-978.

McAuliffe, W. E., Doering, S., Breer, P., Silverman, H., Branson, B., & Williams, K. (1987, June). *An evaluation of using ex-addict outreach workers to educate intravenous drug users about AIDS prevention.* Paper presented at the 3rd International Conference on AIDS, Washington, DC.

McKusick, L., Horstman, W., & Coates, T. J. (1985). AIDS and sexual behavior reported by gay men in San Francisco. *American Journal of Public Health, 75,* 493-496.

Melton, G. B. (1987, June 18). *Prevention of HIV infection among adolescents.* Testimony presented before the United States House of Representatives Select Committee on Children, Youth, and Families, Washington, DC.

Miller, L., & Downer, A. (1987, June). *Knowledge and attitude changes in adolescents following one hour of AIDS instruction.* Paper presented at the 3rd International Conference on AIDS, Washington, DC.

Moss, A. R., Bacchetti, P., Osmond, D., Krampf, W., Chaisson, R. E., Stites, D., Wilber, J., Allain, J. P., & Carlson, J. (1988). Seropositivity for HIV and the development of AIDS or AIDS related condition: Three years follow up of the San Francisco Hospital cohort. *British Medical Journal, 296,* 745-750.

National Academy of Sciences. (1986). *Confronting AIDS: Directions for public health, health care, and research.* Washington DC: National Academy Press.

Nitschke, R., Humphrey, G. B., Sexauer, C. L., Catron, B., Wunder, S., & Jay, S. (1982). Therapeutic choices made by patients with end-stage cancer. *Journal of Pediatrics, 101,* 471-476.

Norman, C. (1985). AIDS trends: Projections from limited data. *Science, 230,* 1018-1021.

Petty, R. E., & Cacioppo, J. T. (1981). *Attitudes and persuasion: Classic and contemporary approaches.* Dubuque, IA: Wm. C. Brown.

Price, R. W., Brew, B., Sidtis, J., Rosenblum, M., Scheck, A. C., & Cleary, P. (1988). The brain in AIDS: Central nervous system HIV-I infection and AIDS dementia complex. *Science, 239,* 586-592.

Quadland, M. C., Shattls, W., Schuman, R., Jacobs, R., & D'Eramo, J. (1988). *The 800 men study: A systemic evaluation of AIDS prevention programs.* Unpublished manuscript.

Ranki, A., Valle, S. L., & Krohn, M. (1987). Long latency precedes overt seroconversion in sexually transmitted human immunodeficiency-virus infection. *Lancet, 2,* 589-593.

Rosenstock, I. M . (1966). Why people use health services. *Milbank Memorial Fund Quarterly, 44,* 94-127.

Schnike, S. P., Blythe, B. J., & Gilchrist, L. D. (1981). Cognitive-behavioral prevention of adolescent pregnancy. *Journal of Counseling Psychology, 28,* 451-454.

Schnike, S. P., Gilchrist, L. D., Schilling, R. F., Snow, W. H., & Bobo, J. K. (1986). Skills methods to prevent smoking. *Health Education Quarterly, 13,* 21-27.

Schowalter, J. E. (1974). Anticipatory grief and going on the "danger list." In B. Schoenberg, A. C. Carr, A. H. Kutscher, D. Petetz, & K. Goldberg (Eds.), *Anticipatory grief* (pp. 187-192). New York: Columbia University Press.

Scott, G. B., Buck, B. E., Letterman, J. G., Bloom, F. L., & Parks, W. P. (1984). Acquired immunodeficiency in infants. *New England Journal of Medicine, 310,* 76-81.

Seibert, J. M., Garcia, A., Kaplan, M., & Septimus, A. (in press). Three model pediatric AIDS programs: Meeting the needs of children, families and communities. In J. M. Seibert (Ed.), *Pediatric AIDS.* Lincoln: University of Nebraska Press.

Sheer, L., & Green, J. (1987, June). *Evaluation of health education in Britain.* Paper presented at the 3rd International Conference on AIDS, Washington, DC.

Simon, K. J., & Das, A. (1984). An application of the health belief model toward educational diagnosis for VD education. *Health Education Quarterly, 11,* 403-418.

Solomon, M. Z., & DeJong, W. (1986). Recent sexually transmitted disease prevention efforts and their implications for AIDS health education. *Health Education Quarterly, 13,* 301-316.

Stehr-Green, J. K., Holman, R. C., Jason, J. M., & Evatt, B. L. (1988). Hemophilia-associated AIDS in the United States, 1981 to September 1987. *American Journal of Public Health, 78,* 439-442.

Tarasoff v. Regents of the University of California, 17 Cal. 3d 425, 551 P.2d 334 (1976). (Tarasoff II).

Temoshok, L., Sweet, D. M., & Zich, J. (1988). A three city comparison of the public's knowledge and attitudes about AIDS. *Psychology and Health, 1,* 43-60.

Wachter, E. H. (1971). Children's awareness of fatal illness. *American Journal of Nursing, 7,* 1168-1172.

Watters, J. K. (1987, June). *Preventing human immunodeficiency virus contagion among intravenous drug users: The impact of street-based education on risk behavior.* Paper presented at the 3rd International Conference on AIDS, Washington, DC.

Weber, J. N., Wadsworth, J., Rogers, L. A., Mosktael, D., Scott, K., McManus, J., Berrie, E., Jeffries, D. J., Harris, J. R., & Pinching, M. (1986). Three-year prospective study of HTLV-III/LAV infection in homosexual men. *Lancet, 1,* 1179-1182.

White, E., Elsom, B., & Prawat, R. (1978). Children's conceptions of death. *Child Development, 49,* 307-310.

Williams, N. B. (Ed.). (1986). *Contraceptive technology 1986-1987.* New York: Irvington.

Index